THE WHITE DEATH

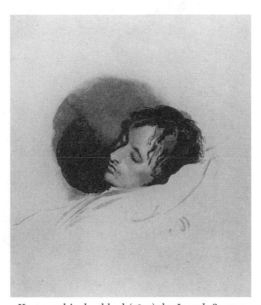

Keats on his deathbed (1821), by Joseph Severn

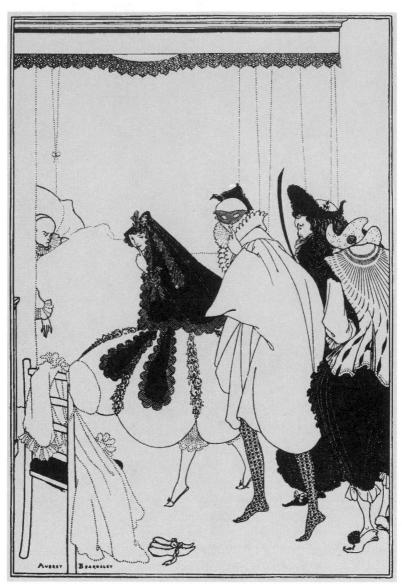

The Death of Pierrot (1896), drawing by Aubrey Beardsley.

The White Death

A History of Tuberculosis

Thomas Dormandy

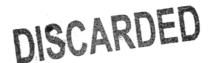

NEW YORK UNIVERSITY PRESS
Washington Square, New York

First published in the USA in 2000 by

NEW YORK UNIVERSITY PRESS
Washington Square
New York, NY 10003

Library of Congress Cataloging-in-Publication Data

Dormandy, Thomas.
The white death : a history of tuberculosis / Thomas Dormandy
p. cm.
Originally published: London ; Rio Grande, Ohio : Hambledon Press, 1999
Includes bibliographical references and index.
ISBN 0-8147-1927-9 (cl. : alk. paper)
1. Tuberculosis—History. I. Title.
[RC311.D67 2000]   99-32169
616.9'95'009—dc21   CIP

Typeset in Minion by Carnegie Publishing, Lancaster
Printed and bound in the UK on acid-free paper
by Cambridge University Press

Contents

Illustrations

Text Illustrations

Acknowledgements

My family have borne with patience the spells of gloom and exhilaration which have seemed inseparable from writing a book on tuberculosis. Dr Caroline Mezey helped me along the byways of nineteenth-century French and Italian literature. Barrie MacKay compiled the index with vigilance, as well as exemplary dispatch. Eva Osborne improved the manuscript by innumerable small corrections. Martin Sheppard, my wonderful editor, has been exacting and critical but always sympathetic, involved and supportive.

The author and publisher are grateful to the following institutions for permission to reproduce illustrations: the Brontë Society, p. 40; the County Record Office, Cambridge, pls 15, 16, 17; the County Record Office, Norwich, pl. 14; Keats's House, p. i; the Louvre, pl. 4; the National Gallery, Budapest, pl. 2; the Munch Museum, Oslo, pl. 6; the National Portrait Gallery, pls 3, 5, 19, 20, 21; the Statens Museum for Kunst, pl. 7; the Wellcome Institute, p. 305.

For Liz

Introduction

The girl sits propped up on pillows. Her face has become almost transparent. She turns towards the window. Cold winter sunlight streams in. Faint dashes hint rather than depict her eyes: yet the wistful gaze is miraculously caught. Her orange hair glows against the white linen of the bedclothes. A green curtain billows into the room. Next to her the mother's head is sunk on her chest, hardly more than a shadow. It is the image of inexpressible grief.

This is the picture of Sophie Munch, aged fourteen, of Oslo, then still called Christiania, a few months before her death from tuberculosis. Painted by her brother, Edvard, it is one of the graven images of what was for millions a personal experience. For Sophie Munch was a member of a sisterhood – and a brotherhood – which knew no geographical boundaries and no barriers of class or rank and which spanned the centuries.

Death is part of life: it is the most predictable and therefore the most humdrum of the great biological milestones. It is also an essential precondition of what – for unfathomable reasons – seems to be the overriding objective of our existence: the survival of the species. In the vast majority of cases this mundane event is preceded by a period hardly less wearisome. Terminal diseases come in a wide range but by definition their outcome is always the same. The Black Death of the fifteenth century is said to have wiped out a third of Europe's population. Many other diseases also had an impact on European and world history. At the time of Sophie Munch's death her father, a district physician, was battling against the annual summer epidemic of cholera. In Oslo, as in most other European cities, it still killed more people than tuberculosis. So probably did infantile gastroenteritis, measles and scarlet fever.

But tuberculosis was wholly unlike any of these. Of course it was a killer like the rest; but it was not just a killer. It transformed the lives as well as causing the deaths of its victims. For a century and a half it became a formative influence in art, music and literature. This was not only because the list of tuberculous artists, poets, philosophers and musicians still reads like a roll-call of genius; the disease also imprinted itself on the creations of the non-tuberculous majority. For tuberculosis affected more than its immediate victims, more even than its immediate victims' parents, brothers, sisters, lovers, enemies and friends. Like no other disease before or since, it compelled doctors to question the very purpose of their calling – or its lack of purpose. It mocked statesmen and social reformers. It challenged the churches and the agnostic scientific establishment equally. It was also "white", not only because anaemia was an almost invariable clinical feature, but also because of its long association with childhood, innocence and even holiness. The last did not seem to conflict with the deeply ingrained notion that it was also the most lecherous of all illnesses: such grand generalisations often appeared to be as true a their opposites.

The past tense may be misleading. *The Triumph over Tuberculosis, The Retreat of Tuberculosis, Requiem for a Great Killer* and suchlike titles make up a significant part of the modern literature of the disease. When these books were written, some less than ten years ago, the implied finality would not have raised an eyebrow. Of course it was known that among the teeming millions of Asia, Africa and South America the disease was still rampant; but that was a political problem: sooner or later it would yield to medical progress. Today few people are so certain.

Time and again in the past – even before chemotherapy was supposed to have delivered the coup de grace – tuberculosis seemed conquered. Time and again it re-emerged with a grin. It may be doing so again today. It is too early to say what new and unexpected guises it will assume. This may, nevertheless, be an opportune moment for a less than triumphalist look at the story so far.

1

The Mists of History

Only births and deaths have shaped human history more decisively than illnesses; yet infinitely less is known about the important illnesses of the past than about many quite trivial political, social, economic and cultural events. This is often attributed to the difficulty of interpreting obsolete medical jargon and the uncertain meaning of popular terms describing common symptoms and signs. Reticence and obfuscation have also frequently surrounded ill-health – as they still do. The main difficulty, however, is that diseases change. Illnesses bearing familiar names and with causes seemingly well established behaved differently in the past from the way they behave today. Before the mid nineteenth century gout was more common and more severe than rheumatoid arthritis. Today the position is reversed. Within living memory scarlet fever and rheumatic fever were serial killers. They are so no longer. Asthma has become more severe. Fifty years ago acute appendicitis was by far the commonest life-threatening surgical emergency. Today it is rare or unrecognisably benign.

The causes for these transformation are usually obscure. Doctors tend to attribute improvements to scientific advances or to their own ever-increasing wisdom. They rarely claim responsibility for the dire effects of medical misconceptions. The evidence is usually inconclusive. This has been especially true of the disease known today as tuberculosis. It can now be defined as an infection caused by the human or bovine strain of the micro-organism *Mycobacterium tuberculosis*;[1] but such a definition has been possible only for the past hundred years. Before then the illness had been known by many names and had undoubtedly been confused with many other conditions. It must often have been missed. Equally, it must often have been misdiagnosed. Most critically, it has frequently and for no obvious reason changed its character. Indeed, it is still changing. None of this makes it a easy subject for historical research.

Yet tuberculosis is one of the most historical – as well as historically im-portant – diseases. A number of characteristic lesions in prehistoric skeletons

---

[1] There are others – porcine tuberculosis in pigs, murine in rats and avian in birds are well recognised – but they have not been established as pathogenic in man.

and in Egyptian mummies have been attributed to it;[2] and some of the lively hunchbacks portrayed in Egyptian tomb paintings look like sufferers from Pott's disease.[3] The Greeks coined the word phthisis (Φθίσις, literally "wasting"), until recently the most widely used medical label. (The lay equivalent was consumption.) A slowly but inexorably progressive and debilitating illness of young people was certainly well known to Hippocrates and his circle. Of course the condition could have been any one of a dozen other illnesses and was most probably a mixture; but the familiarity with which it was described makes one thing clear. Pale, emaciated youths, fighting for breath, coughing up blood and dying young were as common in the Antique world as were the wonderfully fit horsemen who parade on the frieze of the Parthenon.[4]

The Alexandrian physicians added anatomical findings to the clinical descriptions of classical Greece;[5] but it was two Roman doctors (or two Greek doctors practising in the Roman Empire) whose writings became holy writ for a thousand years. Little is known about Aretaeus the Cappadocian – even his dates of birth and death are uncertain – but his extant writings are a monument to acute clinical observation.[6] Nowhere is this more evident than in his terse description of advanced tuberculosis.

> Voice hoarse; neck slightly bent, tender and stiff; fingers slender but the joints swollen; severe wasting of the fleshy parts leaving the bones prominently outlined; the nails crooked or flat and brittle without their normal rotundity ... The nose is sharp and slender, the cheeks are prominent and abnormally flushed; the eyes are deeply sunk in their hollows but brilliant and glittering ... The slender parts

---

[2] Cave, A. J. E., *British Journal of Tuberculosis*, 33 (1939), 142; Cockburn, A., Cockburn, E., *Mummies, Diseases and Ancient Cultures* (Cambridge, 1980). One famous mummy of a high priest of Amon of around 3000 BC still shows evidence of a so-called Psoas abscess – that is of pus tracking from a collapsed vertebra in the thoracic region under the sheath of the Psoas muscle to a point on the surface just below the groin. Today such a lesion would be virtually pathognomonic of spinal tuberculosis (see Chapter 2, below, p. 24) and the same was probably true 5000 years ago. Most prehistoric finds of bone tuberculosis, the form of the infection most likely to be detected in archaeological finds, have been in the skeletons of young men and women, suggesting that the disease was characteristically an affliction of the young in prehistoric days, as it was to remain until recently. The earliest remains found in Britain suggestive of tuberculosis date from the Roman era; but similar finds in Italy and Denmark are at least a thousand years earlier.

[3] The spinal form of the infection.

[4] Adams, F., ed. and trans., *The Genuine Works of Hippocrates* (London, 1849); Manchester, K., "Tuberculosis and Leprosy in Antiquity: An Interpretation", *Medical History*, 28 (1984), 162; Phillips, E. D., *Greek Medicine* (London, 1963).

[5] There is no evidence that post-mortem examinations were performed anywhere in pre-Alexandrian Greece.

[6] The translator of his works, F. Adams (London, 1856), suggested the middle of the second century AD.

of the jaws rests on the teeth as if smiling but it is the smile of cadavers ... The muscles of the limbs all wasted. Only the nipples mark the breasts in women. One may not only count the ribs but also easily trace them to their terminations; for even the articulations of the vertebrae are quite visible as are the connections with the sternum ... The shoulder blades are like the wings of the birds.[7]

Aretaeus also noted the intermittent fever, the sweating and the lassitude but also the occasional bursts of excitement and even of "foolish gaiety".

More information is available about Galen the Pergamite, not a prey to shyness. He travelled widely in the empire but eventually settled in Rome and became the city's most famous physician. He regarded blood in the sputum as the most important early diagnostic sign and was guarded in his prognosis once the patient became hot and perspiring. He recognised the disease as being mildly contagious and wrote with common sense about diet, travel, the value of moderate exercise and the misuse of drugs. He also bequeathed on his profession that faintly hectoring tone of just-you-do-as-I-say-I-know-best which doctors still employ when completely in the dark.[8]

Byzantine, Arabic and medieval western manuscripts are full of interesting and often accurate snippets of clinical lore, suggesting that tuberculosis or a disease very similar to it remained common and widely distributed; but the most persuasive evidence of the prevalence of the illness is the crowds of sufferers known to have sought relief from the King's Evil.

Many people, now mostly in their sixties, seventies and eighties, still bear on the side of their necks a somewhat unsightly scar, usually about half an inch to an inch long, the legacy of an illness from which they suffered in their late teens or early twenties and which often dramatically altered their lives. The illness, tuberculous glands in the neck, was among the commonest presenting manifestations of the disease and was thought to be the result of the bacillus gaining entry through the tonsils and being carried by lymph to the nearest lymph nodes. One of the functions of these nodes is to filter out potentially harmful organisms and expose them to the body's defences, the explanation for the frequency in pre-antibiotic days of painful boils and carbuncles in this region. When the organism trapped was the *Mycobacterium tuberculosis* the enlarged lymph-nodes were usually painless, slow-growing and only slightly tender. They neither burst nor resolved. Occasionally their appearance coincided with spikes of temperature in the evenings. Eventually, in some though not in all cases, the initially somewhat rubbery mass softened and had to be aspirated or drained. The incision and even the puncture

---

[7] In *De causis et signis diurnorum morborum* or the *Causes and Symptoms of Chronic Diseases*. The translation was published by the Sydenham Society, London, in 1856.

[8] Walsh, J., *American Review of Tuberculosis and Pulmonary Diseases*, 24 (1931), 1.

wound often took months or even years to heal and almost always left a nasty, puckered scar. The material collected was sent to the laboratory for culture and some of it was injected into two or three guinea-pigs. Conclusive bacteriological diagnosis took six to eight weeks; but the chances were that both procedures would confirm what had been suspected on clinical grounds. The first grew "acid-alcohol-fast" bacilli. The second induced a virulent form of abdominal tuberculosis in the inoculated animals.

With the diagnosis established, the patient was withdrawn from his or her work-place, school or university, dispatched to a sanatorium or to the country, put on a nutritious milk-based diet liberally laced with cod-liver oil and made to rest for several hours during the day. A year or two later the lucky few, who after half a century are still alive, returned cured. The majority went on to years of ill-health and a host of complications in distant organs and usually died within ten to fifteen years.

The King's Evil began as a similar enlargement of the cervical lymph-nodes, often or mostly – it is impossible today to say which – of tuberculous origin. It could lead to terrible ulceration and scarring. Apart from being called the King's Evil it was also known as scrofula (literally meaning little pigs) and was recognised by the learned commentators of Salerno and Montpellier, the leading medical schools of the early middle ages, as a manifestation of a general disease with a poor prognosis. Why of all the unspeakable ills that beset medieval men and women it should have been singled out as being susceptible to the touch of Kings is uncertain; but it was so identified as early as the fifth century. The touch formed the basis of treatment – and indeed, if contemporary chronicles are to be believed, of numerous cures – in most of Europe.[9] (Oddly perhaps, the fact that royalty themselves were not immune – both England's Edward VI and France's Charles IX were scrofulous and may have died of tuberculosis – in no way diminished the faith of their subjects.) The numbers treated were usually recorded and are probably reliable guides to the prevalence of the condition. It is known, for instance, that Edward I (1272–1307) touched 533 sufferers in one month, while Philip Augustus of France (1180–1223) is credited with 1500 touches in a single ceremony. The practice continued long after the age of the Divine Right of Kings. Charles II during his twenty-five-year reign (1660–1685) is said to have touched 92,102 of his subjects; and Queen Anne (1702–1714), the last English

---

[9] The procedure was described by Shakespeare in *Macbeth*: "strangely-visited people / All swoll'n and ulcerous, pitiful to the eye / The mere despair of surgery, he cures / Hanging a golden stamp about their necks, / Put on with holy prayers; and 'tis spoken, / To the succeeding royalty he leaves / The healing benediction." (Act IV, Scene 3, lines 150–56).

monarch to touch, counted Dr Johnson (as a child) among her patients. Several people were trampled to death on the last occasion. In many countries the practice survived even longer: the present writer's great-great-grand-father's coachman's son was cured by the touch of Hungary's last but one Apostolic King, Franz Josef I, in 1886.

The superstitions surrounding the King's Evil – as indeed most illnesses – should not detract from the astonishing insights shown by some of the leading anatomists, pathologists and clinicians of the sixteenth, seventeenth and eighteenth centuries. The larger than life figure of Philippus Aureolus Theophrastus Bombastus von Hohenheim, known as Paracelsus (1490–1541), is better remembered for ceremoniously burning the books of Galen before starting his course of lectures than for what he actually lectured about; but before settling in Basle he travelled widely and wrote a monograph on miners' phthisis after visiting the tin mines of Cornwall. It is a remarkable work (not published until twenty-seven years after his death), though it is not clear whether his croaking, cyanosed and blood-spitting patients were suffering from tuberculosis, silicosis or both.

Girolamo Fracastoro (1483–1553), physician, poet and philosopher, native of Verona and professor at the university of Padua, was most renowned for his epic, *Syphilis seu morbus Gallicus*, which named the famous illness (often to be twinned with tuberculosis in centuries to come); but his work most relevant to tuberculosis, *De contagione*, was no less prescient.[10] He described how diseases like phthisis are transmitted by invisible particles called *seminaria* which, he postulated, could survive outside the body for several years and still infect. A little anticlimactically perhaps for an *uomo* so *universale*, he has been called the Father of Epidemiology.

For almost two centuries Leyden in Holland enjoyed an unrivalled repu-tation as Europe's leading medical school (eventually to be eclipsed by Vienna). It owed much of its initial prestige to Franciscus de la Boë, better known as Sylvius (1614–1672), professor of clinical and anatomical medicine for thirty years. A much-admired teacher, he attracted students from every part of Europe to his small twelve-bedded hospital. It was he who associated the small nodules – tubercles as he called them – with phthisis, describing their gradual growth and suppuration.

Of Sylvius's English pupils two are still remembered. Thomas Willis (1621–1675), Sedleian professor of natural philosophy at Oxford, related the localised ulceration in the lungs to the pining away of the body as a whole and described

---

[10] It was published in 1546. Though he emphasised the role of contagion, he also discussed the importance of heredity, describing several families of up to six generations whom phthisis always struck at the same age.

galloping tuberculosis as well as the chronic fibrosing disease.[11] The other, Richard Morton (1637–1698), began his career as a clergymen but was deprived of his living for refusing to subscribe to the Act of Uniformity. He turned to medicine as a second career and eventually set up in successful practice in Grey Friar's Court, Newgate Street, in the City of London. His popular *Phthysiologia*, dedicated to William of Orange, remains an admirable compendium of homely common sense, advising temperance in eating and drinking, sound and adequate sleep, moderate exercise, the avoidance of strong purges and, above all, the laying aside of care and melancholy. Like the authors of similarly oracular (and best-selling) guides today, he was less specific about how to achieve these admirable objectives.

More celebrated in his day than either was Thomas Sydenham (1624–1689), hailed as the prince of clinicians and (inevitably) the English Hippocrates. He numbered several distinguished consumptives among his patients, including John Locke and his family;[12] but he wrote specifically about tuberculosis only in a short note, *De phthysi*. Its main interest lies in his warm recommendation of horseback riding as a therapeutic measure: "bark [quinine] is no surer cure for ague than riding is for phthisis". His counsel was endorsed by Locke (who was himself a doctor) and it probably did little harm until carried to insane length by later generations.[13]

[11] His book, *The Practice of Physic*, was published in 1684 and is remarkable for the accuracy of his observations and his lateral thinking; but he is better remembered for distinguishing "sweet" from "non-sweet" diabetes (the latter known today as diabetes insipidus as distinct from diabetes mellitus) by tasting his patients' urines. An important arterial circle at the base of the brain is also named after him.

[12] Locke's father and brother died from tuberculosis and he himself suffered from it all his life. Dewhurst, K., *John Locke, Physician and Philosopher: A Medical Biography* (London, 1963).

[13] Locke was a friend and admirer of Sydenham's and, in his his *Anecdota Sydenhamiana*, he described how the famous doctor cured his nephew:

> Ye Doctor sent him into ye County on Horseback (tho he was soe weak yt he could hardly walk), & ordered him to ride six or seven miles ye first day (which he did) & to encrease dayly his journey as he shd be able, until he had rid one hundred and fifty miles: when he had travelld half ye way his Diarrhoea stopt & at last he came to ye end of his journey & was pretty well (at least somewhat better) & he has a good appetite: but when he had staid at his Sister's house some four or five days his Diarrhoea came on again; the Doctor had ordered him not to stay above two days at most; for if they stay above two days before they are recovered this spoils all again; & therefore he betook him self to his riding again, and in four days he came up to London perfectly cured.

Of course horseback riding was the most widely used form of transport and the easiest way for sick people to get out and about and even perhaps to forget about their ailment. Benjamin Marten a century later also warmly recommended it "not only for their Bodies but also their Minds which will be much better entertained while they are on horseback". In Holland Gerhard Van Swieten, later professor of medicine in Vienna, urged consumptives of the lower

What today would be called morbid anatomy was dominated for most of the eighteenth century by Giovanni Battista Morgagni (1682–1771), professor of anatomy in Padua for fifty-six years and author of the first bible of pathologists, *De sedibus et causis morborum*. He was so firm a believer in contagion that he avoided performing post-mortem examinations on subjects who had died of phthisis but observed and directed proceedings with a silver-headed cane from a specially built gallery. (It is not clear from contemporary accounts who actually performed the dissections and what fate eventually befell them.) Despite his prudently maintained distance, Morgagni gave a masterly account of the cavities formed in the lungs in advanced tuberculosis and of the associated scarring.

Benjamin Marten (1704–1782), "flashed meteor-like across this firmament of theoretical disputations and speculation",[14] but little is known about him other than the title of his book, *A New Theory of Consumptions: More Especially of a Phthisis or Consumption of the Lungs* written in his house in Theobald's Row near Red Lion Square in Holborn. Even that book lay forgotten for the best part of one hundred and fifty years. Marten was in fact more remarkable for the vividness of his descriptions than for the novelty of his views: but he was one of the first to emphasise the need to keep up patients' spirits, "Hope being the greatest Comfort they have and their only source of enjoyment".

The outstanding teacher of the century, drawing to Leyden thousands of young physicians, many of them later leaders of their profession in their own countries, was Hermann Boerhaave (1668–1734).[15] While he wrote comparatively little on consumption, he introduced a tool that would eventually assume almost symbolic significance in the management of the disease. Fever had been recognised at least since the days of Hippocrates as a sign of illness or indeed as an illness in itself; but, until Boerhaave, no attempt had been made to measure it. This was in contrast to the devout attention given to the pulse. Hundreds of eighteenth-century paintings depict physicians delicately fingering the wrists of their patients, almost always comely young women, while gazing raptly at a bottle of urine held up to the light.[16] None

classes engaged in sedentary occupations to seek employment as coachmen or grooms. In America Benjamin Rush described a cobbler patient who found employment as a coachman and recovered but relapsed as soon as he returned to cobbling.

[14] Keers, R. Y., *Pulmonary Tuberculosis: A Journey down the Centuries* (London, 1978), p. 34.

[15] Called by his admirers "The Batavian Hippocrates", what else? See Lindenboom, G. A., *Hermann Boerhaave: The Man and his Work* (London, 1968).

[16] The reason for their absorption has puzzled the present writer for many years. He was eventually enlightened by his learned friend Dr B. I. Hoffbrand, who explained that the diagnosis they were seeking was early pregnancy, believed to cause a slight increase in the pulse rate and a faint haze in the urine.

handles a thermometer. Boerhaave's original instrument was not in fact designed for easy handling. Calibrated in degrees of Fahrenheit,[17] it was fifteen inches long and had to be inserted into the rectum for up to twenty minutes. It was, in other words, what today would be described as a research tool rather than a clinical aid. It established the extraordinary narrow normal range of body temperature and its even more remarkable constancy in any one individual. There is no reference in Boerhaave's writings to the characteristic daily spikes of low-grade fever in tuberculosis; but he did mention the intermittently raised temperature in some chronic diseases. Measuring the temperature also figured prominently in the fifteen-volume *Ratio medendi* by Anton De Haen, one of Boerhaave's prize pupils, who became professor of medicine in Vienna.[18]

Because of the close academic links between Edinburgh and Leyden, clinical thermometry soon found its way to Scotland and spread from there to England and America. (The French did not trust it until it was popularised by Charcot in the mid nineteenth century and recalibrated to the scale devised by the great eighteenth-century French scientist René Réaumur.) The British pioneer, James Currie (who moved from Edinburgh to Liverpool) described gruesome experiments to test the body-temperature response both to drinking and to immersion into very hot and very cold water. The only change occurred in some feverish patients on whom an ice-cold bath had a slight cooling effect. A few felt improved afterwards. He published his findings in 1797. Another Scottish graduate, Archibald Arnott, recorded Napoleon's temperature shortly before the ex-Emperor's death. The subnormal reading convinced him that the illness was *not* consumption.

By the end of the eighteenth century many others had written well and extensively on tuberculosis: William Stark and Matthew Baillie of London, Thomas Beddoes of Bristol, Benjamin Rush of Philadelphia, Pierre Desault of Paris and Adolf Altgruber of Vienna were some. The common technical

[17] A scale devised by the German physicist, Gabriel Daniel Fahrenheit, in 1710 while working in Holland.

[18] De Haen seems to have used thermometry regularly in his wards in Vienna toward the end of the eighteenth century; but the procedure did not become a routine, indeed the most commonly performed, bedside measurement, until Carl Wunderlich, professor of medicine in Leipzig, published his magnum opus, *Das Verhalten der Eigenwärme in Krankheiten,* in 1868. Based on several million temperature readings in 25,000 patients over a twenty-year period, his descriptions of different patterns of abnormal temperature in different diseases have never been bettered. He devoted 200 pages to the regularly recurring spikes of temperature in tuberculosis, toying with the idea that the regularity may be related to variations in daylight or other forms of radiation. Eventually he concluded that the pattern was one of many mysterious temporal cycles to which the human body is heir, a conclusion which could not be significantly bettered today.

terms of today were beginning to be used. "Tuberculosis" was used by Richard Morton, though it did not supplant "phthisis" till the mid nineteenth century.[19] Pierre Manget described tubercles so small that they resembled millet seeds, the origin of "miliary" tuberculosis.[20] Matthew Baillie gave a vivid account of the caseous or cheese-like material of tuberculous abscesses. Physicians and many laymen knew what cavities and fibrosis meant. But after two centuries it is not easy to make a balanced judgement about these texts. Almost all contain impressively detailed morbid anatomical accounts and shrewd clinical passages, and much good practical advice, even when based on fanciful reasoning. There are also long and wordy attempts, often highly polemical, at giving logical accounts of processes which were clearly not understood and indeed incapable of being understood without the techniques which became available only in the last decades of the nineteenth century. Childish hypotheses were often expounded at inordinate length, the questions raised being generally more to the point than the answers given. How did it come about that tubercles could be either chalky or bone-like, full of liquid pus or cheesy? What determined the size of the cavities and the raw or smooth character of their surface? Why did some cavities remain closed and others open into the bronchi or blood vessels? Did the tubercles occurring in parts other than the lungs bear any relation to pulmonary phthisis? Were the swollen lymph nodes that disfigured the neck in scrofula related in any way to the lesions in the chest and elsewhere in the body?

Individual case histories are often more revealing than general medical texts. Of course they shed no light on the millions of victims who lived unsung or died too young to leave their mark on the world. Celebrities, however precocious, generate the false impression that the average onset of the disease was later in life and survival longer than was probably the rule. Nor does it seem particularly fruitful to speculate about such distant figures as St Francis of Assisi, John Calvin or the celestial Simonetta Vespucci, Botticelli's model for Venus. All three may well have been tuberculous; but what is known of their medical histories could fit a dozen other illnesses.[21]

[19] In 1839 J. L. Schönlein, professor of medicine in Zurich, suggested that the word "tuberculosis" should be used as a generic name for all manifestations of phthisis since the tubercle was the fundamental pathological unit.

[20] The grain was so named by Romans (from *mille*, a thousand) because of its fertility. The term miliary tuberculosis was not widely used in clinical practice until attached to the rapidly spreading, generalised and (until the chemotherapeutic revolution) invariably fatal form of the disease by Ludwig Buhl, professor of pathology in Munich in 1872.

[21] Musicologists have been particularly exercised by the cause of the sudden and untimely death of Henry Purcell on 21 November (the Eve of St Cecilia's Feast Day) in 1695, aged thirty-six. Sudden death does not usually raise the suspicion of tuberculosis; but Purcell scholars have recently described a progressive deterioration in the composer's handwriting –

Approaching the second half of the seventeenth century, however, there emerges from the mists the head of that extraordinary procession of artists, poets, writers, thinkers and scientists about whom one can reasonably say that they suffered and died from tuberculosis.

Jean-Baptiste Poquelin, who assumed the name of Molière, was born in 1622 into a family of well-to-do artisans. As a young man he fell in love with the theatre, as well as with a particular star of the theatre, Madeleine Béjart, a double infatuation from which he never recovered. Running a theatrical company was always a risky venture; and at one time the young man had to be bailed out from the debtors' prison by his father. Prisons were insalubrious places and some biographers have suggested that it was during his incarceration that he contracted consumption. It remained with him for the rest of his life, striking him down from time to time with fever, cough and extreme weakness for weeks or months. Despite this, he kept extraordinarily busy: perhaps relatively long periods of quiescence were not uncommon in his day. No kind of social pretence escaped his vitriolic pen; but he was particularly scathing about the murkier side of medicine and pitiless in ridiculing hypochondriacs. He was himself playing *Le malade imaginaire* before the Court in 1673 when he was seized by an all-too-unimaginary fit of coughing and a small pulmonary bleed. He recovered after an unscheduled interval. The King, Louis XIV, urged him to go to his room and rest, but the writer-actor-director insisted on finishing the performance before collapsing with another haemorrhage and dying offstage.

His near-contemporary, Baruch Spinoza (1632–1677), lived a less outwardly hectic life in the well-ordered Dutch city of The Hague, making a modest living from grinding optical lenses and teaching a small but devoted group of disciples. Born into a Sephardic Jewish family in Amsterdam, he had fallen foul of his own religious community (as fierce in anathemising deviations from orthodoxy as were the Catholic Inquisition and Calvinistic theocracies) and had to move to another city. But the Netherlands were still an island

though not in the level of his musical inspiration – during the last year of his life; and this and other circumstantial evidence points to the possibility that he may have died of pulmonary tuberculosis

The uncertainty persists well into the nineteenth century. Much circumstantial evidence suggests that it was tuberculosis which killed Count Giacomo Leopardi (1798–1837), the Italian Ottocento's greatest poet; but in all the extensive correspondence by and about him the only reference is to his delicate health, cough, weak chest, and the need for him to live in a warm climate. The dread word "consumption" was never uttered. By contrast, Alexander Petöfi (1823–1849), one of Hungary's most popular lyrical poets, is usually listed as a famous victim in books which favour such lists. Yet, apart from his dread of "withering away like a flower of a slowly consuming illness" (expressed in a celebrated poem), there is no evidence that he was tuberculous. He eventually died in battle.

of sanity in a Europe torn by religious bigotries and his life was not in danger. His Hebrew learning stood him in good stead in elaborating a philosophical system which inspired thinkers from Leibnitz to Bertrand Russell. His quiet and austere life was shattered by the French invasion of 1672, a time of anguish, grief and physical privation; and he emerged from the ordeal a respiratory cripple. How far the dust of his glass grinding contributed to his breathlessness is uncertain: he himself described his condition as a form of consumption. The disease certainly ran in his family. His most important works were not published until after his death.

When a generation or two later Jean Antoine Watteau (1684–1721) died, he was well regarded by his fellow academicians as an accomplished painter of Arcadias, but he had no pupils and after his death he was quickly forgotten.[22] It was the *nouveau riche* bourgeoisie of the Second Empire, a crudely materialistic class in vain pursuit of eighteenth-century grace, which rediscovered his elegant and melancholic world.[23] He had been sickly since childhood, rarely fit to accept large-scale commissions which might have come his way. Haunted (as many other tuberculous would be in later centuries) by the fear that physical weakness might deprive him of his livelihood before the disease deprived him of life itself, he travelled to England to consult one of the most fashionable physicians of his day. Dr Robert Mead had seen some of Watteau's work in Paris and was a connoisseur as well as a kindly man. He put the artist up for several months trying the effects of wholesome food and a battery of medical concoctions. But London was already a city of damp and smoke – or so it seemed to the painter. Coughing and short of breath he returned to France and spent his last months on the country estate of his patron, the Abbé Haranger. His host later described his last days: semiconscious and mute, probably a victim of tuberculous laryngitis, he went on clutching a brush to the end, painting imaginary pictures in the air.

There were many others and in every part of Europe. In Italy, Giovanni Battista Pergolesi (1710–1736), composer of a short but sensationally successful operatic intermezzo,[24] which brought a breath of fresh air into the solemn world of opera, and of a well-crafted and in style not very different *Stabat Mater*, developed what seems to have been a case of galloping tuberculosis when he was twenty-four. When he could hardly eat or breathe his doctors sent him to the fashionable spa of Pozzuoli, near Naples. He was popular

[22] Except perhaps Jean-Baptiste Joseph Pater (1695–1734), who found the master too exacting, capricious and irritable to stay with him for long. But he went on painting *fêtes galantes* in the Watteau manner until he too died of consumption.

[23] The Goncourts were his most ardent posthumous champions.

[24] *La serva padrone* (*The Servant Mistress*), first performed in 1733. It caused a riot in Paris.

but profligate and penniless: it is not known who paid for the sojourn. In any case it was short: he died aged twenty-six, the brevity of his career contributing to many improbable legends and to an almost inexhaustible supply of pretty concertos, cantatas and concertinos falsely or doubtfully attributed to him.

In England Laurence Sterne (1713–1768), a writer whom Goethe was to rate among the noblest of human spirits, had his first major pulmonary haemorrhage as an undergraduate in Cambridge and was never afterwards entirely free from symptoms. During his stay in Paris in 1761 he was pronounced dead after another bleed – but recovered. With his daughter, also tuberculous, he travelled to the south – to Nice, Montpellier, Bordeaux and eventually to Rome – writing, when he was strong enough to hold a pen, *A Sentimental Journey through France and Italy*. Rome, he thought, might give him another ten years of life; but he was mistaken. He developed a painful pleurisy which did not respond to repeated venesections and which persuaded him to return to England. He made it to London – just. He died alone, his body being snatched from the grave two days later. His remains found their way back to the dissecting room of the Anatomy School in Cambridge, not far from where his career (and probably his illness) had begun.

Contrary to what has been said by some writers on tuberculosis, the disease was generally deeply respectful of wealth and rank; but now and again it played tricks on the mighty. Wilhelmine, Markgräfin of Bayreuth, was the sister of Frederick II (the Great) of Prussia and probably the only woman he selflessly loved. Her last letter reached him on the battlefield shortly after his victory at Leuthen in 1756:

> You ask after me, dear Brother. Like poor Lazarus I lie in bed: it's the sixth month. For the past eight days I have been unable to move on my own: I am being carried around in a wheelchair or on a stretcher once or twice a day. The painful, dry cough never seems to stop: at night it wakes me whenever I doze off after a hefty dose of medicine. My hands, feet and face are all swollen. I have resigned myself to my fate: I shall die happy and in peace so long as I know that you are happy.[25]

She died two weeks later.

---

[25] Voigt, J., *Tuberkulose: Geschichte einer Krankheit* (Cologne, 1994), p. 124.

2

Half in Love with Easeful Death

One winter evening in 1818 John Keats, just past his twenty-third birthday, was returning on the evening coach from the City to Wentworth Place, a modest villa on the edge of Hampstead Heath which he shared with his "capital friend", John Arbuthnot Brown.[1] Because he was hard up and liked fresh air he had been riding cheaply on the outside and the chill air bit him to the bone. Alighting at the stop at the bottom of Pond Street he staggered home and (according to Brown) burst into the house like a man wildly drunk. Brown suggested that he go to bed and Keats meekly complied. "On entering the cold sheets", Brown later recalled,

> before his head was on the pillow he coughed and I heard him say – "This is blood". I approached him and saw that he was examining a stain on the sheet. "Bring me a candle, Brown, and let me see this blood." After I handed him the candle and he examined the blood he looked up into my face with a calmness of countenance that I can never forget and said: "This is arterial blood: I cannot be deceived by its colour. It is my death warrant." [2]

Keats's certainty derived not just from his years as a medical student at Guy's and St Thomas's Hospitals: in fact, though he was a licentiate of the Society of Apothecaries of London and therefore a qualified doctor, he had never shown much interest in medicine.[3] (He wrote one of his best sonnets, "Much Have I Travelled in the Realm of Gold", whilst attending a lecture by Dr George Lucas on the pathology of the hobnailed liver.) Nor did he probably remember the death of his mother from tuberculosis eighteen years earlier. But more recently he had spent a year nursing his younger brother, Tom, through the terminal stages of the disease; and it was only a few

---

[1] Keats has been fortunate in his biographers, none more sympathetic than the most recent ones, Cook, S., *John Keats: A Life* (London, 1995), and Motion, A., *Keats* (London, 1997). Other works which explore his illness in particular are Hale-White, W., *Keats as Doctor and Patient* (Oxford, 1938), and Almeida, H. de, *Romantic Medicine and John Keats* (Oxford, 1991). His circle, including John Arbuthnot Brown, are portrayed in Richardson, J., *Keats and his Circle* (London, 1980).

[2] Cook, S., *Keats*, p. 294.

[3] Despite Keats's professed lack of interest in medicine, his full-length portrait today adorns the Apothecaries' Hall in London.

months earlier that Tom's long-drawn-out ordeal had ended in his brother's arms.[4]

John himself probably had advance warnings of the disease. On his Scottish walking tour, from which he was summoned back after Tom's last relapse, he had developed a sore throat from which he never completely recovered: it was probably tuberculous laryngitis. It is also possible that his periods of profound exhaustion, malaise, depression and insane jealousy, alternating and sometimes overlapping with sublime poetic inspiration, for at least the previous year reflected a slowly advancing illness. Yet both doctors and laymen traditionally believed that coughing up blood was an *early* sign of tuberculosis; and there is no way of proving today that in Keats's case it was not. It would make subsequent events fractionally less horrific.

A second and then a third more violent haemorrhage followed the same night: later he told his betrothed, Fanny Brawne, that he had not expected to live until the morning and that his mind had been filled with her beloved image. Brown summoned Mr Rodd, a surgeon practising in Hampstead High Street, who bled him repeatedly until he fell to sleep from sheer exhaustion. Rodd also put him on a near-starvation diet, the recognised treatment for what was labelled early consumption.

Over the next few months Keats spent long hours in bed or on the sofa in the front parlour gazing out of the window. He was greatly weakened, sometimes it seems nearly delirious, from what must have been partly at least hunger as well as regular bleedings (every time he coughed up blood); but he was still capable of writing long letters to his sister. They are not poetry or even memorable prose but are extraordinary documents of the acutely heightened awareness of many tuberculous patients. A passing pot-boy, the delivery of the coal, a small gipsy caravan, "a fellow with a wooden clock under his arm that strikes a hundred or more", all espied through the window, fascinated him. He watched the elderly Mr Lewis, "a neighbour who had been kind to poor Tom", pass by, noticing for the first time the man's rather unusual limp, and an old French immigrant walking with his hands clasped behind his back "his face drawn into a frown and full of political schemes". Bricklayers, maiden ladies with their dogs and ivory canes were all invested with a vivid present-tense actuality, as were the half-built houses opposite "dying of old age". And as he contemplated the "dingy tinge" of the winter grass, and the few dismal cabbage stalks below his window, his mind turned to the "flower-strewn world of summer": he

---

[4] The intensity of the contagion in such cases must have been intense. Poe, Trudeau. Thoreau and the Brontës were among others who nursed their dying brothers or sisters in small, often hermetically sealed rooms for months.

thought of every type of blossom he had known since infancy and "their shapes and colours were as new to me as if I had just perceived them for the first time". Above all it was the adored Fanny Brawne who obsessed his mind and whom he both longed for and feared to see: "You must believe – you shall, you will – that I can do, say or think nothing but what springs from my love for you". Under the regime inflicted on him he was fast sinking.

A hundred and fifty years later Sir George Pickering, Regius Professor of Medicine in Oxford University, called the history of medicine a monument to human folly. What in particular prompted his remark was the practice of indiscriminate blood-letting. Five years before Keats's illness declared itself, Colonel George McDonald of the Coldstream Guards came across a young army surgeon attending a wounded guardsman on the battlefield of Water-loo. The colonel was impressed by the coolness of the surgeon as he bent over his patient while cannon-balls were whizzing past and exploding around them, and hurriedly dismounted to offer his assistance. He then noticed with horror that the guardsman had a right thigh wound from which arterial blood was spurting unchecked, while, as a first-aid measure, his would-be rescuer was attempting to coax a few drops of blood from a surgically sectioned vein in the left arm. McDonald was unbuckling his belt to use as a tourniquet when the bleeding stopped. The guardsman was dead. Many years later the colonel related this experience to illustrate the mindlessness of overdrilled but inexperienced doctors under stress. In fact tens of thousands of patients had been bled to death for centuries before Waterloo and for at least fifty years after, not only on battlefields by inexperienced doctors working under stress but also in the hushed calm of sick-rooms and in hospital wards.

Nor does folly entirely explain the extraordinary hold the practice had on both doctors and the public. The explanation not grasped by wise men after the event is that at a time when effective forms of treatment were in short supply, blood-letting could produce dramatically beneficial results. Until comparatively recently it was the best first-aid treatment in acute pulmonary oedema – the sudden onset of choking breathlessness with co-pious blood-stained sputum, the face pale and cyanosed, the expression one of intense anxiety, the skin bathed on cold sweat – and tuberculosis was a rare cause of such an emergency.[5] In such cases a sudden reduction of the

---

[5] By far the most frequent cause was a failure of the left ventricle of the heart (in Keats's day probably most commonly due to valvular disease) to pump its load of blood into the peripheral circulation. Intracranial disease, kidney disease, pregnancy and acute fevers were some of the other causes.

circulating blood volume could afford instant (if rarely long-lasting) symptomatic relief.[6]

But in sick people the benefits were usually outweighed by the potential dangers. Most blatantly, if an illness was largely caused by blood loss, further bleeding was madness on common-sense as well as on scientific grounds; and the practice by generations of medical men to match every ounce of blood lost by haemorrhage from the lungs by an ounce of blood withdrawn by venesection remains baffling – and to doctors humiliating.[7]

In his short life Keats had had much to contend with apart from the terrors of a lingering illness. Some of his most ambitious works and some of his most beautiful, *Endymion* among them, were slated by small-minded mediocrities. He had to suffer the agony of Tom's long decline. His relations with his older brother, George, became clouded by unnecessary and petty disputes over their inheritance. His personal finances were always precarious if not catastrophic. Yet he was always surrounded by friends who responded to his generous nature and admired his still developing but incandescent genius. Many of them were concerned about his deteriorating health and, after he suffered an attack of chest pain accompanied by severe palpitations, invited Dr Robert Bree to see him.

Bree was a senior fellow of the Royal College of Physicians who had gained a lucrative reputation as a miracle worker by treating asthma with heroic

---

[6] There was more to blood-letting than providing relief in an acute emergency. Anybody concerned with the provision of a blood-transfusion service soon discovers that many donors become addicted and suffer true deprivation if they are not regularly bled. The explanation is not purely psychological as is sometimes glibly stated. The viscosity or thickness of the blood is one of the main variables which governs the speed and volume of blood flowing through the small arteries and capillaries. The most important variable which determines viscosity is the proportion of red blood cells to plasma (the "haematocrit", normally around 45 per cent): the greater the proportion of cells, the greater the viscosity. After blood-letting the body rapidly restores the total circulating blood volume by transferring fluid from the extravascular to the intravascular compartment; but it takes much longer to replace the lost cells. During this transitional period the haematocrit is low and so is the viscosity. As a result, outweighing the effect of the diminished number of red blood cells, the oxygen supply to the tissues may actually improve and the patient may feel better. In addition, the loss of blood is sensed by the bone marrow which steps up the rate of formation of new red blood cells. As a result the patient may enjoy for some time the benefits of a smaller but more youthful cell population. Modern concepts relating to this are discussed in Chien, S., Dormandy, J. A., Ernst, E., Matrai, A., *Clinical Haemorheology* (Dordrecht, 1987).

[7] Even in Keats's day outstanding physicians like Laënnec railed against indiscriminate blood-letting: "it never cured a single case of consumption"; but he provoked only sarcasm from his younger and more fashionable colleagues like Broussais; and Broussais' camp-followers always outnumbered those of Laënnec.

doses of digitalis.[8] The book in which he described his method and put forward his claims quickly ran through four editions; and since heart disease is one cause of asthma, and digitalis undoubtedly benefits many forms of heart disease, there was probably some substance in his claims. (His recommended dose, however, if carried into practice, must have killed more patients than it cured.) As befits a specialist in diseases of the heart, he was a hearty fellow but, less fittingly, an appalling diagnostician.

A glance at the prostrate patient, and the knowledge that Keats, a licensed doctor, had chosen poetry instead medicine, enabled him to make an instant diagnosis. The foolish young man had plainly no organic disease: his illness was all in the mind. After such preternatural insight it was hardly necessary to carry out a physical examination; but a quick inspection of the patient's chest confirmed that there was "no pulmonary affliction whatever". He then expressed the opinion that the patient had been the victim of his own feverish imaginings, not uncommon in poets, and that if he could not be persuaded to start earning an honest living as a doctor he should at least devote himself to studying an exact science like mathematics.

As often happened (and still does) the misdiagnosis gave the patient a few last happy and productive months. Bree was disgusted with the starvation diet and the unnecessary mollycoddling of the highly-strung young hypochondriac. What the invalid needed was a nutritious and ample diet with a good deal of red meat, an occasional glass of red wine, regular exercise, no bleeding and no drugs beyond the obligatory dose of digitalis. On this eminently sensible regime, Keats began to recover: day by day he looked better, he put on weight, he went for short walks, and, after refusing for months even to think of work, asked for the manuscripts of his poems to set about their final revision. Most importantly to him, he now genuinely hoped – at least at times – that his dream, his marriage to Fanny Brawne, might one day come true.

Of course it could not last. The publication of his next collection of verse was greeted with some of the most venomous criticisms of his poetry yet and gave birth to the legend that it was the poisoned pen of John Gibson Lockhart, the scorpion of the *Edinburgh Review*, which precipitated his relapse. This was almost certainly untrue; but it inspired Shelley's elegy *Adonais*, and much of the poetic mythology of the Pre-Raphaelites. In

---

[8] The discovery in the 1780s of the astonishing cardiotonic properties of digitalis contained in extracts of the foxglove leaf by a Shropshire general practitioner, William Withering, was probably the most important therapeutic advance of the eighteenth century. The dramatic disappearance of oedema and easing of breathlessness in patients with congestive heart failure made it perhaps inevitable that the drug should be tried in other conditions associated with vaguely similar symptoms. It then did no good and in high doses could be dangerous or fatal.

fact, after the first onslaught praise was nearly unanimous: the *Literary Gazette* printed a selection of his work, as did several other journals; Lamb was enthusiastic; and the *Sun* hailed *Hyperion* as "the greatest effort yet of Mr Keats's genius".

By then Keats was barely aware of this. In July 1819 he had suffered another haemorrhage, followed once again by the obligatory blood-letting, and he was under growing pressure not to face another winter in England. Apart from his reluctance to part from Fanny, a host of difficulties – financial and legal – had to be overcome; but his friends once again rallied round. Shelley, with whom he had never had an easy relationship, wrote from Pisa inviting him to stay; and a suitable travelling companion was found in the person of Joseph Severn. Severn, a modestly gifted painter in the early Romantic vein, had recently won the gold medal of the Royal Academy with his picture, *The Cave of Despair*, and was anxious to explore Italy. He was to prove a devoted friend.[9]

There was still the parting from Fanny. In their painful and precious last moments together she and Keats exchanged locks of hair and she gave him a diary, a travelling cap which she had lined, and a piece of smooth marble which she had always used to cool her hands and which would accompany him into his deathbed. He gave her a copy of *The Literary Pocket Book*. After his coach had departed she inscribed it with the date and the words "Today Mr Keats left Hampstead".[10]

The journey was frightful. After ten days in the Channel the overcrowded brigantine was blown back to beyond Gravesend, the first port of departure. The passengers were seasick and irritable. Keats suffered from sweats and bouts of temperature. Before their second departure from Portsmouth he procured for himself a bottle of laudanum "guaranteed to ensure a speedy and painless death if that become necessary". After their arrival in Naples, because of rumours (false as it later transpired) of an epidemic of typhoid in England, they were not allowed to disembark for a fortnight. All this suffering might have been worthwhile had it delivered Keats into the hands of local doctors. In their reluctance to take active measures (other than pray) they were far in advance of their British and French colleagues: indeed, they probably contributed as much as the climate to the healing properties attributed north of the Alps to the air of Italy. Unfortunately, a Scottish

[9] After Keats's death, Severn remained in Rome where he made a modest living as a painter. In 1861 he was appointed British Consul. He lies buried in Rome's Protestant cemetery next to Keats, whose memory he cherished. He well deserved the sympathetic biography by Sheila Birkenhead, *Against Oblivion: A Life of Joseph Severn* (London, 1944).

[10] She was twenty at the time and she wore mourning for Keats for seven years. In 1833 she married Louis Lindo (later Lindon) and had three children by him. She died in 1865.

doctor, Dr James Clark, had been warmly recommended to both Keats and Severn in England; and Clark resided in Rome. The journey there took another five days: only the spectacle of a Cardinal and his retinue in varying shades of purple on a duck-shoot in the Campagna provided light relief.

Clark, who was to return to London a few years later to became a royal physician, arguably the worst in a competitive field, and to end his long life a baronet, was a kindly and cultivated man.[11] He had read some of Keats's poetry and had liked it; and he found comfortable living quarters for the two young Englishmen only two minutes' walk from his own house overlooking the Spanish Steps. Unfortunately, he was also a lamentable doctor. It is almost unbelievable that the appearance of the emaciated, feverish, coughing, staggering young man did not make the diagnosis for him. Even the most cursory physical examination would surely have revealed the dismal state of the patient's lungs. Yet writing to a London medical friend after his first professional visit, Clark stated that "the chief part of the disease seems to be in the stomach and I have some suspicion of disease of the heart ... The lungs appear to be fairly sound and I am confident that I shall give you more reassuring news after the first few weeks of treatment". As in the case of Bree, one might forgive his diagnostic incompetence if his management had been less actively harmful.

The patient, Clark pronounced, needed exercise; and the best exercise was riding. Keats was by then barely strong enough to stand upright and stayed in the saddle for only a few minutes. The same night he suffered a haemorrhage from the lungs. As always, Clark came at once – and bled him. Next day Keats had another haemorrhage and Clark came and bled him again. It would have been kinder to administer the bottle of laudanum or at least a draught of it; but Clark did not believe in pain-killers and forbade Severn to administer even the smallest dose.

Mrs Clark was as tender-hearted as her husband and took on the task of providing the poet with that "dainty diet" which the doctor had prescribed. This was deemed necessary since Clark still regarded Keats's digestive system as the seat of the illness and he had to be nursed back to health by the blandest of food and little even of that. An anchovy a day was supplemented by large doses of antimony as a tonic – almost as if to ensure that if the patient did not perish from blood loss and starvation he would die from chemical poisoning. By the end of 1820 the gravity – indeed the hopelessness – of the situation had dawned even on Clark.

"Poor Keats is in a deplorable condition", he wrote to a medical friend in

---

[11] He died in 1870, aged eighty-two.

London. "Yesterday he had a haemorrhage from his stomach which I partially relieved by a venesection. But his state of mind is the worst possible."

Keats had always been a Grecian pagan professing no religious faith; but he had until his last illness clung to a pantheistic belief in the immortality of the soul. He now began to doubt even that and lapsed into total despair. Severn, a committed Christian, read Jeremy Taylor's *Holy Dying and Living Holy* to him; far from bringing comfort to the sick man, this plunged him into a state of "screaming horrors". "He seemed to be both longing for the end and terrified of death, tortured by his past mistakes, mostly quite trivial or even imaginary, which seemed to crowd in on him like ghosts", Severn was to recall.[12] A century later Sir William Osler wrote that "poor Keats had not even the hope of the tuberculous that often carries them to the very gates of death". It was the so-called treatment – the combination of blood-letting, starvation, antimony and the prohibition of sedatives – rather than the disease which was responsible for his suffering.

This was indeed terrible. During his last fortnight he was unconscious most of the time but sobbed and groaned whenever he regained conscious-ness. It was certainly no easeful death; nor did he "call death soft names in many a mused rhyme"; nor did he "cease upon the midnight with no pain". In the afternoon on Friday 23 February 1821 he turned to his exhausted friend, who had hardly left his bedside: "Severn – lift me up – I am dying – but I shall die easy. Don't be frightened and thank God it has come." Reclining in Severn's arms he stopped breathing a few minutes before midnight. Severn was not a great painter but his sketch of the dying poet remains a poignant memorial of the White Death. So perhaps does Clark's report on the post-mortem: "both lungs had completely gone exactly as I had thought".

Keats's short life-span, at the beginning of the Industrial Revolution, probably marked the first explosive peak in the incidence of pulmonary tuberculosis in England.[13] The man who invited him to stay in Italy, Percy Bysshe Shelley, was a fellow victim. He had had his first intimations of the illness, attacks of pleuritic pain, in 1817, a time when he was also deep in financial worries and tormented by his tragic relations with Harriet

[12] Birkenhead, S., *Against Oblivion*, p. 242.

[13] This is of course impossible to verify since reliable data are not available from before the Industrial Revolution; but over the next hundred years the beginning of industrialisation marked an upsurge in tuberculosis in every other country; and in Britain the incidence slowly but continually declined after 1840 until the First World War. The fact that the upsurge in England was still relatively recent at the time of Keats's death might serve as a slight mitigation of Clark's misdiagnosis and mishandling of the case. Unfortunately, his later career as an authority on tuberculosis was just as bad.

Westbrook. He probably had only a few more months to live when, six months after Keats's death in Rome, he perished in a sailing accident off the coast near Spezia.[14] He was twenty-nine.

Less familiar than the two poets and their promise even less fulfilled were two English painters.[15] Tom Girtin was born in 1775, within a few months and a few miles of another cockney genius, Joseph Mallord William Turner. (Mr Turner senior was a wig-maker in Covent Garden. Mr Girtin senior made brushes in Southwark.) The two young men became friends and rivals: they were both prodigies, making a precarious living as topographical water-colour artists, both determined to reach the top. Only one of them made it. By the time Girtin married and settled with his wife and little daughter in the "health-giving air of Islington" it was too late: he was coughing up blood regularly and so thin that "the slightest gust of wind might blow him away". He went to Paris, planning a huge panorama of the city and hoping perhaps to recover his health as well as make a fortune. Neither expectation was to be fulfilled. Soon after his return he collapsed and died in his studio in the Strand. A few days later his friend Turner, not given to self-deprecation, wrote: "Poor Tom, had he lived I would have starved." Looking at the comparatively few works left behind by Girtin – some of his best, like *The White House in Chelsea*, are in London's Tate Gallery but many may have been lost – it is easy to see what Turner meant.

Richard Parkes Bonington was born in Nottingham in 1802; and he too first became famous cultivating what on the Continent was already known as the English Art, water colour. It was the demand for the genre which took him to Paris at the age of nineteen. He became one of the sensations of the Salon of 1824, the most memorable of the century.[16] When he approached Baron Gros, expressing the wish to become Gros's pupil, the older man sent him packing: there was nothing a living artist could teach the young Englishman. For a time he shared a studio with another youthful genius, Delacroix, who both loved and admired him. "You are the king, there has been nobody like you since Watteau", the Frenchman wrote when Bonnington voiced his concern that his paintings were too small to attract

---

[14] When his decomposed body was washed ashore he was identified by two books found in his pockets, a volume of Sophocles in Greek and Keats's last published volume of verse.

[15] Short biographies of both are included in A. Wilton, *British Water Colour Artists* (London, 1978).

[16] It was the beginning of the Romantic era in painting with Delacroix's *Massacre of Chios* and Géricault's *The Raft of the Medusa* on show. The English contingent was also remarkable, showing Constables's *The Hay Wain* and *A View on the Stour* as well as Bonington's brilliant water-colours.

attention. The reference to another tuberculous master not yet widely known was probably no accident: Bonington was already ill and, like Watteau, became quickly exhausted when attacking a large canvas. For a few years he divided his time between Paris and London, equally sought after by connoisseurs in both cities, but fast using up his reserves. In 1824 his doctors sent him off to recuperate in the south of Italy. For some reason he only got as far as Venice. The city, beautiful but cold and damp in the early spring, did his lungs no good but carried his art to its peak. His intimate interiors, suffused with light but oddly claustrophobic, were the only ones which Turner later accepted as the equals of his own. A few months after he painted his last Venetian scene, a shimmering view of the Piazza San Marco,[17] he returned to France. He was barely strong enough to hold a brush. His father brought him back to London and installed him in a Harley Street nursing home. There he was bled of what little life there was left in him. To Delacroix he was "carried away like a young god by his own genius". He was twenty-six.

What then was the disease which claimed some of the finest of England's artists and poets at a time when in the applied sciences and technology the country was racing ahead, set to become within fifty years the world's greatest power?

Pulmonary tuberculosis, known as phthisis, consumption, wasting disease, weakness of the lungs, graveyard cough and a host of other more or less descriptive synonyms, was probably the commonest and certainly the most emblematic form of the illness. It could be acute or galloping (the term "miliary" came into general use in the early twentieth century),[18] but classically it was chronic and even intermittent, with seemingly miraculous remissions and startling improvements followed by terrible relapses. Until the 1950s informed opinion – that is standard textbooks – reckoned that it was fatal in 80 per cent of cases in five to fifteen years; but in all periods cures or apparent cures were well recognised and kept hope and a staggering number of therapeutic regimes alive.[19] In the early stages the symptoms were vague; but in the days (or centuries) when tuberculosis was in everybody's mind lassitude, a poor appetite, a declining performance at school or at work, loss of weight, pallor (which often contrasted with an unhealthy flush of the cheeks), night sweats, a chronically running nose and especially a cough in a child or young person previously fit instantly raised fears. If the

---

[17] Now in the Wallace Collection in London with other examples of Bonington's art.
[18] See note 20 to Chapter 1.
[19] See also section of successor diseases, below, Chapter 33, pp. 379–82.

fears were well founded other symptoms singly or in combination soon appeared: a harsh cough, hoarseness or loss of control of the voice, an audible wheezing sound, shortness of breath on exertion and, most dramatically, haemoptysis or the coughing up of blood. Perhaps the most constant manifestation was fever, usually slight but characteristically recurring in the late afternoon or at night. As the temperature dropped after a few hours the patient became drenched in sweat and felt physically exhausted though mentally alert. The end could be painful and messy; but the ethereal way of going was not entirely operatic fiction.

Tabes mesenterica, which had nothing to do with the tabes of tertiary syphilis,[20] was tuberculosis of the small intestine and lymph nodes in the abdomen and, sooner or later, of the peritoneum which in turn matted together loops of bowels and caused intermittent, usually subacute obstruction. Colicky pain, vomiting and diarrhoea were the chief symptoms. Because abdominal tuberculosis could become chronic with striking physical signs, it was a favourite short case in medical examinations. Medicine is beset with clichés. Candidates were expected to lay their hands on the patient's irregularly swollen abdomen and pronounce the sensation as "doughy". Together with scrofula, it was the form of tuberculosis most commonly caused by the milk-borne bovine strain of the organism.[21]

Lupus vulgaris, "the common wolf", was tuberculosis of the skin, pink or brown nodules appearing anywhere on the body – the face was a particularly common site – growing slowly but eventually ulcerating and often causing terrible destruction. This was the form of disease which most resembled another worldwide infection caused by a cousin of the *Mycobacterium tuberculosis*, *Mycobacterium leprae*. The culinary cliché to be applied by medical students to the early nodules was redcurrant jelly, which the early nodules were supposed to resemble when pressed down with a glass slide.

More even than tuberculosis of the lungs, tuberculosis of the bones and joints was a disease of childhood. It most commonly began with a painless swelling of a knee or with a limp if the affected joint was the hip. It seemed a mild illness at first, but the ultimate prognosis in most cases was poor; and often the infection was associated with tuberculosis of the kidneys and bladder, a particularly painful and demoralising complication. But the disease *could* be arrested for many years and even cured. Hugh Owen Thomas treated thousands of sufferers in the slums of Liverpool. The son, grandson and great-grandson of Welsh bone-setters, he wrote little and badly; but, as his fame spread, rich and titled patients came to consult him in his surgery in

---

[20] *Tabes* means wasting in Latin: linguistically it is synonymous with the Greek *phthisis*.
[21] See below, Chapter 29.

Nelson Street, open twenty-four hours a day, seven days a week. The poor he looked after free of charge. The cardinal tenet of his creed was that inflamed joints needed rest – "enforced, uninterrupted and prolonged" – and to this end he devised his famous splint, one of the simplest and most effective surgical appliances ever invented. (The Zimmer frame runs it a close second.) He prolonged the life – and perhaps saved – thousands of tuberculous patients; and after his death his splint proved no less useful in transporting the wounded on the battlefields of two world wars.[22]

In English-speaking countries tuberculosis of the spine was named after the eminent eighteenth-century surgeon, Percival Pott (1714–1788) – knighthoods did not come to surgeons, however eminent, for another hundred years – but it had been for centuries before Pott one of the best-known forms of the illness. It also provided a striking demonstration that left to itself the infection would occasionally burn itself out: there was no other explanation for elderly hunchbacks like Victor Hugo's famous bell-ringer or, in a more friendly English incarnation, Mr Punch. The deformity – still a common enough sight in the streets of Delhi and Jakarta – was the result of the softening of one or several vertebrae by tuberculous abscesses and their wedge-shaped collapse. Healing was by calcification and, in a growing child and unless prevented, it led to the formation of the permanent angle or gibbus.[23] Self-limitation was the exception rather than the rule. If the abscess burst into the spinal canal, it could compress the spinal cord and cause paralysis and death; or it could burst sideways, track along the sheath of the Psoas muscle and present as a fluctuating swelling below the groin. As in all tuberculous infections, the final event was often a secondary infection with pus-forming organisms. The list could be continued: there was almost no organ or tissue in the body which was immune. Tuberculosis of the cortex of the adrenal glands, named after the Guy's Hospital physician, Thomas Addison, probably killed Jane Austen. Tuberculous meningitis was the most feared acute form of the disease, often killing children in less than forty-eight hours and, when not killing them, leaving them permanently brain-damaged. Tuberculosis of the choroid in the eye could lead to blindness, of the inner ear to deafness, of the Fallopian tubes to painful chronic

[22] Thomas died in 1891 aged fifty-seven. His recognition as a benefactor of mankind owes much to his nephew and pupil, Sir Robert Jones, and to the opportunities provided by the First World War. Thanks largely to the use of the Thomas splint on the battlefield, the mortality from wounds involving bones fell from 80 per cent in 1914 to 7.3 per cent in 1918. Aitken, K. M., *Hugh Owen Thomas: His Principles and Practice* (Oxford, 1968).

[23] This could be avoided by timely recognition (almost impossible before X-rays) and immobilisation in a plaster of Paris bed. As Lord Dunglass, heir to the earldom of Home, Sir Alec Douglas-Home, Prime Minister in 1962–63, spent three years in such a cast as a schoolboy.

pelvic inflammation and sterility.[24] Accompanying every localised manifestation were the famous general signs – wasting, anaemia, tiredness and fever.

Treatment in the days of Keats added its quota to the suffering. It was rooted in ignorance. Despite the achievements of earlier centuries, there was, as the eighteenth century turned into the nineteenth, still a yawning gap in the minds of doctors between the clinical symptoms and signs on the one hand and the underlying pathology on the other. To bridge that gap would not necessarily bring relief, but without it any advance in that direction was impossible. Almost a century separates the diagnostic revolution in medicine which began that progression from Koch's historic discovery of the cause; and another fifty years would pass before the cause would yield to treatment; but the three milestones are inseparably linked. Compared to the blood, gore and clamour of Paris's Place de la Révolution, and the endlessly mulled over Napoleonic marches and countermarches, the diagnostic revolution in medicine lacked instant drama. It certainly gets short shrift in history books if it is mentioned at all. Yet in the long term it affected the human condition more deeply than the orations of politicians and the toings and froings of Kings and Emperors.

---

[24] No generalisation was ever absolutely true about tuberculosis. One of the puzzling features of the illness was that some organs were frequently affected while others virtually never. Tuberculosis of the cortices of the adrenal glands was relatively common and often bilaterial while the anatomically adjacent medullae were hardly ever involved. Though tuberculosis of the epidydimis was often referred to by patients (including Frank Muir in his autobiography, *A Kentish Lad*) as "tuberculosis of the testis", the testes were virtually immune.

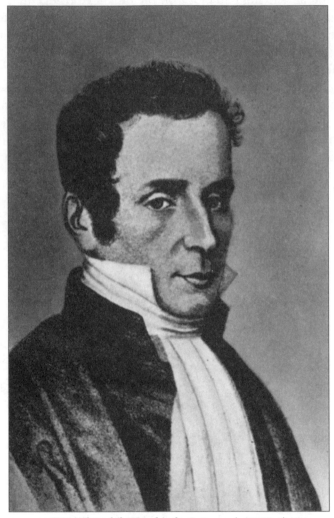

Réné Théophile Hyachinthe Laënnec (1781–1826)

3

The Sounds of Tuberculosis

The man who started that revolution was Leopold Auenbrugger (1722–1809), the son of an Austrian innkeeper, blessed with a musical ear. The legend, if it is a legend, that he first discovered the diagnostic potential of percussion by observing his father tapping caskets in the inn's wine-cellar stems from Observation III in his own book: "and the cause which occasions this diminution of resonance, whether by liquid or solid, is similar to that which occurs when a cask is being filled with wine".[1] The hostelry must have prospered for Leopold was sent to study medicine in Vienna. There, under the solicitous eye of the Empress Maria Theresa and guided by her medical and musical factotum, Baron Gerhard van Swieten,[2] the medical school was entering its first golden age. Leopold did well and eventually became physician to the city's Spanish Military Hospital. Little else is known about his private life or personality. He married the aristocratic Marianna von Priesterberg who died in her thirties. He mourned her; but, presided over by the elder of their two accomplished daughters, the family house on the Mehlmarkt, next to the Capuchin church, was for some years celebrated for its musical soirées.

Professionally he began to study the sounds that can be elicited by tapping the chest soon after establishing himself in practice; and he spent the best part of two decades exploring this ludicrously simple manoeuvre. Ludicrously simple to perform, that is, but far from simple to interpret. To understand the resonances and dullnesses and their relationship to other clinical findings and the underlying pathological processes required extraordinary perseverence: many of his patients Auenbrugger followed up for years and sometimes into the post-mortem room. He also performed experiments on

[1] *Inventum novum in percussione thoracis humani ut signo abstrusos interim pectoris morbos detegendi.* It was first translated into English by John Forbes in 1824 under the title *A New Invention for Percussing the Human Chest to Detect Hidden Signs of Disease.*

[2] A Dutchman who had looked after Maria Theresa's much-loved sister, Marianne, wife of Charles of Lorraine, Stadholder of the Netherlands, in her last illness. After her death he was summoned to the imperial court and became effectively the founder of the medical school of Vienna (modelled on the Dutch schools), as well as a patron of music, the librettist of Haydn's *Creation* and the dedicatee of Beethoven's first symphony.

cadavers. When he was fifty he published his observations in what is not only a medical classic but still a readable and clear exposition of the art of percussion.

Like countless clinical teachers who have since tried, more or less successfully, to convey similar messages to groups of medical students on their introductory ward round, he emphasised the importance of the surface markings of organs inside the living chest (as distinct from post-mortem appearances and illustrations in anatomy textbooks) and the changes which occur during the normal respiratory and cardiac cycle. His insistence on comparing corresponding spots on the two sides of the chest rather than percussing a rib on one side and an intercostal space on the other and declaring the first to be abnormally dull has lost none of its relevance. He demonstrated how percussing the same place while the patient is instructed to assume different positions can help to distinguish dullness due to underlying fluid in the pleural space (which shifts with posture) from dullness due to consolidation of the lung (which does not); and how far the persistence of a dull area in expiration can help to assess the depth of the lesion. Unlike casks, the chest can hyperresonate as well as sound dull; and the book showed how to distinguish between the hyperresonance of a zone adjacent to fluid from other causes such as a tuberculous cavity.[3]

In general what Auenbrugger discovered was that by percussing the chest wall a perceptive and mentally prepared listener could obtain almost as much information about physical events inside the chest as if he or she were looking through it (which did not become possible for another hundred and fifty years). It was possible to diagnose abscesses and areas of collapse, air in the pleural cavity, different kinds of enlargements of the heart or its displacement to one side or the other, dilatations or aneurysms of the great vessels, consolidations – that is the filling up of the air spaces with inflammatory fluid or pus – and the formation of air-filled or partially air-filled cavities. Nor was this all. Percussion was so quick and simple that small changes could be monitored daily or indeed several times daily, something few X-ray departments would countenance today, and related to the patient's general progress.

Auenbrugger's avoidance of unnecessary jargon – as well as his exposure of more than one venerable misconception – may not have endeared him to some of his colleagues. In the introduction to his great work he stated

---

[3] The name attached to this sound today is "skodaic resonance" after Joseph Skoda (1805–1860), the first in Vienna to appreciate fully and carry forward Auenbrugger's work, and one of the outstanding figures of the second generation of the Viennese School. His *Abhandlung über Percussion und Auscultation* (*Treatise on Percussion and Auscultation*) established physical diagnosis in German-speaking countries, just as Corvisart's translation did in France.

that in, placing the fruits of his labours at the disposal of his professional brethren, he was "not unconscious of the dangers he must encounter ... since it has always been the fate of those who tried to improve their arts or sciences to be beset by envy, malice, hatred, detraction and calumny". This might seem a fairly comprehensive list of misfortunes; but he omitted the gravest risk of all: that of being ignored.

In fact he may have been (like many an original thinker) a little paranoid: his rejection was far from complete. Maximilian Stoll, de Haen's successor as professor of medicine at the university,[4] mentioned "tapping" as a clever device "popular with some" and "wholly without risk to the patient" in his widely-read *Aphorisms*. There was even a much-abridged and heavily distorted translation of the *Inventum novum* into French before Corvisart's.[5] At court Auenbrugger must have been popular, since he was ennobled in 1784 – he signed himself *Edler von* Auenbrugg after that – though this may have been in recognition of his musical rather than his medical accomplishments. The former must have extended well beyond distinguishing between high-pitched and low-pitched dullnesses in the lung. At the Emperor's behest he wrote the libretto for a comic opera, *Der Rauchfangskehrer (The Chimney Sweep)*, for the court composer Salieri. (The first performance was *ein kolossales Succes* about the same time as Mozart earned modest plaudits for *The Marriage of Figaro*.[6] The Auenbrugger text is not available for comparison; but the Emperor never considered ennobling Mozart's somewhat disreputable librettist, Lorenzo da Ponte.)[7] It is true nevertheless that percussion did not become a widely performed bedside art until espoused by a more commanding figure.

The year of Auenbrugger's death was not a happy one for Austria. After the battle of Wagram the man who occupied Maria Theresa's beloved castle of Schönbrunn was not her grandson, the Emperor of Austria,[8] but the Corsican parvenu who now styled himself Emperor of the French. It was of course only a temporary occupancy (while negotiations were proceeding about the price of peace, the terms including a marriageable Habsburg Princess); but, as always on his campaigns, Napoleon was accompanied by

---

[4] He was the first native Austrian to occupy the chair in Vienna.

[5] By Rosière de Chassagne of Montpellier who recommended it, though he had "not had occasion to try it himself". Since he seems to have confused percussion with Hippocratic succusion (from which it is totally different) this was perhaps just as well.

[6] Neuburger, M., biographical note to facsimile edition of Auenbrugger's *Inventum novum* (Vienna, 1922), p. 242.

[7] The approximate date was 1786. By then the Emperor was Joseph II (1780–1790), who had succeeded his mother, Maria Theresa.

[8] Francis I (1792–1830), the first to be styled Emperor of Austria.

his personal physician, Baron Jean Nicolas Corvisart (1775–1821).[9] Three times a week the Baron would enter the imperial dressing room after the Emperor's early-morning bath, feel the great man's pulse, gaze at his urine, prod his abdomen and palpate and then carefully percuss his chest. This was unusual but in character: even after acquiring in middle age the professional gravitas befitting a court physician, Corvisart was an unusual person. In fact, in some respects he was not unlike his master. Both had been among the new men who had emerged from their country's revolutionary upheavals, not extreme revolutionaries in politics or sentiment but artists, writers, scientists, soldiers, thinkers and doctors, impatient with old shibboleths and eager to explore new, even dangerous paths.

Originally intended for the law, he had run away from home in 1789, the year of the fall of the Bastille, and had become an orderly at the Hôtel Dieu, Paris's oldest hospital. There he attracted the favourable attention of such influential members of the staff as Antoine Petit and Desbois de Rochefort and in due course presented a thesis for the title of doctor regent to the faculty of medicine. It was highly commended, but he was dissatisfied both with the teaching he had received and with the clinical practice he had observed.

Paris at the end of the eighteenth century had a galaxy of fashionable physicians and its citizens took pride in its hospitals for the poor, but it had no clinical tradition comparable to that of Leyden, Bologna or Vienna. Whether young Corvisart personally visited these centres – it would have been difficult since during most of his apprenticeship France was at war with half of Europe – or merely sought out works published abroad is not known; but he certainly acquired Auenbrugger's treatise, tested its claims and was convinced by their validity. In 1791 his refusal to wear a powdered wig still cost him a staff appointment at Paris's new Hôpital Necker; but when the wigs (with many of the heads they had once adorned) were swept away, his advancement was rapid. In 1795 he became professor of medicine at the Collège de France and the first professor of medicine at the Hôpital de la Charité; and everywhere he preached Auenbrugger's gospel. He also became the personal physician to the First Consul, General Bonaparte, advancing with his patient to become court physician to His Imperial Majesty and His Imperial Majesty's siblings, wives and more important mistresses.[10]

Corvisart was as naturally an authority as Auenbrugger was not, and his

---

[9] Beeson, B. B., *Annals of Medical History*, 2 (1930), p. 300.

[10] Josephine, Marie-Louise and Marie Walewska were all devoted to him. "I do not believe in medicine", Napoleon himself confided in Eugène de Beauharnais, "but I believe in Corvisart."

pupils included such influential future medical and surgical teachers as Cuvier, Piorry, Laënnec and Dupuytren. He was also an honourable man who never tried to appropriate Auenbrugger's great discovery for himself even though his "translation", five times the size of Auenbrugger's modest seventy-five-page offering, was full of useful additional observations and instructions. In particular, he advocated a recent innovation which proved to be almost as significant as the original discovery.

Reading Auenbrugger's account of his invention, the modern medical reader may be bemused by the author's instructions about shoulder and elbow movements and even more by the injunction to hold the wrist steady: how did the writer get any sound response at all? The answer is that Auenbrugger and his early followers percussed the chest directly with the tip of the right middle finger (much as one would percuss a cask of wine). This is still a possible technique but far more difficult than indirect percussion. The first important development in that direction was the introduction of a pleximeter, a thin disc made of bone or ivory, which somewhat distorted but also amplified the sound. The perfected instrument, complete with angled and prettily carved wooden handle, was described by Pierre Adolphe Piorry,[11] professor of medicine at the Hôpital de la Pitié; but the critical step was taken by a visitor to Piorry's clinic about whom nothing is known except that he was an Englishman and that he must have been both absent-minded and inventive. Having mislaid his pleximeter and being unable to make sense of the sounds elicited by direct percussion, he pressed his extended left middle finger to the patient's chest and, lifting off the other fingers so as not to deaden the sound, tapped it from the wrist with the middle finger of his right hand. This was an inspired substitution since it added touch to sound and made the procedure many times more intelligible to unmusical clinicians. Corvisart immediately adopted it; and everybody copied Corvisart.

Useful as Corvisart's advocacy of indirect percussion was, his most important innovation was placing the examination of the whole patient at the centre of the art of diagnosis, indeed of the practice of medicine. To his elderly contemporaries – he called them the Gothics – this seemed eccentric bordering on the outrageous: they rarely ventured beyond the fingering of the pulse and a learned scrutiny of the tongue, regarding undressing patients as both unnecessary and immodest. Corvisart insisted that even the most high-born should divest themselves of all clothing and be examined from

---

[11] A deeply religious man, after a visit to Laënnec's clinic he prayed long and hard to be granted the joy of discovering something as useful and important as the stethoscope. His wish was granted a few months later when trying to percuss the chest of a patient covered with a painful skin eruption. He found that percussing indirectly by tapping on a thin silver medallion laid on the chest not only eased the patient's discomfort but also improved the sound quality.

top to bottom. The excitement of this approach, as rousing in its day as the first bars of the *Marseillaise*, is hard to recapture, not because the practice has become so universal but because it is so rapidly going out of fashion. Of course lip service is still being paid to Citoyen (as he was when he first spelt it out) Corvisart's great principle – that it is a whole individual and not a lung or a knee which is sick and needs help – but in practice examining the whole patient now usually means the filling in of a questionnaire and the dispatching of an assortment of blood samples for laboratory tests. It was Corvisart's approach, nevertheless, which established that, irrespective of the site of the primary lesion and of the dominant symptoms, tuberculosis was a general disease.

Auenbrugger and Corvisart were pioneers, forerunners of the greatest medical revolutionary, René Théophile Hyacinthe Laënnec (1781–1826).[12] Yet though Laënnec's statue now stands in front of the cathedral in Quimper, his birthplace in Brittany, few passing tourists recognise the name. A local political worthy perhaps or a collector of Breton folklore? Even among medical men and women the memory of great doctors rarely survives as vividly does the memory of great artists and writers. Hospitals, bacteria, anatomical structures, diseases and surgical operations may recall a few names; but no practising clinician communes with them in the way that every painter still tries to winkle out the secrets of Titian, every music-lover still finds enchantment in Schubert and every Christian still draws strength from the Gospels.[13] Laënnec was probably as great a genius as Beethoven, Byron, Goethe and Goya (to pick out at random four of his contemporaries); but none of his books are read today except by scholars, and his eponymous fame rests on Laënnec's cirrhosis of the liver – a form of cirrhosis associated with alcoholism – to which his contribution was marginal. But in one respect his legacy lives on: despite hundreds of more sophisticated diagnostic aids,

---

[12] Kervran, R., *Laënnec: médecin Breton* (Paris, 1955); Rouxeau, A., *Laënnec avant 1806* (Paris, 1920); Rouxeau, A., *Laënnec après 1806* (Paris, 1921).

[13] The main reason is that the arts and literature grow but do not in any real sense *advance*: Beethoven never tried to supersede Mozart and Picasso never set out to eclipse Rembrandt. In the sciences, by contrast – and in this respect medical science does not differ from other scientific disciplines – the more important the development the more rapidly it is further developed. The discoveries of the past do not of course disappear, any more than the inside stones of a pyramid disappear, but as individual creative acts they become difficult and sometimes impossible to trace. Nor, as a rule, do scientists and doctors exert themselves trying. A few names – Newton, Volta, Harvey, Faraday – are regularly intoned like tribal incantations; but, while the memory of dozens of the lesser contemporaries of Mozart and Rembrandt are still cherished by music and art lovers, a professor of medicine would be hard put to name a single contemporary of Harvey's and might resent being asked silly questions.

his gadget, the stethoscope, remains the trade-mark, prop and prayer-bead of doctors everywhere.[14] (Until the Second World War nurses were not allowed to take patients' blood pressures because the measurement involved the use of a stethoscope and the use of a stethoscope was deemed to be an exclusively medical skill.)

Laënnec's mother died giving birth to a stillborn fourth child: she is said to have been tuberculous and her disease may have been activated by her last pregnancy.[15] René was then five and his brother, Michaud, three; about a sister, Marie-Anne, little is known. Laënnec *père* was an advocate of some distinction but judged to be too morally irresponsible to look after his children. All three were farmed out first to an uncle, a *curé* in a nearby parish who had to flee to England from the Revolution,[16] and then to another uncle who was in medical practice in Nantes. It is there that at the age of fourteen and a half René first entered a medical school.

These were grim times in the west of France. After the royalist rebellion in the Vendée and during the Terror more than 3000 people were put to death in Nantes alone – many more in the countryside around it. Because the guillotine had been erected in front of Dr Laënnec's house,[17] the children had to leave for school by the back door. (Soon the guillotine proved too slow: the condemned – men, women and children – were then mown down by chain-shot or drowned in the Loire.) Robespierre's fall came just in time to save René's uncle, by then rector of the university and in line for the guillotine;[18] but the young man's studies were soon interrupted by military service. Eventually the boys' father was constrained either by the authorities or by his conscience to provide modest financial support; and this allowed the elder son to move to Paris and enrol once again as a medical student.

During the next five years Laënnec came under the influence of Corvisart, whom he admired but did not like, and formed a lifelong friendship with Gaspard Laurent Bayle (1774–1816), a former army surgeon from the Midi, who had become obsessed with the pathology of tuberculosis. Laënnec's own professional preeminence was soon recognised. In 1802 he was awarded both the chief prizes instituted by the Ministry of the Interior for papers on diseases of the lung; he became editor of the prestigious *Journal de médecine;*

[14] For a Greek scholar the word, coined from στῆτος (chest) and σκοπειν (to view), was a curious misnomer since the latter means only visual examination.

[15] It had long been recognised that pregnancy can affect the progress of phthisis in either direction (as it can many other chronic diseases): unpredictably the illness may either rapidly deteriorate or dramatically improve.

[16] He died of phthisis in exile.

[17] Still standing in the Place de Buffai.

[18] On 26 July 1794.

he was appointed to the staff of the Hôpital Necker; and Corvisart recommended him to his rich clientele.

It was while examining one such patient, Mlle de Surenne, in the spring of 1818 that he made his historic discovery; contrary to legend, it was his young patient's plumpness rather than her aristocratic birth which created the need.

> As I realised that both percussion and direct auscultation were almost useless through the layer of fat I recalled from boyhood a familiar fact of acoustics, namely that if one places one's ear at the end of a piece of timber one can hear very distinctly the scratch of a pin at the other end ... I therefore took a paper notebook, rolled it up tightly, applied one end to the precardiac region and listened at the other. I was as surprised as I was pleased to hear the heartbeats much more clearly and distinctly.[19]

After painstaking further experiments to establish the best material, the most useful length, the best proportions of the internal canal and the exact shape, he developed the first stethoscope, a hollow wooden tube about a foot long and two inches in diameter, widening into a funnel at one end and fitting into the physician's ear at the other. It was – and remains – a brilliant device, a compromise (like Bach's *Well-Tempered Clavier*) for the transmission of an extraordinarily wide range of sounds, from the sibilant susurration of air passing through a narrowed bronchus to the motoric lub-dub of the normal heart.

Inevitably Laënnec's first report to the Académie des Sciences was greeted with polite scepticism; but most of those prepared to try his novel method of eavesdropping were impressed; and within a few years several hundred stethoscopes, mostly home-made and therefore varying widely in shape, size and elaboration, were in use in France and not only of France. Among Laënnec's admirers was a young English physician on a visit to Paris, John Forbes, who, on his return, translated the French doctor's recently published book. But though enthusiastic, Forbes was not sanguine: "I am sure", he wrote in his preface,

> that Monsieur Laënnec's ingenious instrument will never come into general use in this country ... not only because its beneficial application requires a good deal of trouble and skill but also because its whole character is utterly foreign ... To Englishmen there will always be something ludicrous in the image of a grave physician listening to the chest through a long wooden tube as if the disease were a living thing in communication with him ... Besides, there is in this method a sort of bold faith in the physical examination of patients wholly alien to English medicine, more accustomed to calm cautious philosophical musings.[20]

---

[19] See Laënnec, R. T. H., *A Treatise on Diseases of the Chest and on Mediate Auscultation*, translated by J. Forbes (London, 1827), p. 3.
[20] Forbes, J., introduction to Laënnec, *A Treatise on Disease*, p. 2.

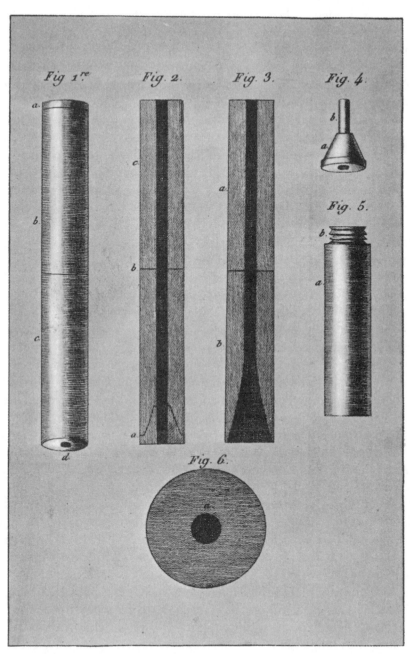

The first drawing of the stethoscope. Like most great doctors, Laënnec was a man of many parts: an accomplished draughtsman and engraver, he illustrated his own paper describing its invention.

Forbes was an acute observer of the English character and an excellent translator but crystal-gazing was not his forte.

In itself, the stethoscope was, of course, only a toy: what mattered in Laënnec's day (as it still does) was the understanding of the sounds reaching the doctor's ear. In describing them – râles, rhonchi, wheezes, tell-tale silences and the grating of the inflamed pleural layers – Laënnec combined them with his extensive clinical knowledge and post-mortem observations and expounded the correlations with great clarity. Of the 393 pages of his treatise the lungs take up only about a hundred: but it is the section which most impressed his contemporaries – rightly so. The proportion was also in keeping with his and Bayle's estimate that a quarter of the people who died in Paris every year died of pulmonary disease. After the turgidity of medical texts of pre-revolutionary days his descriptions were marvels of concision and his interpretation of the physical signs of tuberculosis in pathological terms masterly. And not only of tuberculosis.

In some respects his descriptions of what he recognised as non-tuberculous lesions seem today even more impressive. There is a strong inclusive tendency in medical research. A postgraduate student engaged in a project about a rare heart condition will gradually tend to recognise it as a factor in an increasing number of wholly unrelated illnesses. A surgeon who has spent years devising a new operation for hammer toes will come to regard the whole field of surgery as an extension of this important but essentially localised and rarely life-threatening deformity. This was true of many of the best workers interested in tuberculosis. Bayle was a painstaking investigator and his book, *Recherches sur la phthisie pulmonaire*, published in 1810, was based on no less than 900 post-mortem examinations. It is full of acute observations; but his findings led him to postulate the existence of six different categories of *phthisies* into which all his cases could be – or had to be – fitted. This in practice implied a single underlying pathology for all diseases of the lungs. Largely because of this tendency to unify, his diagnoses today are almost impossible to understand. How did his *phthisies granuleuses* (183 cases) differ from his *phthisies tuberculeuses* (624 cases)? What did his three cases of *phthisies cancereuses* mean? Did he believe phthisis to be precancerous? Or that cancer of the bronchus was a form of phthisie? Even allowing for the likelihood that cancer of the bronchus was less common 200 years ago than it is today, is it conceivable that there were only three cases in a series of over 900 deaths from wasting associated with lung disease? It is such excessively comprehensive classifications which make the reading and understanding of the works not only of Bayle but of most of his contemporaries such an uphill task today.[21]

---

[21] Discussed in the section on the successor diseases, below, Chapter 33, 379–82.

This was – and is – not true of Laënnec's writings. He too described what can still be recognised and accepted as almost certainly tuberculosis; but he also identified other and rarer forms of lung pathologies. In today's terminology what he called *bronchorrhées purulentes* would be called bronchiectasis, a condition in which a localised segment of a bronchus loses its elasticity and becomes dilated and infected. Many causative factors have been suggested; but the aetiology is still uncertain.[22] Severe forms of the disease are comparatively rare: they are characterised by large volumes of foul-smelling sputum which seem to well up from the chest on changing position rather than being coughed up. Such cases are usually accompanied by a general decline in health and the condition is probably precancerous. Mild forms are common and may disappear clinically without treatment; but they are often associated with a blood-stained sputum. For centuries this was the alarm bell signalling phthisis or, in later parlance, pulmonary tuberculosis. Indeed, how common bronchiectasis is did not become apparent until the decline in tuberculosis in the 1950s in response to the first wave of effective antibiotic therapy. Bronchiectasis then emerged as the most common cause of haemoptysis in otherwise fit young people. This last experience does not mean that bronchiectasis was equally common in Laënnec's day or during the century and a half between Laënnec and the discovery of streptomycin; but the disease probably always accounted for some cases of haemoptysis and was usually misdiagnosed.[23]

Laënnec's medical and scientific achievements, as well as the relentless tempo of his daily life as teacher, author, editor and clinician, might suggest a robust and obsessive worker exclusively focused on medicine. In fact, even in youth he was frail and thin to the point of emaciation with prominent cheek-bones and hollow cheeks. One obituarist, and a life-long friend, the painter Lefair, likened him to the young Bonaparte on the Bridge of Arcola in Gros's famous battle-scene.) But his stamina was extraordinary. He conducted a daily two-to-three-hour teaching round in Latin so as to be understood by foreign visitors who flocked to Paris to hear him. He had a large private practice and never gave up research. Nor did his profession monopolise his interests. Even during his military service and in all his later travels he carried with him his flute; and composers dedicated chamber works

[22] In particular the question whether the bronchial dilatation is secondary to infection or to the focal collapse of the surrounding lung remains unsettled.

[23] Goethe is one of many famous people who have been included from time to time among victims of tuberculosis on the grounds that he occasionally coughed up blood-stained sputum as a young man. Although he himself certainly suspected that he had (like his friend Schiller) phthisis, after his return to Weimar from Italy he remained in good health and lived to the age of eighty-three. It is much more likely that he had mild bronchiectasis.

to him.[24] He was an accomplished draughtsman illustrating his own medical papers, including his classic description of the stethoscope. He translated Hippocrates from the original Greek.[25] Above all, he was a Celtic scholar whose studies of Breton dialects are still admired. The last accomplishment reflected his attachment to his native province and its people. Despite his mastery of literary French, he always considered himself a Breton. In 1814 he organised at the Hôpital de la Charité a special ward for wounded Breton soldiers who spoke no French. He visited them every day to comfort them in their native tongue. In 1824 he married a relative, Marie Argou, with whom he had been living for some years, perhaps with the idea of starting a family; but by then he was hopelessly ill.

What were probably not the first but the first unmistakable signs of tuberculosis – paroxysms of "asthma", attacks of fever and periods of extreme lassitude – struck him soon after his appointment to the chair of medicine at the Collège de France in succession to Corvisart. He may have had a high degree of immunity from exposure to the illness in childhood; but with hindsight his lack of precautions during thousands of post-mortem examinations conducted on cases of virulent infection can only be described as suicidal.[26] In 1804 alone he infected his fingers eight times with what he himself realised was pus from bodies dead from phthisis; and he soon had attacks of diarrhoea which he attributed to contamination from the same source. What is almost inexplicable is that neither he nor his friend Bayle, nor their brilliant colleague and near contemporary Bichat, drew the obvious conclusion.[27]

Both Bayle and Laënnec also ignored warning signs that the disease was

---

[24] None seems to have survived. Corvisart too was a lover of music and looked after artists and actors free of charge.

[25] Earlier translations were from Latin texts.

[26] The cavalier attitude of dissectors to the possibility of transmitting diseases from dead bodies either to themselves or to their patients continued almost till the end of the century (except in Italy). Ignaz Semmelweiss's heroic advocacy in the 1850s of washing hands between the post-mortem room and the wards went almost entirely unheeded. Apart from causing puerperal fever (which was Semmelweiss's concern), the practice must have been particularly fraught with danger in dealing with an organism like the *Mycobacterium tuberculosis* which could survive in dead tissue for weeks or months.

[27] In a detailed assessment of Laënnec's illness (about which a great deal is known), S. Lyle Cummins came to the conclusion that "it was the reinfections of the post-mortem room, frequently repeated in the course of hundreds of autopsies ... that led to his early death ..." Tuberculosis contracted in the same way almost certainly crippled and eventually killed both Bayle at the age of thirty-nine and their colleague, the great histologist Marie François-Xavier Bichat, in 1802 aged thirty-one. The sheer volume of achievement of all three during their short careers constantly plagued by ill-health is extraordinary.

gaining a grip on them; but a few uncharacteristic passages inserted into the second edition of Laënnec's book make one suspect that by 1822 he was beginning to realise the truth. While he still professed to agree with Bayle and his own earlier statement that "a cure of consumption in its early stages is perfectly illusory", he now stated that once the tubercles have coalesced and have become soft "nature and art may retard or even arrest their progress". In another newly-inserted passage he wrote: "I am convinced from a great number of observed facts that in some cases the disease is curable after the softening of the tubercles and the formation of ulcerous cavities". The passages are uncharacteristic because there were no such facts: there could not have been. But they enshrine what was soon to become known as the *spes phthisica*, "the hope of the tuberculous", an irrational optimism which many patients themselves recognised as irrational and which tended to alternate with troughs of deep depression. Laënnec himself was to prove the fallacy of the famous hope as well as its sustaining force.

For some years, whenever he had driven himself to the verge of collapse, he left Paris for a period of recuperation in Brittany where "invariably I recover simply by going on long exhausting walks and breathing the region's incomparable air".[28] But after his return to Paris sooner or later there was another relapse; and from his last escape in 1826 he never returned. When even in the health-giving air of Kerlouarnec he developed a high fever, and his sickness and diarrhoea did not improve, he added to his will detailed and updated instructions about the disposal of his unfinished manuscripts. Coughing and fighting for breath he went on dictating a chapter for the new edition of his book until the day before he died.

[28] He was impressed by the virtual non-existence of tuberculosis among the peasantry in Brittany (in sharp contrast to the inhabitants of Paris) and attributed this to something in sea air which protected against the disease. Inventive as ever, he even had seaweed brought from Brittany to Paris and had it spread on the floor of his wards. Two generations later Dr Robert Mariotte found that phthisis was, in fact, more common in Brittany than in most other provinces in France. By then – but not before – Brittany was also among the poorest of France's regions, as it indeed has remained until comparatively recently.

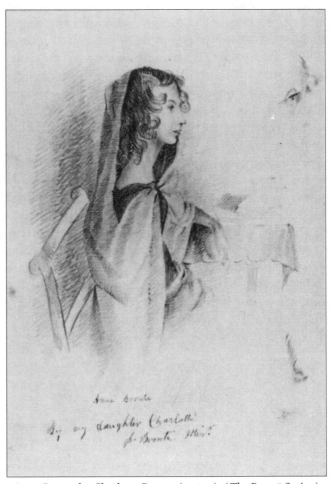

Anne Brontë by Charlotte Brontë (*c.* 1840). (*The Brontë Society*)

4

The Diathesis

Scientifically and medically the decades between Laënnec and the rise of the sanatorium movement were among the most sterile. They were also the most clamorous: disputes among baffled doctors are always intemperate and often hysterical. While doctors argued, the illness continued to kill men and women of all ages, but especially the young: it wrecked hopes, it broke courtships and it struck down bread-winners leaving large families destitute. Even as it declined slowly after the mid nineteenth century – on the Continent and in the United States it peaked several decades after England – it remained until the 1940s the commonest cause of death among those about to enter the most productive period of their lives – or what should have been the most productive period of their lives. What then was this disease as it appeared not to the high-powered but impotent specialists but to ordinary people and their family doctors?

Faced with such a daunting diversity of clinical presentations, the question which dominated scientific discussion was how this terrible affliction arose and why it singled out some individuals and spared others. More precisely, there was in most countries north of the Alps not a great deal of discussion: more a determined effort to suppress the few dissenting voices and any evidence which cast doubt on the doctrine of the tuberculous diathesis. This meant that, while one might argue about the relative importance of precipitating, contributory and environmental factors, the illness was essentially the product of an inborn – usually familial – disposition. "Tradition and common observation clearly show why some individuals rather than others become consumptive", wrote Sir James Clark in his textbook which became known as the tuberculosis doctor's bible. "These unfortunates are instantly recognisable by their scrawny body, flat, narrow or concave chest, fair freckled skin, red or very pale hair and eyes, irregularly harsh instead of silky breathing and of course the high probability that they had had elder tubercular kin with similar characteristics." The irregular harsh breathing was particularly important because it indicated a "weak circulatory system incapable of flushing out the tubercular poison".[1]

[1] Clark, J., *A Treatise on Pulmonary Consumption* (London, 1835), p. 128.

Nor was the accursed diathesis confined to humans: tuberculous lesions in cattle were similarly the products of an inborn constitutional defect, scraggy, doomed animals being more often than not the offspring of scraggy, doomed parents. The occurrence of the disease in some but not in other species lent support to this idea: consumptives who could afford it would be ordered to drink asses' milk because asses were believed not to be prone to the diathesis.[2]

The diathesis alone was never of course enough to explain the occurrence of clinical tuberculosis in some but not in other members of a family, all presumably carrying the same burden of inheritance;[3] nor, in the Victorian high noon of bourgeois morality, would an explanation devoid of an ethical dimension have been acceptable. While not disputing the importance of inheritance, Dr James Copland in 1869 enumerated the eighteen most important precipitating causes which allowed the diathesis to become manifest. (Over the next half century the list inevitably became a favourite with medical examiners while ribald mnemonics circulated among the students.) Most of the items represented more or less culpable deviations from healthy living, the term "health" embracing – as it did to most of Copland's readers – moral as well as physical attributes. "Ill-regulated studies and an incontinent search for pleasure ... sapped nervous power which controlled cell growth and thereby allowed anarchic cell proliferation which in turn accelerated the deposition of tubercles." (While commending Copland's exposition, another sage, Dr Simon Bullstrode of the Brompton Hospital, added that "on rare occasions even constitutionally healthy individuals could develop the disease during periods of depravity or spiritual anguish".) Further down on the Copland list came "improper clothing of several regions of the body [which could] precipitate consumption because they lowered body heat: immodest dress in women in particular could fatally expose their respiratory system". Then came the dread triad of sexual indulgence, masturbation and celibacy, all requiring detailed exegeses and telling illustrations. "We need look no further than the Catholic nunneries in France where not more than one in

---

[2] Asses are relatively resistant to tuberculosis and their milk is the closest in composition to human milk. It was recommended by the School of Salerno in the eleventh century; and in England *The Family Oracle of Health* (first published in 1824 and later vying in popularity with Mrs Beeton's *Household Management*) printed a recipe for preparing an artificial asses milk to be used by consumptives. "Bruise eighteen garden snails with one ounce of heartshorn shaving, an ounce of eryngo root ..." and so on.

[3] Before Mendel invented genetic inheritance (making his famous sweet peas obey the laws he had wisely conceived well in advance), this burden was regarded as a kind of amorphous soup or rather two lots of soup, one lot from each parent, which got mixed up in each individual.

ten entrants survive their period of novitiate." But alas, if the British were temperamentally less given to religious excesses, they were more drawn to physical self-abuse. In women Copland attributed this to an early addiction to riding: he could think of no more certain way of inducing the vice and thus paving the way for phthisis.[4]

The close link between sexual irregularities and tuberculosis spawned a large literature, capped by the discovery of a distinctly syphilitic form of tuberculosis by Dr Henry Green of Northampton (but anticipated in fiction by George Meredith in *The Ordeal of Richard Feverel*). Alcoholism too was as inevitable an entry on every list as smoking would be today; and it inevitably generated another distinct and easily recognisable form of the illness, alcoholic phthisis. It was described in astonishing detail (considering that it does not exist) by Dr J. B. Bradbury of Addenbrooke's Hospital in Cambridge, as impressive a hodge-podge of fact, fiction, limping statistics and religious moralising as any modern antismoking tract. Indeed the *Boston Medical and Surgical Journal,* an otherwise serious organ, published a note in 1851 on the *Diary of a Tobacco Smoker and Chewer,* purporting to be the journal of the Reverend Solomon Spittle. The physician who performed the post-mortem examination on the unfortunate Spittle was in no doubt that the cleric's death was due to "phthisis caused by the inordinate use of tobacco". In the same minatory vein when waltzing became the rage on the Continent in the 1820s it was regarded by many as an ally if not the cause of consumption, Dr Ferdinand Hahn of the University of Graz even suggesting that the disease should be renamed *Polka morbus* because of the frequency of relapses induced by too vigorous an indulgence in the *Dreitakt.*

Awareness of the importance of poverty, overcrowding, lack of hygiene and occupational hazards in causing diseases in general, but especially consumption, did not become widespread among the professional and middle classes till comparatively late in the nineteenth century; and then in response to the horrific pictures painted by popular novelists like Charles Kingsley, Disraeli and above all and incomparably by Dickens rather than as a result of medical agitation.

If the hereditary diathesis had a rival as the primary cause of tuberculosis it was foul air. Florence Nightingale had no doubts – she rarely had any on matters of health – and her words, almost invariably reinforced by strong though entirely circumstantial evidence, carried enormous weight. She professed to be convinced that air rebreathed by too many people for too long could by itself generate tuberculosis; and her conviction was seemingly

---

[4] Riding was strongly recommended for men and its ill-effects in women could be mitigated by riding side-saddle.

vindicated when the incidence of the disease in the army fell after barracks were enlarged and new and stringent rules for ventilation embodied in Queen's Regulations. But Miss Nightingale's followers did not always help her causes. One of her ardent admirers, the fashionable Belfast physician Dr Henry McCormack, not only asserted that the genesis of tuberculosis by foul air was "as true as that the stars shine in Heaven" but also declared on first principles – that is having taken no steps to ascertain facts – that "consumption must be rife in Iceland because the country's inhabitants have to breathe each other's spoiled air while living huddled together through the cold and dark winter months". As luck would have it his article in the *Lancet* was read by a proud Icelander who was stung into a devastating rebuff, asserting (wrongly as it later transpired) that consumption was unknown in his country except when introduced by drunken English, Irish and Scottish sailors.

Antituberculous regimes were as dismal as speculations about the causes of the disease. The mania for bleeding happily waned by the mid century (though Dr Copland was still bleeding patients who were "strong enough to withstand this powerful remedy" in the 1860s); but "cupping" continued in most countries for much longer. The object of this horrific procedure was "to draw out deep-seated infections" (and any other buried mischief) by making a small incision in the skin over the suspected site,[5] and then applying to the area a preheated glass cup with slightly rough edges. As the cup and the air within it cooled and contracted, blood and tissue fluid and sometimes pus and other necrotic material oozed out through the incision, hopefully carrying with it the causative noxious agents. It was still practised in field ambulance stations on the Russian front in the First World War in treating gunshot wounds.

Lesions already open were attacked with a fantastic variety of infusions, incrustations, ointments and poultices. Iodine became popular in the 1840s, its near-miraculous properties having been discovered by Jean Guillaume Auguste Lugol (1786–1851) of the Hôpital St-Louis in Paris. (Rediscovered would perhaps be more accurate, since Hippocrates advocated the burning of sea sponges in sick chambers, an excellent way of combating iodine deficiency.) His famous solution, still in use after Second World War though for the entirely different purpose of preparing patients with toxic goitres for operation, was taken by mouth, rubbed in, added to bath water, mixed with food or given in combination with mercurial pills. Dr John Savory of the Edinburgh Royal Infirmary noted that, in the last formulation and in the doses recommended, it usually caused "serious derangements of the nervous system" but "the beneficial effects outweighed the disadvantages". In contrast

[5] A specially designed pointed scalpel was used for this purpose.

to such dangerous and usually expensive remedies, cod-liver oil, popularised by Dr D. J. Blasius Williams, physician to the Brompton Hospital in the 1850s, was both cheap and harmless.[6] It became in every civilised country the prime restorative of the physically enfeebled and the invariable adjunct to any kind of treatment of tuberculosis (and of almost anything else): it continued to hold sway for a hundred years though most patients, especially children, found it revolting – as indeed it was. Blasius Williams never divulged what had inspired him; but its scientific rationale was explained by Dr Theophilus Thomson of Bath: "The oil combines with the albuminous element of chyle – that is the milky fluid generated by the small intestine composed of tissue fluid and fat absorbed from food – so as to form health-giving chyle granules which feed and purify the blood". He was widely quoted: so it has to be assumed that some readers understood this.

Continental countries were as fertile in trashy and sometimes dangerous invention as was Britain: only in retrospect do such luminous intellects as Corvisart, Laënnec and Bayle dominate the crowd of crooks, ignoramuses and charlatans. Of the last Jean-Paul Marat, gutter journalist and revolutionary martyr, can serve as the representative. A native of Cagliari he had studied medicine in Bordeaux, Paris and Amsterdam before setting up in practice in London, specialising in diseases of the eyes. In 1775 at the age of thirty-two St Andrews University bestowed on him the degree of Doctor of Medicine. Back in Paris he was appointed physician to the guards of the Comte d'Artois (the future Charles X); but, more importantly to him, he launched his patent cure for phthisis, *L'eau antipulmonaire du Docteur Marat*. Despite its exorbitant price (or perhaps because of it) – a bottle cost as much as a bottle of vintage calvados – it sold in vast quantities. He was clearly an accomplished publicist, as he was to prove again as the voice of the Paris mob.[7] The liquid was later analysed and proved to be dilute calcium phosphate.

Charlatans may have done less harm than pillars of the medical establishment. S. Jaccoud, the author of *The Curability and Treatment of Pulmonary Phthisis*, was a professor of medical pathology in the faculty of

---

[6] Fish-liver oils, rich in vitamins A and D, had in fact been used in many parts of the world – notably in India and Burma – since time immemorial; and there are numerous references to their curative properties in the European medical literature before the nineteenth century. Most importantly, they were recommended against rickets (caused by Vitamin D deficiency) by Francis Glisson in 1650, presumably with excellent results. But it was the introduction of cod-liver oil at the Brompton Hospital which sanctified its use in tuberculosis.

[7] In the latter capacity he was largely responsible for sending the greatest chemist of his age, Lavoisier, to the guillotine. He was killed by Charlotte Corday in his bath and transformed into an appropriately fraudulent ikon by Jacques-Louis David.

Paris, a member of the Académie de Médecine, physician to the Laribosière Hospital and (in the words of his English translator) "generally recognised on the Continent as one of the greatest authorities on pulmonary disease").[8] He wrote enthusiastically and at length on an extensive variety of medicaments to which he ascribed "some of the most brilliant successes of my practice". He was a particularly fervent believer in counter-irritation for every form of fever but especially for consumption, "provided that the treatment was perseveringly employed even in the face of occasionally considerable discomfort".[9]

> Of the different forms [already considered] the successive application of blisters seems the best. In many cases it will be useful to provoke and maintain suppuration at the surface ... The practice is undoubtedly painful; but when the local lesions are recent, large in size and threaten to remain in the acute condition, such treatment is more beneficial than any other ... The only contraindication is extreme constitutional debility.[10]

More gruesome than blistering was the widespread use of fresh blood in Mediterranean countries, usually but not always of animal origin. A report of a crime committed in Andalusia printed in the *Presse médicale* concerned a boy of eight who was kidnapped and taken to the room of a noble patient dying of tuberculosis. "Unmoved by the boy's cries and prayers the attendant quack plunged a knife into his left axilla and the patient drank the blood while the boy was dying."[11] Compared to such practices Thomas Young's advocacy in England of the daily consumption of half a pound of mutton suet boiled in a pint of milk as a certain cure for phthisis seems anodyne.

As the century progressed, so did the complexity and uselessness of the remedies. For "patients who looked healthy enough", Dr John Travers

[8] Translator's introduction, Jaccoud, S., *The Curability and Treatment of Pulmonary Phthisis*, translated by M. Lubbock (London, 1855).

[9] The principle of counter-irritation in its original form is of course sound and is one reason why even small children exert pressure on any site which hurts. The effect is almost entirely psychological: the vast medical literature on the various forms of surface irritation to neutralise or to draw to the surface a deep-seated pathological process was totally without merit and undoubtedly responsible for much suffering.

[10] Jaccoud, S., *The Curability and Treatment of Pulmonary Phthisis*, 235. Having devoted a long chapter to itemising the effects of various mineral waters (with Vichy already in the ascendant) and three to the effects of climate, Jaccoud introduced his speciality, his recommendations regarding the consumption of milk. "Not only should milk be drunk fresh but it is essential that this should be done in the cowshed. Milk taken in this way will immediately diminish the frequency and intensity of cough and has an undoubted long-term effect on nervous and vascular excitability ... Patients should remain in the cowshed for at least a few minutes but for up to two hours depending on the severity of their condition."

[11] Bercher, J., *Presse médicale*, 1 (1939), 606.

of the Brompton Hospital recommended two grains of antimony tartrate dissolved in gentian water and "as soon as nausea commences a nutmeg size electuary of quinine, sulphurous sublimate, potassium nitrate and antimony sulphate kneaded together with gum". Hydrocyanic acid was deemed "most useful for asthenic patients". Dr Samuel Fillimore of Glasgow found creosote in various forms "a most serviceable standby". None of these preparations were ever subjected to anything resembling a controlled trial: when in the 1880s Austin Flint of New York first suggested that some "of our cherished remedies" should be subjected to such an investigation, his proposal caused great hilarity among the grandees of Harley Street.

Dramatic results with new and bizarre treatments based on the flimsiest of evidence were by contrast widely publicised, especially when expounded by qualified and socially well-connected practitioners. Having observed the relative immunity of butchers to consumption, Dr Edgar Spilsbury of Walsall achieved "total success" with four advanced phthisics by rubbing lard into their bodies. Chaulmoogra oil, a foul-tasting, foul-smelling brownish mess imported from Burma, had several vogues both applied externally and given by mouth: many patients presumably felt (as many would today) that a remedy so obnoxious had to be effective. Dr John Hastings reported instant relief of chest pain and cough obtained with a preparation of boa-constrictor excreta, half a tea-spoonful in a gallon of water (the stuff was virtually insoluble). Dr Joseph Pick announced that aluminium and its compounds were most effective. Dr Albert Broster advocated a mixture of Indian hemp, quinine, mercury, beef tea and cod-liver oil. He reported in 1871 that, after five weeks, a woman patient originally classified as "far gone" was restored to being "only delicate".

For almost a century doctors both in Britain and on the Continent sought to get "at the very seat of the disease" with inhalations.[12] Dr Reid Clanny of Sunderland pumped twelve cubic inches of sulphuretted hydrogen and coal gas into a woman patient four times a day for six weeks: after a fortnight all her symptoms disappeared. (A rival practitioner informed readers of the *Lancet* a week later that the patient had never had phthisis in the first place;

---

[12] The man whom the "inhalers" acknowledged as their forerunner was Dr Thomas Beddoes of Bristol, founder in the 1790s of the Pneumonic Medical Institution. Beddoes, an excellent chemist as well as a caring physician, was fascinated by the potential healing powers of pure gases (many, such as oxygen, nitrogen, carbon dioxide and nitrous oxide only recently isolated) not only in tuberculosis but also against various forms of rheumatism and even obesity. He enjoyed the enthusiastic support of the beautiful but profligate Duchess of Devonshire (*née* Georgiana Spencer, daughter of the first Earl Spencer), and later of the scientist and inventor James Watt, who had lost a much-loved daughter to tuberculosis. Beddoes had little success with the disease but became the unwitting pioneer of general inhalation anaethesia.

but his corrective efforts were put down to professional jealousy.) This form of treatment served a twofold purpose: the gas would expand the bronchi and thereby "enliven the circulatory system in the lungs", while the active ingredients, most commonly iodine, sulphuretted hydrogen, creosote, turpentine and (after Lister's publications in the 1880s) carbolic acid acted as a stimulant on the "indolent masses of the tubercle and thereby promoted their absorption".

Inevitably, as the gas mixtures became more complex, the paraphernalia for their administration and the routes by which they were introduced began to resemble Heath Robinson fantasies. Patients lay immersed in gas-filled rooms for hours or used complicated (and dangerous) inhalers resembling steam engines. Dr Robert Hunter of Ipswich charged a guinea a time for pumping a litre of his patent gas mixture into his patients' rectum "whence they were sure to reach the lungs" and half a guinea for the monthly refill. His method was adopted by no lesser a personage than Dr Burney Yeo, senior physician to King's College Hospital, London; while the British Pharmacopeia Commission, citadel of the great and the good, admitted "vapores" in 1888 to the ranks of officially approved remedies. The section was not expunged till 1932. In German-speaking countries the emphasis was more on the temperature of the gas than on its composition; after it was shown in the 1880s (and confirmed by reputable German scientists) that most pathogenic micro-organisms cannot survive at high temperatures, the pumping of air superheated to 150 degrees into the rectum became fashionable and was claimed to produce excellent results.

Country folk, too, though they could not afford such complicated remedies, believed in the inhalation of the exhaled warm breath of healthy beasts.[13] In Suffolk the source had to be a stallion, in Herefordshire a piebald horse, in the Scottish Lowlands a cow and in the Highlands a sheep. In *La peau de chagrin* Balzac described a Swiss peasant who cured himself of consumption by breathing in the thick air of his cowhouse. The effluvium of maggoty meat was a popular folk remedy in many parts of France, Austria, Hungary and Poland well into the twentieth century; and wave after wave of poor immigrants to the New World carried with them their homely cures as they tracked west in their covered wagons or squashed into the ethnic urban ghettoes of the cities.

In contrast to the plethora of useless panaceas – or at lest of panaceas which depended entirely on the faith of the consumer – there was one which in its limited purpose never failed and which in a crisis even its enemies recognised as a blessing. The name "laudanum" is said to have originated

[13] Rolleston, J. D. (1941) "The Folklore of Pulmonary Tuberculosis", *Tubercle*, 55 (1941), 3.

with Paracelsus;[14] but he clearly referred to a solid as did Le Mort of Leyden in the eighteenth century. Sydenham's celebrated elixir was a vinous drink.[15] Who first prepared the magical brown tincture of macerated opium in dilute spirit, which patients could instantly recognise as their one ever-dependable friend by its sheen and smell, is uncertain.[16] Its quality throughout western Europe varied – it contained anything between 0.0075 and 0.0125 per cent (weight per volume) of morphine – and so did its price; but it was never exorbitantly expensive.[17] It was only a mild soporific and pain-killer but as a sedative it was supreme, allaying fear and making sufferers tolerant of physical pain, resigned to their fate, even happy. It helped hundreds of thousands of tuberculous to die in peace and comforted those who held them in their arms.

In the context of tuberculosis few worried about the risk of addiction. If the drug had a recognised drawback it was its tendency to cause constipation. But purgation was one field in which doctors and nurses of the nineteenth century excelled; and laudanum gave them a chance to demonstrate their virtuosity Of course the fact that a stupefying agent was the greatest thera-peutic stand-by throughout these decades was as much a reflection on the bleakness of the state of medicine as the rise of alcoholism in the towns was a reflection on the quality of life in the industrial slums. Yet there were a few even then who preached sanity; and, though they cried in the wilderness, their voices deserve to be heard.

[14] "Ich hab ein Arkanum, heiss ich Laudanum; ist über alles wo es zum Tod reichen will", he rightly claimed. Michael Scott in about 1200 used the term to mean a "humour of the air in the Orient", possibly referring to the strong and sweet scent of the poppy. Quercetanus, a pupil of Paracelsus and physician to Henri IV of France, was the first to suggest the derivation of the name from *laudo*, I praise.

[15] Probably an equal mixture of opium and saffron extracted with canary wine.

[16] When the famous Brown Mixture was described by Barton of Philadelphia the tincture was already widely known on both sides of the Atlantic.

[17] This was remarkable since, when poppy cultivation was tried in the United States in the early years of the nineteenth century, it was found that it took 283 hours' labour to collect one kilogram of opium: even on the slave plantations this was considered uneconomical.

5

Three Heretics

Dr William Budd (1811–1880) lived and practised in Bristol, a city which had more than its fair share of tuberculosis. His own clientele came from two backgrounds. His more affluent and genteel patients (of whom he had many) had been largely drawn to the kinder climate of the south west from the midlands and the north of England. In this group tuberculosis was the sad, chronic illness with its remissions and recrudescences which Dr Budd had learnt about as a medical student and which was enshrined in his well-stocked library.[1] More puzzling were the black seamen who arrived in the city's busy port in large numbers to stay only until they had spent – or frittered away – their wages and were ready to offer themselves for rehiring on their endless journeyings over the Seven Seas. Not all of them were able to do so. Some fell ill with symptoms and signs which initially resembled ordinary consumption but which quickly became more severe and then fulminating. They died within two to three weeks. Dr Budd performed several post-mortem examinations on these unfortunates and found evidence of widely disseminated tuberculosis.

He was also fascinated by the gruesome story of the schooner *Farah* of the Bristol Oceanic Trading Company. While in harbour on a Pacific island – probably one of the Gilberts – one of the crew suffered a massive pulmonary haemorrhage. What might have happened on the high seas was anybody's guess; but the man begged the master to be left behind in the care of a tribe of immensely hospitable natives in a setting that approximated to the Garden of Eden before the Fall. The master was a kindly man: he not only agreed to the sick sailor staying on the island but allowed a volunteer to remain and look after him. Eight months later – either by luck or by phenomenal navigational skill – the *Farah* found its way back. Her crew were glad to see the sick sailor recovered and his friend well; but almost the whole of the

---

[1] He was one of six sons of a wealthy surgeon – five of his brothers became doctors and two were elected to the Royal Society – and he himself received an excellent medical education in London, Edinburgh and Paris before settling down in Bristol and being elected to the staff of the Royal Infirmary.

tribe who had greeted them with such joy were now dead; and the few who had survived had fled to another island.

"While I was walking on the Observatory Hill at Clifton in the second week of August, 1856", Budd wrote later,

the thought came into my mind unbidden, so to speak, that what I had observed among my patients and what I had learnt by reliable hearsay could be explained by assuming that phthisis is a self-propagating zymotic disease disseminated through society by specific germs in the tuberculous matter cast off by persons already suffering from the disease.[2]

His reliable hearsay included a friendly exchange of letters with the celebrated Dr David Livingstone, who assured him that phthisis was unknown in the interior of Africa where no other Europeans had yet penetrated. Budd was not a person to rush into print: he did not publish his memorandum of which the above is the opening sentence till eleven years later, in October 1867. But if he spent a long time pondering, he pondered to good effect. Purely from clinical observations and the occasional post-mortem examination – he had never had time nor perhaps the inclination for experimental work and it is not certain whether he ever looked down a microscope – he outlined the manner of the spread of tuberculosis with startling clarity. His clarity was also a little naive, since he was apparently unprepared for the storm of indignation his assumption would raise. "We are not of course unaware of the 'germ theory' prevalent among the people of some Mediterranean countries", Sir Joseph Benham, a fashionable London physician, remembered today chiefly for misdiagnosing the last illness of the Prince Consort,[3] wrote with ponderous wit, "but it is lamentable to see such a figment of hot air promoted in our 'cooler' climate." Some readers of Budd's memorandum in the Lancet did rise to his defence, but Budd was not by nature a fighter; and while he never recanted he found other things to interest him.[4]

The egregious Sir Joseph Benham was not the first to contrast the superstitions of the south with the scientific outlook of the north. The divide was centuries old. During a concert tour in 1818 Niccolò Paganini suffered a relapse of his tuberculosis in Naples. As soon as the landlord guessed the nature of the illness he turned the celebrated violinist into the street, hurling

[2] Budd, W., "Memorandum on the Nature and Mode of Propagation of Phthisis", Lancet (1867), 451.

[3] The honour was evenly shared with Sir James Clark.

[4] His main epidemiological interests were typhoid and cholera and he made important contributions to the understanding of both. In particular, he recognised the importance of water in the transmission in cholera about the same time as John Snow but took a little longer to publish his findings and recommendations. He was elected a Fellow of the Royal Society in 1871.

all his possessions after him.⁵ The prospect of having all his and Severn's possessions burnt after his death because they might harbour germs (as they probably did) added to the despair of Keats's last days in Rome. A few years later René de Chateaubriand had great difficulty in the city finding a house for his friend, Madame de Beaumont: it had transpired that she was suffering from phthisis. When compelled to put his equipage on sale to raise enough money to bribe the owner of a secluded villa, he was mortified to discover that there would be no takers because the signora had been seen riding in it on two or three occasions. In fact, despite the intervention of the French Ambassador and the somewhat half-hearted pleas of a Cardinal, he was ordered to burn his carriages.

This was not just popular superstition – or perhaps wisdom. Chateaubriand's reference in a letter to "this insane law dating back to the Goths" was a slight exaggeration; but as early as 1699 the republic of Lucca had enacted a decree directing citizens "to burn all objects remaining after the death of a person suffering from phthisis" and ordering physicians to notify the occurrence of the disease to the authorities without delay. Over the next hundred years most Italian states (and later the Spain of Ferdinand VI) followed suit, the last and perhaps strictest edict being issued in Naples in 1767.⁶

The doctrinal divide did not follow precise geographical or political boundaries. In Vienna, where Italian influence was always strong, Panarolli, a Venetian physician much in demand, reported having seen a man fall dead after stepping on the sputum of a consumptive. Another of his patients contracted the illness after inhaling the fumes emitted by sputum expectorated by a phthisic on burning coal. Even the expatriate Dutchman, Van Swieten, described (though in a literary rather than a medical context) how the tender kiss of a loving wife dying of phthisis could transmit the disease to her husband. Prague too had strict quarantine regulations and medical opinion in Munich fluctuated. Florence, by contrast, though south of the border, was traditionally sceptical, as was Nice on the Riviera. It was one reason why so many northern consumptives took up residence there.

By and large, nevertheless, the further north one travelled, the more contemptuously contagion was rejected as a southern superstition; and in

⁵ Fortunately for Paganini one of his admirers happened to be passing by and took him to more hospitable lodgings outside the city, "not without first beating the frightened landlord with his stick".

⁶ Ironically, while strict legislation based on the idea of contagion remained in force on paper in many Italian states throughout the nineteenth century, enforcement of the regulations became progressively more lax. By the time Koch's discovery proved the transmissibility of the disease they had practically lapsed.

Paris, and wherever the writ of its Académie de Médecine ran, the germ
theory was anathema. This was true even of Parisians who had originally
come from the Midi like Bayle: indeed, nothing illustrates the sharpness of
the divide more clearly than comparison of Morgagni's dread of touching a
phthisic corpse with Bayle's crazy insoucience in handling infected material.
Although with characteristic moderation Laënnec had written that "while
contagion seems to be important in some countries, this did not seem to
the case in France", Gabriel Andral, the editor of the fourth edition of his
book, changed the passage to "contagion is never seen in countries north of
the Alps".

In England and Scotland too official opinion was firmly wedded to the
idea of the unhappy diathesis – that is a predisposing inherited constitution,
aggravated by an unwholesome life. The relative importance of the two was
the only question worthy of rational scientific debate. In his *Phthisiologia*
Richard Morton told the story of a Mr Hunt, a citizen of London, who "had
lived almost from his youth in a consumptive state doing his business well
enough by taking care and by moderation". He had four sons all of whom
at the age of thirty "were inevitably seized by the inheritance, precipitated
in each by Passions of the Mind and the immoderate drinking of Spirituous
Liquors ... the Distemper carrying them all off before the emaciated old
man died".

In 1830 William Cullen, a well-respected Edinburgh physician, summed
up medical opinion in Scotland, stating that while contagion could conceivably lead to consumption, such an occurrence was quite exceptional; and
John Forbes added a footnote to his translation of Laënnec's great book
saying that "the opinion of the great majority of medical men in this country
is opposed to contagion: and I think this opinion is justified equally by
statistical facts, by the truth of pathology and by analogical reasoning". It
was against such a consensus that Budd of Bristol had tried to advance his
crackpot idea of a zymotic disease; and it was this doctrine which, on the
other side of the Channel, another heretic, Jean Antoine Villemin (1827–1892),
set out to challenge.

Villemin was born in Prey in the Vosges, a poor farmer's son. He lost his
father when he was ten and his studies were financed by a more prosperous
uncle. He originally intended to be a teacher but changed his mind when,
during his military service, he was persuaded by his commanding officer to
take up military medicine instead. He acquired a loan from another uncle
and qualified after three and a half years as an army doctor (This, until 1872,
qualified him to look after soldiers and horses but not civilian patients.) He
was then posted first to a cavalry regiment and then to the Val de Grâce

military hospital in Paris. The latter was recognised as a quiet and desirable posting; but Villemin was not a quiet person. His interest had been aroused by the apparent similarity between tuberculosis and a disease familiar to him both from his boyhood on his father's farm and from his stint as a cavalry medical officer.

Glanders was first described by a fourth-century horse trader, Publius Vegetius Rinatus, a contemporary of Galen's, in a book called *Ars veterinaria*. Although primarily a disease of horses (hence its official name, *equinia*), Paracelsus among others recognised that it could be transmitted to men. Its acute human form was a pustular eruption of the skin and infection of the nose and lungs: it was in Villemin's day rapidly fatal. The chronic form, also known as farcie, was in many ways similar to chronic tuberculosis, affecting the lungs, joints, bones, glands and skin in addition to the lungs. What interested Villemin was the fact known since the early years of the century that the disease could be transmitted not only by handling affected horses but also by inoculation from one animal to another: it was, in short, caused by some kind of a germ. He approached his colonel who assigned to him a corner of a laboratory and a few rats and rabbits. Thus equipped, in March 1865, he began his experiments.

Through small subcutaneous incisions he introduced into two rabbits a small quantity of pus recovered from the lung cavity of a tuberculous patient who had died thirty-three hours earlier. The other two rabbits were inoculated with tissue fluid from a burn blister and acted as his controls. Two months later, when the rabbits were killed, Villemin found widespread pulmonary and lymph-node tuberculosis in the two animals inoculated with tuberculous pus and no evidence of the disease in the other two. This encouraged him to continue, performing altogether six series of experiments using human tuberculous material with similar results and six more with material derived from the udder of an infected cow. In contrast to most laboratory work at the time, his experiments were carefully controlled and his documentation was meticulous.[7] Eventually he was left in no doubt that tuberculosis was a specific infection transmitted by an agent present in necrotic tuberculous material. He also noted that the disease was much more acute and severe in rabbits which had been inoculated with tuberculous pus from a cow than when the inoculum was from a human source. This made him "suppose that, like all other virulent substances, tuberculosis acts with

---

[7] He must have been (like Pasteur and Calmette) one of nature's born experimenters, as distinct a species as are gardeners with green fingers; but this is not always allied with a gift to communicate the results.

greater intensity when there is a physiological affinity between the creature that furnishes the virus and that receiving it".[8]

Two years after embarking on his project he was ready to report his discoveries to the Académie de Médecine. His communication was given the most tepid of receptions – a vote of thanks for his intriguing contribution to veterinary science. This was partly because his audience, mostly elderly and successful clinicians, could not easily relate to experiments involving rabbits, cows and horses; but it did not help that the next item on the agenda was the presentation of a prize of 10,000 francs to Professor Jean Pidou, who in his monumental *Etudes sur la phthisie* had established the familial character of phthisis, the famous *diathèse*, "beyond any reasonable doubt". As for contagion, Pidou could only echo his master Brichetau, who felt that "cette conception n'a pu naître que dans l'imagination fiévreuse des méridionaux". Villemin had a somewhat abrasive personality (especially when he felt slighted by civilians) but he did not lack courage. When the Académie refused to publish his paper he proceeded to publish it himself privately. This elicited a mild rebuke from his commanding officer: for a major he was "a little too inclined to seek the limelight".

While Villemin achieved no recognition in his own country, his work did not pass unnoticed in England. There the late 1860s witnessed one of those waves of popular interest in tuberculosis (to recur at regular ten to twenty year intervals over the next eighty years) which were always coupled with a vociferous demands in the press for immediate government action. Dr John Burdon-Sanderson, physician to the Brompton Hospital and Medical Officer to the Privy Council, was accordingly charged by Disraeli's administration to go to France and collect first-hand information about what *The Times* described as the "bizarre claims of the veterinary major which we can nevertheless not wholly ignore". Burdon-Sanderson, who was not bigoted about germs and had a genuinely inquisitive mind, got on well with the crusty and opinionated Frenchman – both by and large preferred the company of horses to that of most humans – and on his return, in collaboration with Dr John (later Sir John) Simon of the Local Government Board, he repeated Villemin's experiments. Their report confirmed Villemin's findings – with one crucial reservation. Although they succeeded in transmitting tuberculosis to a large number of rabbits and guinea-pigs by inoculating tuberculous material from a recently dead tuberculous individual, they also produced in one of their control animals similar lesions by inoculating normal tissue fluid from a body unsuspected of having died from the disease. It is still uncertain how

[8] His observations were correct but his conclusion was mistaken, since he did not realise that the human and bovine strains of tuberculosis are distinct. It is now known that rabbits happen to be more susceptible to the bovine than to the human organism.

this happened: there could have been an error in the experiments themselves, but more probably it was a product of the perfunctory documentation; neither Burdon-Sanderson nor Simon were experienced laboratory scientists and they had busy lives outside the animal house.[9] Whatever the reason, they reported back to the Privy Council that the infection could not be regarded as necessarily dependent on a tuberculous source. This was a serious setback not only to Villemin but to all those inclined to take the contagion idea seriously. Villemin's work was repeated again in the early 1880s by W. (later Sir William) Watson Cheyne and Dawson Williams, who showed that Villemin had been entirely correct both in his findings and in his conclusions;[10] but it is difficult to resurrect a medical concept once it had been deemed unsound.

The veterinary major had by then given up experimental work, advancing up the professional ladder of military medicine, eventually succeeding his old chief, Godelier, as professor of medicine at the Val de Grâce and as a General. His idea that tuberculosis might be catching was remembered, if at all, as a youthful and pardonable indiscretion. Then, twenty years after his pioneering experiments, and to his infinite chagrin, it was resurrected and proved right but on the wrong side of the Rhine. To a true patriot it was a denouement worse than oblivion.[11]

A third heretic was Dr George Bodington (1811–1882), one of a species endangered even in his day and even more today, an independent-minded general practitioner removed both geographically and in spirit from the fashionable centres of learning, impatient with pontifical pronouncements handed down from on high and sceptical about medical dogmas based on

---

[9] A third possible explanation is that the "tuberculous" control animal died not of tuberculosis but of a disease of rodents closely resembling it, *pseudotuberculosis rodentium*. This was not recognised at the time.

[10] See note 15 to Chapter 9 below.

[11] In 1887, on hearing of the reception to be given by the Académie des Sciences to Koch, he could not refrain from writing to Pasteur:

> I do not hope to gain a place beside you but – you will see that I am less modest than I appear – I have been so much attacked that I suffer some distress that our Académie still gives shelter to my enemies. Twenty years have passed and all this is now ancient history, but Koch's bacillus of which the Germans are so proud, is being allowed to obscure all memory of the achievements of French scientists and Koch will enter the Académie through widely flung doors with all the honours of our country.

Quoted by S. Lyle Cummings, *Tuberculosis in History* (London, 1949), p. 234. Pasteur's answer has been lost but, though he was generous in his praise of Koch, he also remained a staunch champion of Villemin.

revelation. Early in his career he wrote a peppery article condemning the then current trend of treating cholera patients with blood-letting and large doses of calomel, acquiring the reputation of an eccentric and preparing the ground for the reception of his most ambitious work, his *Essay on the Treatment and Cure of Pulmonary Consumption: On Principles Natural, Rational and Successful.*

The *Essay* is remarkable for the humanity and common sense of its message; but dealing with his professional brethren Bodington showed a deplorable lack of respect. He began with an attack on the

> helpless and meagre system of medical treatment of consumption in general use in the present day, the utter uselessness of which is so well known and so obvious that members of the medical profession are in the habit of sending their patients to distant sea-ports or watering places where, falling under precisely the same mode of treatment, they commonly die.[12]

Such an opening was unlikely to endear him to his colleagues; but worse was to come. He vehemently condemned the two most popular drugs of the day, digitalis and tartar emetic, as useless in tuberculosis and the standard practice of imprisoning patients in hermetically sealed rooms as abominable.

More important and heretical were his positive recommendations. He proposed that the most effective remedial agent in consumption was fresh air, out of doors,

> best early in the morning ... walking if that is not too exhausting and gradually increasing the length of the walk until it can often be maintained for several hours ... The weather is almost never too severe for a consumptive patient in our benign climate: the cooler the air which passes through the lungs the greater will be the its healing power ... sharp frosty days in the winter, provided only that the rest of the body is well protected and there is no sweating, will prove to be the most powerful sedative that can be applied and does more to promote the healing of cavities and ulcers of the lung than any other measure currently employed.[13]

He rented a house at Maney, close to his home, for patients "who are desirous or who are recommended to remove from their homes for the benefit of the dryness, freshness and purity of the air, constant and watchful care, exercise and a varied and nutritious diet". He advocated the stimulus of small quantities of wine with meals but he had little use for drugs except for morphine hydrochlorate when a sedative was needed, especially at night.

These principles now seem so mild and commonsensical that the outrage they provoked in 1840 is hard to understand. His "very crude ideas", an

---

[12] Bodington, G, *An Essay on the Treatment and Cure of Pulmonary Consumption* (1840; reprinted London, 1906), p. 16.

[13] Ibid., p. 38.

anonymous leader-writer wrote in the *Lancet*, "are best left to fall into rapid and well-merited oblivion". This was supported by letters from many of the most eminent doctors of the day: Sir James Clark, recently knighted, was particularly vitriolic in his condemnation. Bodington continued in general practice for some years, but tuberculous patients who sought his advice or who were referred to him became fewer and fewer and he had to give up his sanatorium in Maney. He was also under continuous attack by his local fellow practitioners for criticising their practices and his private life seems to have become overcast. In the late 1850s he went insane and died in an asylum.

The *Lancet* made posthumous amends in its obituary notice on 11 March 1882, expressing surprise that

> a simple village doctor in the 1840s should have arrived at conclusions which anticipated some of our most recent teachings. It is alas less surprising that he met with the usual fate of those who question authority. He was so severely handled by the reviewers that he was discouraged from pursuing his observations and perhaps driven to give up general practice ... But we are glad to claim for this obscure practitioner the credit of having been among the first to advocate the more rational, scientific and successful treatment of pulmonary consumption which we now practise.[14]

It was a generous, if sadly belated, tribute – though how rational, scientific and successful the treatment of pulmonary consumption was at the time the obituary was penned is questionable.[15]

---

[14] *Lancet*, 11 March 1882, p. 417.

[15] Not many people read old obituary notices in the *Lancet*; but G. B. Shaw's reference to Bodington in Act I of *The Doctor's Dilemma* will perhaps be heard for longer. Chiding his former pupil, Sir Colenso Ridgeon, for claiming to have discovered a new treatment of tuberculosis, Sir Patrick Cullen, doyen of London's medical knights, says: "Ah yes. It's very interesting. What is it the old cardinal says in Browning's play? 'I have known four and twenty leaders of revolt'. Well, I've known over thirty men that found out how to cure consumption. Why do people go on dying of it, Colly? ... There was my father's old friend, George Bodington of Sutton Coldfield. He discovered the open-air cure in eighteen-forty. He was ruined and driven out of practice for only opening the windows; and now we won't let a consumptive patient have as much as a roof over his head."

6

Sacrifice and Atonement

In 1800 the European middle classes (or the bourgeoisie as they were beginning to call themselves) were still hardly more than the troublesome inhabitants of a narrow strip of No Man's Land between the nobility and the masses. By the end of the century they effectively ruled Europe and very nearly the world. Nor was this all. No ruling class in history had ever been so numerous and yet had a better expectation of a long and fulfilled life. Yet no ruling class had ever lived in such constant dread of disease.

In part this was the result of the new class ethos. Illness is an intensely individual experience and reverence for individuals rather than for families, clans or lineages was a bourgeois invention. The death from tuberculosis of the Princesse de Broglie, the last of the Ingres's society sitters, soon after the great portrait was completed, was no doubt mourned by her family and friends; but, having given birth to an heir and a second-in-line to the dukedom, her earthly destiny was probably regarded by the family as having been satisfactorily fulfilled. The death of Sophie Munch, the child of a typical middle-class family, from the same disease, by contrast, was an irreplaceable personal loss which her father and brother would never forget.

There were other reasons too. Private wealth and public virtue were not only the ideals but also the almost, but not quite, invincible defences of the new ruling estate. It is true that many of the pestilences of the past had been overcome or banished to the industrial slums, but not all. Pillars of bourgeois probity were haunted by the spectre of madness from tertiary syphilis. The effects of alcoholism could destroy whole families. But the disease which most cruelly mocked material advances and moral precepts was tuberculosis.

There had to be an explanation, a reason for the devastation. One could understand the prevalence of the disease among the poor: it was regrettable but it was the destiny of the poor to suffer. It could also be the result of a profligate life. That, too, could be understood. But neither virtue nor wealth guaranteed protection against tuberculosis, so the disease acquired one of its most persistent and characteristic attributes: an aura of sacrifice and atonement. Sacrifice for whom? Atonement for what? The questions were rarely asked and the answers did not much matter. It was the aura itself, with its optional religious overtones, which provided an explanation. It justified what would otherwise have been unbearable: the suffering and deaths of the pure, the innocent and the beloved. Inevitably, it also inspired luminous literary creations.

Few consumptive destinies stirred the emotions of generations – and not only in France – more deeply than that of Napoleon II, *l'Aiglon*, the Eaglet, King of Rome, Duke of Reichstadt.[1] He was two overlapping characters. The historical character always remained a little opaque. But even before he died another personality had been created by the poets, dramatists, political pamphleteers and dreamers of the age. It was that second incarnation which was eventually immortalised by Edmond Rostand and made its first and most memorable appearance on the stage on 15 March 1900. He was a youth of twenty-one played by the divine Sarah Bernhardt well past fifty. In a country where history had often been made or at least rehearsed in the theatre – with memories of Beaumarchais' *Marriage of Figaro* and Victor Hugo's *Hernani* stirring – it was to be a long-remembered first night.[2]

More than one Napoleonic scholar has suggested that the Emperor's divorce from Josephine was one of his fateful mistakes: not only did he lose a trusted friend – and by 1808 he had few left – but he also severed for all to see the last of his own revolutionary roots. His marriage to a Habsburg Princess did not establish him within the tight inner circle of the divinely ordered ruling dynasties (as he was soon to learn to his cost): it merely transformed a man of destiny into a still dangerous but faintly ludicrous character out of Molière, an upstart. This was not immediately apparent and, within a year, his second marriage did give him what he desired above all: a legitimate heir.

Few royal births can ever have been greeted with such ostentatious rejoicing. The *Moniteur*, France's official newspaper, reported that no fewer than 2000 celebratory odes in eight different languages (which did not include English) were composed within a few days to commemorate the event. More tangibly, using France's and conquered and subservient Europe's foremost artists and craftsmen, a whole wing of the Tuilleries was refurbished to receive the infant. Hardly out of the womb, he was created King of Rome, the first since Tarquin the Proud in 600 BC,[3] and frescoes representing

---

[1] Creston, D., *In Search of Two Characters* (London, 1945); Masson, F., *Napoleon et son fils* (Paris, 1922).

[2] "Rostand could have been carried to the Elysée that night by the smartest mob Paris had ever seen on the barricades", Anatole France later wrote.

[3] The heir to the Holy Roman Emperor was styled King of the Romans (Rex Romanorum, Römischer König), not King of Rome.

twenty-four views of his kingdom appeared on the walls of his apartment. Still in his silver cradle created by Prudhon, a present from the city of Paris (costing 300,000 francs), a library of 6000 instructive books specially printed and bound by the doyen of royal bookbinders, Didon, was waiting for the day when he would open his eyes to the charms of the printed word. A Sèvres table service of 234 pieces, emblazoned with the imperial eagle and embellished with vignettes representing the pure and the applied sciences, was in readiness for his future delectation. Most importantly, everything was to be done to safeguard his physical health.

The search for safety had begun even before the imperial birth or indeed marriage. Over a period of several months, before the engagement was formally announced, Count Laborde, France's ambassador in Vienna, and Marshal Berthier, the Emperor's personal representative, had scoured the royal archives and interviewed Archdukes, Archduchesses, royal mistresses, courtiers, physicians, nurses, midwives, servants, tradesmen and the swarm of professional spies and informers who always buzzed around the Hofburg, researching the intimate bodily functions and the health of the family of the mother-to-be of Napoleon II. Embodied in an eighty-two-page secret document dispatched by courier to their imperial master, their conclusions were by and large reassuring. At seventeen and a half the Archduchess Marie-Louise, twelfth child and ninth surviving child of their Imperial and Apostolic Royal Majesties, Francis I of Austria and his consort Maria Carolina, was nubile: she had been since 4 February 1808 (26 March, according to one chambermaid, Berthier added in his own hand on the margin of Laborde's report), when she had had her first menstrual period; and she was certified by three royal physicians, one of them dispatched from Paris expressly for that purpose, as a virgin. She was sturdily built; in particular her hips and her bosoms were well-formed for future child-bearing and motherhood: she had no history of throat infections, scrofulous swellings, cough, unnatural bleedings or abnormal joint enlargements. Her appetite was hearty and her bowel movements regular. The Princess's skin was flawless; there was no history of rashes; and by all accounts her breath smelled fresh and sweet. She was placid by temperament and not prey to metaphysical speculations, torments of the mind and fanciful flights of the imagination. Her apprehension at being sent as a bride to one who for years had been referred to at her father's court as "The Monster" (and worse) was perhaps forgivable, especially bearing in mind the unfortunate fate of the Princess's great-aunt, the Archduchess Marie-Antoinette, also dispatched to share the throne of France and seal a political rapprochement.

The family history too was explored in depth. On the side of the Princess's imperial and royal father there was, in Laborde's and Berthier's opinion, not much cause for concern. Of course there was a strain of madness in the Habsburgs – both the mad Joanna and the eccentric Emperor Rudolf II were more or less direct ancestors – and, closer to the present, one of the Princess's paternal uncles and one great-aunt were said to be feeble-minded even by royal standards. But there was no dynasty in Europe wholly devoid of this trait. It was also true that at one critical point in history – on the death of the Emperor Charles VI in 1740 – the legitimate male Habsburg line had flickered to extinction; but Charles's daughter and the Archduchess Marie-Louise's great-grandmother, the great and good Empress Maria Theresa, and her lusty consort, the Emperor Francis of Lorraine, were beautifully procreative, producing eighteen children of whom no fewer than sixteen survived infancy and fourteen childhood.

On the Archduchess's mother's side the Bourbons of Naples presented a rather more worrying conspectus. In addition to the usual strain of eccentricity, two of the Empress's sisters, one brother, at least one uncle and two cousins had died in their teens from what the best medical opinion obtainable in Vienna described as consumption. Another cousin was still alive but about to die. This still left a large and healthy family; but the message was clear. The as yet unborn heir to the throne of France should be specially guarded against that most dangerous of afflictions.

This Napoleon was determined to do. Though consumption was not regarded as contagious in French academic circles, the Emperor was Corsican enough to want to take no risks. Every one of the infant's attendants was rigorously checked and his wet-nurse, Mme Moipou, selected only after the most careful scrutiny for any suspicion of consumption in her family. In choosing the infant's playmates aristocratic lineage was jettisoned in favour of a physically robust parentage. After a period of feeds prepared from ass's milk, two carefully selected cows were kept at the Tuilleries to provide all the milk required for the child. (The practice of relying on one or two selected cows to provide milk for royal infants was to be adopted decades later by Queen Victoria at Prince Albert's suggestion.) In opposition to much conservative medical opinion, tinged with a no less traditional suspicion of any advance originating across the Channel, the King of Rome was vaccinated against smallpox at the age of three months. Fresh air was highly regarded by Corvisart as a prophylactic against many disorders but in particular against consumption; and, whatever the weather, every day for two hours in the morning and one in the afternoon, the King of Rome was taken for a ride in the Tuilleries Gardens and up the Champs Elysées in his gold-and-white miniature barouche pulled by two white goats. For five years there can have been no infant in Europe whose future health was watched over with such vigilance and devotion.

Napoleon saw his son for the last time at dawn on 25 January 1814, three months before setting out for his first exile to the island of Elba; but not till after Waterloo did he abandon hope that the Empress and the boy would rejoin him. He implored her in letter after letter, deluding himself that she was being kept in Vienna on Metternich's orders and against her will. In fact, Marie-Louise was determined never again to get embroiled in high politics, conjugal or otherwise: she was perfectly content to exchange her title of Empress for that of Grand Duchess of Parma and the pomp and circumstance of her former imperial station for the dash and charm of Count Adam Neipperg. As for her son by the man who was once again restored to the status of Monster and Antichrist, she was tender-hearted enough to secure for him the title of Duke of Reichstadt and the rank of an imperial Archduke – but wished to see of him in the flesh as little as possible.

He could not be disposed off quite so easily. The sovereigns, ministers and plenipotentiaries who assembled in Vienna for the second time after Waterloo squabbled endlessly over Italian duchies, Slav provinces and German titles but on one overriding principle, legitimacy, they were more firmly united than Europe's rulers had been since the First Crusade. With the Bourbons back in France (having, according to Talleyrand, learnt nothing and forgotten nothing), with their cousins back in Naples and Spain (having forgotten nothing but having learnt many new tricks of misrule), with such Revolutionary or Napoleonic figments as Poland, Germany and Italy consigned to the dustheap forever, the clock was put back to exactly where it had stood before the diabolical interlude of Revolution and Empire. Although the brainchild of Alexander I of Russia, the effective guardian of the Holy Alliance dedicated to the Divine Right of Kings and reaction was Prince Metternich, Chancellor of Austria; and the most painful thorn in his flesh was the boy growing up as an Austrian Archduke in Schönbrunn.

At this point history and legend begin to part company. It is quite probable that the Duke of Reichstadt did in fact – at least until his late teens – grow up as a charming and cosseted Habsburg Prince, eldest and much-loved grandson of the Emperor (a benign old gentleman and passionate cook), something of a playboy in what was still Europe's gayest and most frivolous city, the Vienna of Schubert and of the elder Strauss as well as of Metternich's secret police. He spoke, like all the Habsburgs, broad Viennese; and, since his entourage and tutors were strictly forbidden to make even passing reference to his father, he probably knew little about the circumstances of his birth. He was handsome in a delicate sort of way, a success with the ladies both of the Court and of the Prater: a real *amitié amoureuse* (if no more) linked him to another royal orphan, the Archduchess Sophie.[4] There is no hard evidence, however, that even after his father's death in 1821 – "a news item, no longer an event", as Talleyrand summed it up – or even after the fall of the Bourbons in France in 1830 he seriously plotted to regain what could be regarded as his paternal inheritance or that he did anything to constitute a menace to the divinely ordered status quo.

But he did not actually have to *do* anything. The more repressive the *système Metternich* became not only in Austria but in most of continental Europe, the more "Napoleon II" became a symbol of the revolutionary freedoms which his father's eagles had once carried to the most backward parts of the Continent. His idealised portrait, surmounting an N or an eagle, was secreted in the bindings of books and inside the double lids of snuffboxes and *poudriers* across frontiers and was treasured in tens of thousands of households. Thousands of secretly printed pamphlets spread the news that the eaglet was chaffing in his gilded cage, ready to break out: both in Poland and in Hungary plots were afoot to liberate and abduct him and crown him King of Poland or King of Hungary.

If Edmond Rostand rather than dry-as-dust archives are to be believed (and "to us French", Jean Delcassé was to pronounce in 1905, "*L'Aiglon* will always be the historic truth"), the Prince was far from unaware either of his glorious origins or of his manifest destiny. He knew from books smuggled into his apartment about every stirring event of his father's reign; for every one of Metternich's informers he had his own secret source which kept him abreast of developments in Europe; even his ostensibly amorous revels were in fact devoted to secret preparations for his escape and imperial future. If that had been all to Rostand's Prince, the play today would be no more than a sentimental period piece woven around the premature death of a glamorous but sadly tuberculous prince. But the real climax of Rostand's creation is not the Prince's death but the penultimate scene on the battlefield of Wagram.

In that scene the Prince and his band of conspirators, ready to set out for France, arrive on this historic site, the field not far from Vienna where Napoleon I had won one of his decisive victories over the Austrians in 1808. Here they realise that their plans have been betrayed and that they are surrounded by the Austrian gendarmerie. A bullet kills Flambeau, the

---

[4] A Wittelsbach princess married to the Emperor Francis's younger son, the kindly but notably ineffectual Archduke Francis Charles: she was the mother of the future Emperor Franz Josef and of Maximilian, the future Emperor of Mexico. Rumour long circulated that her first-born child, Franz Josef, was in fact the son of the Duke of Reichstadt. All reliable evidence is against this but the Emperor did retain a fond memory of the Duke, whose portrait was (and is) the only picture allowed to adorn the austere imperial bedchamber in Schönbrunn.

Prince's valet and (unbeknown to Metternich) a former guardsman in the Imperial Guard. The Prince is left alone to await the arrival of a coach which will convey him back to his cage. But not quite alone. Suddenly the battlefield comes alive: he is surrounded by the sounds and voices of the wounded and the dying – their cries, their groans, their calls for help, their screams of despair, their sobs for their families. He tries to still them but in vain. He implores them to stop accusing him and then – if they can – to forgive him. In response the battlefield erupts in the shout: *Vive l'Empereur!* The Prince then realises that his mission in life is not to recreate the Napoleonic Empire but to atone for it. He collapses in a fit of coughing, his blood adding a few fresh drops to the bloodsoaked earth.

The last scene is the death of *l'Aiglon*, the greatest dramatic – though not operatic – representation of the consumptive death. It is of course deliberately lachrymose: "there was not a dry eye at the Châtelet last night", Michel Larousse reported after the first performance, "and the last line, Metternich's chilling 'dress him in his white uniform', was drowned in a chorus of sobs". However calculated the effect, and however obsolete and indeed tarnished the Napoleonic legend had by then become, Anatole France, a hard-bitten critic, still found the scene infinitely moving. What moved him (by his own admission) was not the wafting memory of Bonapartist *gloire* or even the sadness of a young consumptive death but the message of individual sacrifice to atone for the cruelties of history.

Another account of *l'Aiglon*'s illness and death exists, however, unearthed by the Hungarian historian Géza Supka.[5] One of the Archduchess Sophie's ladies in waiting and governess to her two sons, Baroness Sturmfeder, wrote regularly to her sister, Countess Batthyáni. The Duke of Reichstadt was a central character in her and her mistress's life and therefore in her correspondence. At sixteen he was indeed a strikingly handsome youth but a year later he developed scrofula, presumably the swelling of the cervical lymph nodes, and started to have trouble with his teeth, something which plagued him for the rest of his short life. He also developed a rash which healed but recurred. More ominously, he began to cough up blood and foul-smelling matter and had several major pulmonary bleeds. After his death rumours of poisoning (as well as of suicide) were current enough throughout Europe to call for an official denial. They remain highly improbable; but it is undoubtedly true that as a matter of deliberate policy he was encouraged in his friendship with one of Vienna's most notorious reprobates, Dom Miguel,

---

[5] Supka, G., *Habsburg Kronika* (Budapest, 1954).

Pretender to the Portuguese throne, who in turn needed little persuasion to introduce the prince to his debauched life-style.[6]

After his nineteenth birthday the Duke's health seems to have deteriorated further, though there were intermissions when he invariably overtaxed himself, especially in drilling his personal regiment, the Thirteenth Dragoons of Gyula. By then his mother was busy pursuing her own amours in Parma and rarely visited Vienna: it was only the Archduchess Sophie who surrounded him with *tendresse* and looked after him when he was ill. Some of the Archduchess's letters survive: "mein guter lieber Alter" was the way she generally addressed him.[7] It was also the Archduchess who was asked to suggest to him without alarming him that he should partake of the Last Sacrament when the doctors felt that his death could not be long delayed (a common problem in Catholic countries).

Spanish etiquette prescribed that Habsburg Archdukes and Archduchesses should die in public; and to that extent the last scene in Rostand's play is true. It was also true that by chance the room where the Duke lay dying was the one that had been occupied by his father in 1808, and that next to his bed stood his silver cradle which his mother had sent to him as a present from Parma a few weeks earlier. He may even have said at some stage "so small is the distance between birth and death". But for the last forty-eight hours of his life he was too ill to speak and in almost constant pain. The cause of this was probably tuberculous enteritis, almost continuous bloody diarrhoea, despite heavy doses of opium, medicinal spirits and other powdered medicaments (probably calomel). Much of his face and body had to be covered with a soothing white paste to relieve irritation and his hands were heavily bandaged. "His suffering was so terrible", the Baroness wrote to her sister, "that I could not bring myself to pray for anything but that it should not be for much longer: God forgive me." Soon the air in the room was so thick and malodorous that ladies kept fainting and were sent away to recover. "During the night even the men kept disappearing and the six Capuchin monks who prayed at the bedside had to take it in turn to do so, silently changing over every hour." Marie-Louise arrived from Parma only the day before her son's death and then only in response to a peremptory note from the Ballhausplatz.[8] (The Archduke was popular with the sentimental Viennese public and Metternich feared a riot if he should die without

---

[6] Several liaisons of the Duke (in addition to his most famous one with the dancer, Fanny Elssler) are documented. Self-styled illegitimate offspring turned up regularly for many decades after his death.

[7] The '*Alter*' was a Viennese endearment: she was four years older than the Duke.

[8] Then Metternich's Chancellery, later the Foreign Office where the fatal telegram to Serbia was drafted in 1914.

his mother being summoned to his bedside.) In the event, she spent only a few minutes in her son's company: the smell, she protested, gave her an excruciating headache and threatened to give her a heart attack. ("Somebody should have had the *nous* to start burning myrrh or incense", she later wrote to Count Neipperg, "but of course nobody thought of that. Typical of the Viennese bunch of layabouts.")[9] Only the Archduchess Sophie, though she had only just recovered from the birth of her second son,[10] the Baroness and the court physician, Malfatti, stayed throughout the last night. Shortly before the Duke breathed his last – he died at 5 o'clock in the morning on 23 July 1832 – Malfatti, who had been keeping his fingers on the dying man's pulse, must have sent out word because (as in Rostand's play) the doors were thrown open and a concourse of Archdukes, Archduchesses and their retinues crowded in. A few minutes later Malfatti announced: "Er is tot". But instead of a hush interrupted only by Metternich's command, the announcement triggered off a frantic rush to the bedside: "it very nearly swept the exhausted Archduchess and me off our knees". Imperial Highnesses, courtiers and even servants, brandishing knives and scissors, "jostled to get near the body to collect a lock of the dead Prince's golden hair until he was very nearly bald".

The message of atonement did not need a historic context. On 1 June 1847, when Verdi arrived on his first visit to Paris, Marie Dupléssis – or Alphonsine Pléssis to give her the name which is engraved on her tombstone in the cemetery of Montmartre – had been dead for over three months: he never therefore met his Violetta. But Giuseppine Strepponi, the singer who was settled in Paris and would eventually become his second wife, had seen her at the Opéra and the Théâtre Italien, making an entry into one of the great proscenium boxes, "ravishingly young and beautiful, always with a fresh bouquet in her hand, her lustrous hair entwined with diamonds and flowers, her arms and bosom almost bare but for necklaces, bracelets, emeralds". Verdi must also have walked past Marie's handsome town house opposite the Madeleine where a few weeks after her death her belongings, even her pet parrot, were auctioned to one of the most fashionable crowds ever seen in Paris to attend such a function.[11]

Alexandre Dumas *fils*, young, penniless and Romantic, the legitimised son of the immensely successful author of the *Three Musketeers* and the *Count*

---

[9] Later her second husband.

[10] Maximilian was born two weeks before the Duke's death.

[11] The sale was attended by Charles Dickens on a visit to Paris. "One could have believed", he wrote, "that Marie was Jeanne d'Arc or some other national heroine, so profound was the general sadness".

of Monte Cristo, was among Marie's lovers: for how long and how significantly
for Marie is not known. Young Dumas thought that it had been significant
for her as well as for him and later wrote that "she was the last great courtesan
who not only had a heart but also had great nobility.[12] This is no doubt why
she died young and penniless in a sumptuous apartment about to be seized
by her creditors". Whatever the real background, he immortalised her – and
with her tuberculous death as an act of self-sacrifice – first in a novel and
than in a play.[13] *La dame aux camélias* had its first performance in the Théâtre
de Vaudeville on 2 February 1852. Théophile Gautier, who reviewed the event,
summarised the plot. "At the beginning Marguérite [Marie Dupléssis had
become Marguérite Gauthier]

> is not yet transformed by passion: she manoeuvres her army of admirers like
> Celimène coolly: she has the insolence of beauty, the cruelty of youth, the selfishness
> of success. But then, as is she begins to be troubled and then filled with real love,
> she becomes humble, shy, tender – and ill. She is consumed not only by love for
> Armand but also by the disease which consumes her body. And she knows it. But
> she does not care so long as Armand loves her and she can love Armand. Now
> the courtesan is stripped away and she becomes an innocent young girl!" [14]

Of course it is not to be. Enter young Armand's father, the embodiment of
bourgeois convention, propriety and virtue. The liaison – let alone the
marriage of which Marie dreams – would destroy the future of Armand's
sister, an innocent young virgin reared with infinite parental love presumably
for the supreme role of becoming the wife of another respectable and successful bourgeois and, it is to be hoped, the mother of many more.

Marguérite not merely complies with Germont senior's wish to break off
the liaison but is determined to leave no scar of regret in Armand's soul.
She pretends to reject him and accepts his anger as atonement for her own
unworthy past. Only in the last scene, as she lies dying, are the protagonists
brought together in reconciliation, remorse and forgiveness. "Never have I
seen a death scene so painful and yet so uplifting", Théophile Gautier wrote,

[12] She was born in Normandy in 1824 and the name given to her at birth was Alphonsine.
She changed it to Marie in veneration of the Virgin and because she thought it was well
suited to the expression of her own beautiful eyes. It was under the name of Marie Dupléssis
that she married a young and wealthy Englishman who died shortly after of tuberculosis.
Unable to claim her inheritance because of sinister legal machinations by her late husband's
family, she embarked on her glorious but brief career as queen of the Parisian demimonde.
She was twenty-three when she died.

[13] Dumas *fils* later wrote a number of successful plays (as well as novels), mostly of great
seriousness and moral uplift, a striking contrast to the *oeuvre* of his rumbustious parent. He
was eventually elected to the Académie Française (unlike the author of *The Three Musketeers*)
and died in 1895, aged seventy-one. See Claretie, J., *Alexandre Dumas fils* (Paris, 1882).

[14] Quoted by Toussaint, P., *Marie Dupléssis: la vraie Dame aux Camélias* (Paris, 1958), p. 62.

"her pale face set off by the lace pillow, her soul shining through ... grace and sacrifice to ravish the soul". It is one of those scenes which justifies the seemingly crazy conventions of opera. There is very little to say on such occasions and yet an infinity of feelings, memories and even hopes to convey; and while Dumas *fils'* well-crafted dialogue rarely succeeds in capturing the undivided attention of a modern audience,[15] Verdi's music set to the inane repetition of one or two deeply unoriginal sentences almost always does.[16] Violetta-Marguérite is mourned – even though some medical know-all will usually explain that such a death-scene is physically impossible.

The medical know-all (who has probably never seen a tuberculous death) will be wrong. Sixteen hundred years before Marie Dupléssis *alias* Marguérite Gauthier, Aretaeus the Cappadocian wrote about phthisis: "What is most astonishing is that in a case when blood comes from the lung ... where the disease is most serious ... patients do not give up hope ... and the strength of their body holds out to the moment of death ... and the strength of the mind even surpasses that of the body". Eighteen-year-old Virginia Poe, Edgar Allan Poe's bride, continued to attend social functions in the evenings while coughing up blood and being too exhausted for much of the day to get off her day-bed; and she attended her last dance the night when she suffered her last and fatal haemorrhage. It was not perhaps typical but it was possible.

The cult of sacrifice and atonement, so widespread and so powerful during the plentiful years of the Long Peace – the good old days to the generation which saw its passing and mourned it with deep nostalgia – did not survive the sacrificial orgy of 1914–1918. Nor was it capable of resurrection. Dumas'

---

[15] When first produced the play was a resounding success; and, after its initial run, it was performed and regularly revived throughout the century in most European capitals. It was seen in Paris soon after its first performance by an American actress, Jean Davenport, who insisted that it be immediately translated so that she might take the leading role. Under the title of *Camille: or The Fate of a Coquette*, it was an even greater success in New York. There was (according to a 1948 guidebook to the cemetery of Montmartre) never a time until the Second World War when Marie's grave was not covered with fresh bouquets of camelias deposited there by young lovers, even though the flower motif (according to Dumas *fils* himself) was pure invention.

[16] The inanity and repetitiousness was in the nature of opera: the libretto by Francesco Maria Piave was effective, though it greatly ennobled the heroine of Dumas' play. The opera was a dismal failure at its first performance in 1853 at the Fenice Theatre in Venice (where, in deference to the moral susceptibilities of the Austrian censor, it had to be performed in early eighteenth-century costume). After much toing and froing between Verdi and various theatrical managements and impresarios it received its second and successful production again in Venice at the Teatro San Benedetto less than a year later. Since then, and soon restored to its contemporary setting, *La Traviata* has never looked back.

play is still occasionally staged in France; and Verdi's *La Traviata* remains popular in the international repertory; but Greta Garbo in the role of Marguérite Gauthier on the screen in the dismal 1930s was achingly beautiful but painfully unconvincing and the film was a box-office flop.

7

The Poor

Tuberculosis picked out and killed a few Princes and it carried off more than one bejewelled, tender-hearted courtesan; but it slaughtered the poor by the million. Most common diseases have an economic dimension; and most epidemics have social and political causes and consequences; but, as in so many other respects, tuberculosis was unique. With poverty, malnutrition, overcrowding, vice, crime, and moral degradation it became not just a cause or consequence but part of the landscape of the Industrial Revolution.

It is possible though blinkered to write a social history of modern England or Europe without mentioning tuberculosis; but the reverse would be meaningless. Tuberculosis had been around for centuries and in every age it could cross frontiers and transcend social barriers, but it only became a mass killer, especially a mass killer of the poor and the young in England, during the first quarter of nineteenth century. Indeed, the retreat of tuberculosis since 1840, a dogma among epidemiological historians, was almost certainly a slow return to the pre-Industrial Revolution level from an explosive increase and a peak between 1790 and 1840. These dates are transposable with the appropriate adjustments to countries like France, Germany, Scandinavia and those of eastern Europe where the Industrial Revolution was delayed or more protracted or both. When in Germany Käthe Kollwitz began to draw her searing images of poverty, disease and death of women and children, in the 1880s, the bleakest decades of her country's Industrial Revolution were still within living memory.[1] In Norway, Poland and Hungary the revolution was just beginning. In Russia there was as yet barely a sign of it.

Child labour in factories became common in England around 1800, something as relevant to the history of tuberculosis as are the discoveries of Auenbrugger and Laënnec and the therapeutic practices of doctors attending those who could afford them. To quote from one report (published in 1796) "children of five, six and seven are now being collected from the workhouses in London and Westminster and transported in crowds to mills and factories many hundreds of miles distant to work in closed crowded rooms ... the

---

[1] Her first series dates from 1893–1894 when she was only seventeen. Her immediate inspiration was attending Gerhart Hauptmann's play, *Die Weber* (*The Weavers.*)

air they breathe from the oil employed in the machinery injurious ... no regard paid to their cleanliness and frequent changes from hot and dense to cold and thin atmospheres predisposing them to sickness and debility and the epidemic fever which usually kills them within a few years ..."[2] What fever? Nobody tried to put a label on it; and, so long as supplies kept up with the wastage and the profits were satisfactory, nobody much cared.

The supplies did keep up with the wastage and the profits were very satisfactory indeed. By the early decades of the nineteenth century they led to the practice of night working: having worked to exhaustion one set of pair of hands throughout the day, factory owners had another set ready to go on working throughout the night, "the day gang getting into the beds that the night gang had just quitted ... and in turn the night gang getting into the beds that the day gang had quitted in the morning". In this way in Lancashire, as the saying went, the beds never got cold.[3] They probably never got free of tuberculosis either.

All this was not a transient aberration; nor of course was it confined to Lancashire. Forty years later the Children's Employment Commission on Trades and Manufacture in England still reported on children starting work, sometimes at the age of six but regularly at seven or eight, "stunted in growth, their aspect pale, delicate, sickly, presenting the appearance of a race which has suffered from gross physical deterioration ... The diseases most prevalent being of the nutritive organs, curvature and distortion of the spine, deformity of the limbs and especially disease of the lungs ending in atrophy, consumption and death." Was this consumption tuberculosis? It is impossible to say for certain; but tuberculosis must have contributed its quota.[4]

[2] Dubos, R. and J., *The White Plague: Tuberculosis, Man and Society* (London, 1953), p. 198.

[3] Drolet, G. J., "The Epidemiology of Tuberculosis", in *Clinical Tuberculosis*, ed. B. Goldberg (Davis, California, 1946).

[4] The first Act of Parliament to set a legal limit to the working hours of children and young persons (ten hours plus or minus, depending on conditions) was not passed until Lord Althorp's Factory Act of 1833. The Act also set up a factory inspectorate with powers to enter and inspect any factory above a certain size. (The appointment of inspectors had been urged by some of the more humane employers. They had argued – truthfully – that it was not only employers but also parents living off their children's earnings who needed watching.) Out of this "Children's Charter" grew the Ten Hours Bill of 1844–47, more or less contemporaneously with the repeal of the Corn Laws. This measure had been a storm centre for several years and eventually produced the pattern of cross-voting in Parliament characteristic of much Victorian social legislation. (Some leading liberals, Melbourne, Cobden and Bright among them, voted against the Bill; Russell, Palmerston and Macaulay for it.) Over the next decades the principle of factory regulation was gradually extended. Revelations of the unspeakable conditions of female and child labour in the coal mines (several centuries old) led to Lord Shaftesbury's Mines Act which forbade the underground employment of women and children under ten. But the ill-usage of boy-sweeps continued till the 1870s, despite the public outcry in the wake

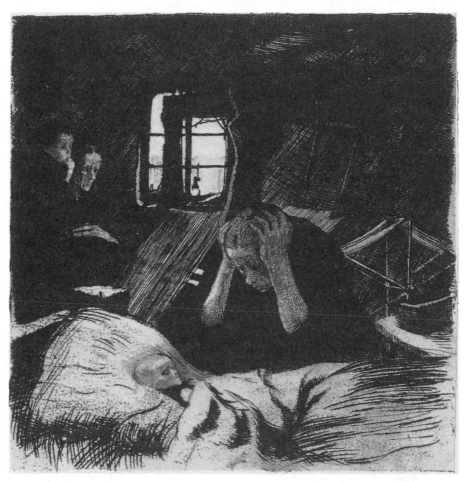

Poverty, drawing by Käthe Kollwitz. Many of the great and good died of tuberculosis; but the illness was always, above all, a disease of the poor. Kollwitz was perhaps their greatest chronicler in the visual arts.

Malnutrition among the young was rife even outside factories. "The bowls never wanted washing. The boys polished them with their spoons till they shone again; and when they had performed this operation ... they would sit staring at the copper with such eager eyes as if they could have devoured the very bricks of which it was composed; employing themselves meanwhile in sucking their fingers most assiduously, with the view of catching up any stray splashes of gruel that might have been cast thereon ..." Was Oliver Twist tuberculous? Very likely. If he was not, many of his fellow inmates at the table certainly were. By the age of eight many of them had probably lost three or four younger siblings from tuberculosis.[5]

The fact that tuberculosis transcended barriers of class and rank did not mean that it ignored social divisions. Indeed, the divergence between the rich and the poor started even before birth. Meaningful statistics for much of Europe and the United States dating from the early nineteenth century are few; but there is a surfeit of evidence of a different kind. The poor of the world's poor countries today are not much better off than were the destitute of Britain, Europe and the United States in the glory days of industrialisation – except in one respect: their destitution, especially in such comparatively simple matters as their exposure to tuberculosis and its consequences, is better documented. Numerous concerned reports and surveys bear witness to the fact that physically enfeebled tuberculous mothers are likely to undergo prolonged labour and die from exhaustion and blood loss. The disease is without a doubt a common cause of still-births, perinatal mortality and the convulsions and vomitings and diarrhoeas which kill babies of the shanty towns of South America soon after birth. Nobody questions the contemporary evidence that tuberculous mothers who survive labour are often too enfeebled to feed their infants and that unboiled cow's milk contributes to the postnatal devastation of gastrointestinal tuberculosis.

In contrast to earlier periods, from about the middle of the nineteenth century for most of Britain, Ireland and much of continental Europe and North America there exists a large body of statistical data – of sorts. It is known, for instance, that at least one in every four hospital deliveries in

of Charles Kingsley's *Water Babies*. Lord Shaftesbury eventually succeeded in getting an Act through Parliament "one hundred and two years after the good Jonas Hanway brought the brutal iniquity before the public". Like the Industrial Revolution itself, similar legislation in other countries was delayed, the time-lag between the two remaining about two generations.

[5] Those who reached adulthood were well described by Friedrich Engels in *The Condition of the Working Man in England* as "the pale, lank, narrow-chested, hollow-eyed ghosts riddled with scrofula".

Manchester between 1829 and 1835 were still-births and that in over half of the still-births the mothers were delicate in the chest, consumptive or scrofulous. It is known that convulsions caused by water on the brain were the assigned cause of death of 52 per cent of children under five who died in St Bride's parish in London in 1844: it is reasonable to assume that tuberculous meningitis was the underlying pathology in a significant proportion of these.[6]

More telling are the differences recorded using the same statistical methods between more or less adjacent impoverished and better off neighbourhoods. Areas recognised even in their day as "heavy with consumption" or "highly insanitary" had infant death rates three to five times higher than those recorded in nearby more salubrious areas; and at least half of the infant deaths in the former were ascribed to phthisis or lung disease. To pick out two examples, the earliest systematic records for England based on the 1841–42 returns show a mortality rate from phthisis four times higher in the poor parishes of St Giles Cripplegate and Whitechapel than it was in Westminster; and three times higher in the poor parish of St Saviour than in Hampstead. In some respects personal experiences provide the most convincing evidence. In the 1870s Dr D. R. Drysdale, physician to the North London Consumption Hospital, wrote that "while detailed estimates would probably differ among members of [my] profession, in my own experience mortality from consumption is about five times higher among the poor than among the rich"; and "none of my colleagues would put the difference at less than threefold".[7] There were similar differences in Glasgow, Liverpool, Birmingham and Dublin; and the differential mortality between the rich and the poor districts of Paris, Lyon and Vienna did not after the mid century lag behind those of British cities.

One of the many and almost insuperable difficulties of interpreting early statistics is that names conceal as much as they reveal. In many parts of Europe doctors avoided attributing any death that was doubtful to tuberculosis: the disease was widely regarded as hereditary with a distinct stigma attached to it. Outside hospitals and other institutions most English parish registrars depended on the testimony of the deceased person's kin, who generally avoided the term "consumption". Such vaguely descriptive catch-alls as "nervous decline" and "respiratory weakness" – "convulsions" in children – were convenient alternatives. After 1870, when death registration rules in England and Wales were tightened up, "bronchitis" emerged as a meaningless but popularly acceptable cause of death in childhood; and

[6] Smith, F. B., *The Retreat of Tuberculosis, 1850–1950* (London, 1988), p. 24.
[7] Drysdale, C. R., *Lancet* (1896), no. 2, 427.

mortality from this cause doubled almost from one year to the other. Once established, such usages are difficult to eradicate: in 1931 bronchitis as an alleged cause of death in childhood was still twice as common in Britain as it was in continental countries or in the United States. This was patently nonsense. (It is more than likely that many deaths registered today as due to coronary disease in elderly people who die without having been seen by a doctor within forty-eight hours of death, and therefore require confirmation by a coroner's post-mortem, represent a similar verbal convenience and the basis for similarly misleading statistics.)

There is in fact no real need to try to interpret early and perhaps less than reliable statistics to prove the class differentials. While overall mortality from tuberculosis fell more or less continuously in Britain (but not in Ireland) after about 1850, the differential mortality between the rich and the poor (later labelled Classes I to V) did not alter much at least until the 1930s: it was still stark by the end of the Second World War. In Liverpool the reported differentials between "fair" and "bad" artisan areas in the years before 1934 varied between 80 and 120 per cent. In Birmingham in the 1930s unskilled artisans died from consumption at twice the rate of skilled artisans and at three times the rate of the professional middle class. In impoverished Dublin the mortality rate from phthisis in the 1880s was almost twice as high as the overall mortality rate in London.[8] Even more striking and persistent were the differential ages of death: well into the twentieth century the poor tuberculous died ten to twenty years younger than the rich tuberculous.[9]

Large-scale and reasonably standardised post-mortem surveys began to be published in England and Scotland during the last quarter of the nineteenth century; and by and large they confirmed the statistics of the living. Of 1420 consecutive post-mortem examinations on children dying of all causes at the London Hospital for Sick Children in the 1880s, tuberculosis was recorded as the principal cause of death in about 45 per cent: nearly all the victims were under five and more than 80 per cent were of the labouring or domestic service class. In a comparable post-mortem series at the Royal Hospital for Sick Children in Edinburgh the figures were similar: 39 per cent of all death were described as tuberculous; 78 per cent of the tuberculous death were under five; and 98 per cent of the patients had been admitted on public assistance. Casting a forward glance beyond countless great advances and

[8] Forbes, T. R., *Journal of the History of Medicine*, 27 (1972), 24.

[9] In 1931 Dr Letitia Fairfield contrasted fifteen- to eighteen-year-old girls from a poor background in paid employment, who were "quickly ravaged by consumption", to their middle-class contemporaries enrolled in secondary schools with only two cases of tuberculosis reported in 90,000, *Transactions of the National Association for the Prevention of Tuberculosis* (1931), 34.

breakthroughs, let alone the natural decline of the disease, in Newcastle-upon-Tyne in 1947 tuberculosis still accounted for 24 per cent of hospital deaths of children under ten, over 90 per cent belonging to the "poor" classes.

By the end of the nineteenth century in most of western Europe tuberculosis was as endemic in the countryside as it was in the cities; but during the first half century of industrialisation its upsurge was an urban phenomenon. In North America, more than in the tightly packed mother countries of Europe, "the terrible distemper could be seen advancing as frontier life receded". Until the mid century the climate of southern California was widely held to be proof against pulmonary disease: "in the 1850s if somebody coughed in church all eyes turned on that person in amazement". By the 1890s the consumptive cough was as common in the cities of the Pacific coast as it was on the eastern seaboard.

What urban life added to malnutrition and other old-established guises of poverty was overcrowding. In the last year of Queen Victoria's reign 36 per cent of Dublin's dwellings consisted of one room only, compared to Glasgow's 26 per cent, the next most crowded city in the United Kingdom. Over 98 per cent of Dublin's single rooms housed at least five occupants, twice as many as Glasgow's and eighteen times as many as London's.[10] The chances of massive and repeated droplet infections were further increased by the exclusion of hopeless cases from workhouse infirmaries and general hospitals and the popular preference (abetted by out-of-hospital poor relief) for keeping the sick at home. It is surprising that Dublin's mortality rate from phthisis was only around twice that of Glasgow's and only ten times that of London's.

The most extreme cases of overcrowding were in prisons. Between 1870 and 1880 half of all prisoners in Chatham Naval Prison developed galloping tuberculosis every winter and died.[11] No lifer in an American prison survived for more than twelve years before 1910 and between 1890 and 1895 tuberculosis was the assigned cause of death in three-quarters of the prison population in Massachusetts.[12] Nine hundred and seventy young soldiers who had fought in the Hungarian War of Liberty of 1848/49 against Austria were sentenced to life imprisonment by courts martial and transported to the fortress prison of Kufstein in Austria. By the time of the first general amnesty in 1861 only 245 were still alive: the rest were reported to have died from phthisis. To make the leap in time to the infinitely more civilised twentieth century: in 1945, 88 per cent of the survivors of Buchenwald concentration camp showed

---

[10] Grimshaw, T. W. (Registrar-General for Ireland), *British Medical Journal* 2 (1887), 23.

[11] *British Medical Journal* (1882), no. 1, p. 630.

[12] *British Medical Journal* (1882), no. 2, p. 1257.

at the time of their liberation evidence of *active* tuberculosis. (How many had had the disease among the piles of rotting corpses which left an indelible impression on the liberating armies will never be known.) Even nearer in time, of the 26,000 refugees who arrived in Aldershot in England by airlift from Austria after the Hungarian uprising of 1956, the first transport of which included a large proportion of prison inmates and gipsies, 36 per cent showed on X-ray screening evidence of *active* disease.[13]

Next to prisons on the scale of endemic tuberculosis were the houses of some continental female religious orders. Nunneries had of course been staples of Protestant demonisation for centuries; but this was not just fevered Calvinistic imagining. Laënnec was a child of the Enlightenment and anti-clerical, but he was a truthful recorder of facts. He wrote in 1819 that he had

> under my own eyes during a period of ten years members of a religious association of women, of recent foundation, and which had never obtained from the ecclesiastical authorities any other than provisional toleration, on account of the extreme severity of its rules. The diet of these persons was very austere yet by no means beyond what nature could bear. But the ascetic spirit which regulated their lives was such as to give rise to consequences no less serious than surprising. Not only was the attention of these women habitually fixed on the most terrible truths of religion, but it was the constant practice to try them by every kind of contrariety and

[13] Nor does this mark the chronological end of the relationship between prison and tuberculosis. In 1988 Nelson Mandela, then an inmate of Pollsmoor Prison, developed a bad cough and became too weak for his daily exercise. After vomiting and fainting in the visiting area he was secretly and under heavy guard transferred to the Tygerberg Hospital, part of the University of Stellenbosch. (Not just the ward but the whole floor to which he was admitted had been evacuated of other patients.) After an initial negative misdiagnosis by a charming but inexperienced junior doctor, he was visited by the head of internal medicine, "a no-nonsense fellow [who] tapped me roughly on the chest and then said gruffly, 'there is a lot of water on your lungs, Mandela' ". He asked the nurse to bring him a syringe and without further ado demonstrated the accuracy of his diagnosis by aspirating some brownish liquid. The patient was then taken to the operating theatre and had the rest of the fluid removed under a general anaesthetic. The bacteriological tests confirmed the diagnosis of tuberculosis.

Mandela was assured that the infection had been caught early and that two or three months' treatment would see him right. In fact, the illness had almost certainly started while he was incarcerated in Robben Island (where tuberculosis was endemic); and in pre-chemotherapy days the prognosis would have been poor. Fortunately, by 1988 negotiations with President Botha and other government emissaries were well advanced and the end of Apartheid was in sight. After six weeks in hospital the patient was transferred to the luxurious Constantiaberg Clinic, the first black patient to be admitted there, where he made a good recovery. Characteristically of the man, barely two pages (pp. 646–47 in the paperback edition) of his 747-page autobiography *Long Walk to Freedom* (London, 1994) are devoted to his brush with what could have been, and twenty years earlier would undoubtedly have been, a rapidly fatal illness. One prisoner was saved, others were not: it was from prisoners that in the 1980s multidrug resistant tuberculosis emerged (see below, Chapter 33, 387).

opposition, in order to bring them, as soon as possible to an entire renouncement of their proper will. The consequences of this discipline were the same in all: after being one or two months in the establishment, the catamenia became suppressed; and in the course of one or two months thereafter phthisis declared itself. As no vow was taken in this society, I endeavoured to prevail upon the patients to leave the house as soon as consumptive symptoms began to appear; and some of those who followed my advice were cured ... During the ten years that I was a physician of this association, I witnessed its entire renovation two or three times owing to the successive loss of all its members, with the exception of the superior, the gate keeper and the sisters who had charge of the garden, kitchen and infirmary.[14]

The situation did not change significantly as the century progressed. Nearly two-thirds of the deaths in Prussian nursing orders in thirty-eight convents between 1864 and 1889 were officially attributed to tuberculosis. The nuns were examined before their admission to the novitiate and had to be declared healthy. Their mean life expectancy after that date was three years. As recently as 1949 a study of more than 50,000 workers in various tuberculosis institutions in Italy showed that the lay medical and nursing staff had an annual morbidity rate of 8.7 per thousand, whereas that of the nuns in the same institutions was 18 per thousand.[15]

At the spiritual level the association between convent life and tuberculosis was not entirely negative: indeed, the disease became an integral part of the Catholic religious revival in France toward the end of the nineteenth and beginning of the twentieth century. The exact cause of the death of St Bernadette Soubirous, the peasant girl whose visions established Lourdes as the most popular of modern Catholic shrines, is not known; but she died a nun in an enclosed order in 1879, at the age of thirty-four, of chronic lung disease. Better documented is the consumption of that other emblem of the religious resurgence, St Thérèse of Lisieux: her moving autobiography, *L'histoire d'une âme*, which became a sensational best-seller, chronicles her physical as well her spiritual struggles in authentic detail.[16]

Some of the blackest spots of the disease, nevertheless, were often far away from densely populated conurbations. Wales remained a redoubt of tuberculosis throughout the nineteenth and the best part of the twentieth century – almost as impregnable as Ireland – and some of its most heavily tuberculous areas were sparsely populated mountain districts in the north and west. In Ireland too the death rate from tuberculosis in impoverished rural regions

[14] Laënnec, R. T. H., *A Treatise on Diseases of the Chest and on Mediate Auscultation*, translated by J. Forbes (London, 1927), p. 83.

[15] Sossi, O., Gaeta, A. P., *Proceedings of the 7th National Congress on Tuberculosis* (Rome, 1948), p. 342.

[16] She died in 1897, aged twenty-four, and was canonised in 1925 by Pope Pius XI.

continued to rise for at least a decade after it had at last begun to fall in Dublin and Belfast. Norway, one of the least densely populated countries in Europe, was also one of the most heavily infected with tuberculosis; and the disease was entrenched in the widely separated villages and farmsteads of the Great Hungarian Plain until the 1930s.

In Britain, as in other countries, consumption was closely linked not only to poverty and overcrowding but also to patterns of employment. Metal workers, tailors, shoemakers, masons, printers, bakers and seamstresses were traditionally high-risk occupations. Many laboured in cramped, dimly-lit and ill-ventilated workshops (beyond the reach of the Factory Acts when the Factory Acts eventually came), hunched in fuggy atmospheres, often inhaling irritating organic vapour or dust. Compositors traditionally threw the remains of their meals into a corner of the printing room where the food rotted into stinking messes: "a deplorable custom", the London Society of Compositors reported in 1883, "but not one which is capable of being altered without causing aggravation among the most experienced of our craft". The seemingly unalterable custom probably explained why a third of the society's funeral allowances had to be set aside for victims of phthisis.[17] Hot, dusty environments in general encouraged spitting, the most effective means of spreading the organism.

Much of this was common knowledge by the time the first great epidemiological studies of occupational hazards were published in Britain in the 1890s; but neither John Tatham of the Registrar General's Office nor Arthur Ransome, a leading consumption specialist, could suggest much in the way of improving practices. As for their readers, what displays of debating skill the reports provoked were largely expended on pointing to the fallacies inherent in such jugglings with figures. Some of the objections were of course valid. Workers whose health became too poor to cope with recognised high-risk trades often drifted into casual employment: general labourers had a mortality rate from phthisis three times higher than that of any specifically named occupation. Or they moved into ill-paid sedentary occupations and helped to inflate the apparent occupational risks of bookbinders, law and railway clerks, servants in public houses, musicians, tobacconists, drapers, street hawkers and messengers. Between 1890 and 1900 all of these had a roughly one in four chance of dying from phthisis, compared to the one in twenty-seven chance of clergymen and the one in twenty-two chance of doctors.

Britain pioneered the Industrial Revolution and many of its attendant miseries. It also created the first hospitals dedicated to the care of

---

[17] *Lancet* (1884) no. 1, p. 265.

consumptives. The impulse behind their foundation makes a fine story. Reality was sometimes less edifying. The Brompton Hospital, the oldest of London's four, was founded in 1842: it remained the most prestigious and, with a nominal 300 odd beds, the largest. But bed numbers are deceptive and have in fact deceived several historians. For most of the nineteenth century at least half the beds were habitually empty for lack of funds or lack of nursing staff or both. The City of London Hospital for Chest Diseases was a Quaker foundation: established in 1848, it had 160 beds. The North London Hospital for Consumption and the Royal National Hospital for Chest Diseases were both founded in the 1860s: the first was a doctor's racket where large grants from the Hospitals Sunday Fund went missing for decades before the scandal broke in 1899. The second had a variable twenty beds.

Writers on public health in Victorian England liked to expatiate on the pioneering role of these institutions in the care and treatment of consumptives. Both the Queen and Prince Albert took great pride in them. State visitors or their consorts were occasionally treated to a tour of the Brompton or the London Hospital for Chest Diseases. It was pointed out to them – truthfully – that London was the only capital city in the world to boast free hospitals dedicated to tuberculosis. They expressed their imperial, royal or serene approval in a suitable inscription in the visitors' book as well by a donation to the hospital's benevolent fund. While it would be wrong to underestimate the value of such charities because more was always needed, or belittle the dedication of some of their staff, a few corrective facts need to be recalled. Once specialist hospitals were established in a city, few others would accept consumptives except to provide material for teaching purposes. The four London specialist hospitals could also only house at their theoretical maximum one thousand patients, when the death rate from consumption in England and Wales ran at over 50,000 a year and in London at over 15,000.

In fact the pressure on beds at least until the 1920s was never great; and this was not perhaps surprising. The more prestigious a hospital, the harsher was the regime for its inmates. After the mid 1860s, when the senior staff became converted to fresh-air theories, the wards at the Brompton were unheated and ventilated with fresh air throughout the year. (Even so, the hospital air vents were a useful source of live tubercle bacilli for experimental purposes in the late 1890s.) Erysipelas and throat infections were endemic, with severe outbreaks every four to five years. Bedding was not disinfected till 1900. The hospital fare was generally described as "standard": it was reinforced with large doses of arsenic, atropine and strychnine to combat night sweats (in addition to the ubiquitous cod-liver oil). Many physicians prescribed antiseptic or hot air inhalations. The patients hated them: the threat was often enough to empty wards of all who could move. But "many patients materially benefited", the hospital reported annually. It never said *how* many. The overall cure rate for in-patients claimed by the reports varied between 3 and 5 per cent. Even 3 per cent was probably too sanguine. The death rate was never officially stated but in the 1880s it was probably around 20 per cent of annual admissions.

8

The Romantic Image

An unbridgeable gulf seems to separate the child labourers of Lancashire and sweat shops of Boston from the Romantic image of consumptive poets, musicians and artists of the same generation: yet the disease which imprinted itself on their lives – often brief – was recognisably the same.

The change from the rationalist ideal (not of course always translated into practice) of the Enlightenment was surprisingly sudden. Melancholic meditations over the transience of youth, doomed beautiful maidens, mouldering tombs, abandoned ruins and weeping willows suddenly became popular everywhere in Europe during the last third of the eighteenth century, as if in response to some fresh revelation about the evanescence of human existence. Ever since the Renaissance poets had sung about the joys and wonders of this world: now, with Thomas Lovell Beddoes (whose father had written a famous essay on consumption), it became – almost as it had been in the middle ages – a "grave-paved star". Since Antiquity autumn had been in literature the time of bountiful harvests, the mellow season after the hard labours of the summer and before the privations of winter when men rejoiced in health and abundance. Now falling leaves became the metaphor for failing hopes, the destruction of young lives. The German poet Ludwig Hölty, dying of consumption at twenty-nine in 1776, compared his life to a leaf "withered and carried by the wind", an image irresistible to the sixteen-year-old Franz Schubert. Hölty was only the first in the long line of consumptives who supplied the words for that uniquely tuberculous flowering of the Romantic spirit, the German *Lied*.

Christian Fürchtegott Gellert, the son of a Protestant pastor, found solace during his long illness in God and the contemplation of God as revealed in Nature, and his prayerful odes provided Beethoven with the words he needed to express in music his own profound if tormented faith.[1]

Friedrich von Schiller was, like Keats and later Chekhov, a doctor before

---

[1] Including "Die Himmel rühmen des Ewigen Ehren" and "Die Ehre Gottes an der Natur". Gellert died in 1769, aged fifty-three.

he became a writer, poet and dramatist.[2] Persecuted in youth by a petty tyrannical prince, Karl Eugen of Württemberg, he celebrated his release and the hospitality of his friend and fellow poet, Christian Gottfried Körner, with his the *Ode to Joy*.[3] In 1794, when he was thirty-five, he met Goethe in Weimar, a union of opposites except in their nobility of spirit; and there followed an outpouring of ballads, lyric poetry and philosophical works. Schubert set to music no less than forty-eight, including *Die Hoffnung*, the most tuberculous of titles, twice.[4] Weimar saw the beginning of Schiller's illness, not yet incapacitating but worrying enough for Goethe to secure for his friend what he hoped would be a tranquil academic position, the chair of history in the University of Jena. Schiller, however, did not regard the appointment as a sinecure; during the next few years he completed his most important historical and philosophical works, as well as some of his historical plays. Having disregarded warning signs – night sweats and blood-stained sputum – since his mid twenties, his health broke down in 1792, two years after his marriage to Charlotte von Lengefeld. He gave up his teaching post and accepted a pension offered by two Danish patrons for three years. It was during his slow and never complete recovery that he wrote his best reflective poetry, progressing from the youthful celebration of physical freedom to the exploration of the freedom of the soul, moral grace. To his long-standing gastrointestinal symptoms – bouts of colic, vomiting and diarrhoea – there were soon added a painful cough, occasional pulmonary bleeds, headaches and insomnia. Between acute episodes, even confined to bed, he completed *Wallenstein, Mary Stuart, Die Jungfrau von Orleans* and *Wilhelm Tell*, always trying to finish just one more work before the inevitable end. When the end did come – on 9 May 1805 – it cut short *Demetrius*, a last noble fragment.

A tuberculous poet stands both at the beginning and at the end of Robert Schumann's *Lieder* decade, a revelation of romantic beauty comparable only to the miracle of Schubert. He composed the song-cycle, *Frauenliebe und*

[2] He was born in 1759, the son of an army surgeon. He was ennobled – hence the *von* – in 1802. Unlike Keats, Schiller was interested in medicine and left behind not only important psychological works but also a collection of clinical notes, several excellent medical and pathological essays, dissertations and post-mortem reports. The last include a detailed necropsy report, dated 10 October 1778, on a young soldier, Johann Christian Hiller, who had died of disseminated tuberculosis. See Dewhurst, K., Reeves, N., *Schiller, F.: Medicine, Psychology, Literature* (Oxford, 1978).

[3] Used by Beethoven in the choral movement of his Ninth Symphony, now the official anthem of the European Union.

[4] Hope was not a feature of syphilis of which the greatest composers (as distinct from the poets) of the *Lieder* died – Schubert, Schumann, Wolf, perhaps Beethoven.

Leben (*A Woman's Love and Life*), in 1840, shortly after his long delayed but ardently hoped for engagement to Clara Wieck. The words had been written twenty years earlier by Adalbert von Chamisso, the scion of a refugee French aristocratic family who had settled in Berlin. A gifted linguist and botanist as well as a writer and poet, the seemingly artless sentiments expressed by the *Frau* had a personal significance for him too: the poems were written shortly after his own marriage to Antonie, a young woman from a humble family,[5] twenty years younger than himself (as was Clara Schumann when she married Robert). It was also a time when he was beginning to show the first sign of pulmonary tuberculosis, a painful cough, and realised that his happiness would not last long. For most of his marriage he was in fact ailing, filling a whole cup with horrible purulent phlegm every morning, spending much of his days in the little summer house in the garden, writing poetry, letters and philological works, being looked after with great devotion by his wife. Soon after their marriage she too developed the first tell-tale symptoms (though concealing them as long as she could); and, belying the sequence in *Frauenliebe und Leben*, "Nun hast du mir den ersten Schmerz getan" ("Now you have hurt me for the first time"), it was he who mourned her death (after a massive pulmonary bleed in 1837), not she his. It was only for another eighteen months, just time enough to write his last and best poetry. It included one of the most memorable tuberculous farewells, addressed to his children (now looked after by his sister-in-law), dated 5 May 1838:

> So hat euch wohl die Angst zu mir getrieben?
> "Wir sind um dich ersammelt". – Alle? – Gut!
> Lasst mich euch überzählen: sechse, sieben –
> Und – sagt mir – eure Mutter? "Mutter ruht". –
>
> Das will auch ich: bin müde, meine Lieben.
> Drum, fahret wohl! wir sind in Gottes Hut.
> Fährt wohl, ich geb euch allen meinen Segen.
> Ich will bequemer mich zur Ruhe Legen.[6]

Frauenliebe und Leben stands near the beginning of Schumann's career in song: the words of a dying woman marked the end. Few appreciated the

---

[5] A way of saying in his day that she was an almost illiterate servant girl in the von Chamisso household.

[6] "Was it fear which drove you to me? / 'We are assembled around you.' – All of you? Good. Let me count you then: six, seven – / And tell me, where is your mother? 'Mother is resting'. – That is what I want to do too: I am tired, my dears. / Therefore farewell! We are in God's care. / Farewell, I give you all my blessing. I will be happier when I rest."

poetry of Elisabeth Kulmann in her day (or since) but the composer, haunted already by the spectre of his own death,[7] responded with deep feeling to her simple art.[8] She was a real-life incarnation of the frail, doomed Mignon, especially of the Mignon dressed like an angel who foresees her early death in Goethe's "So lasst mich scheiden". Russian-born, she was only seventeen in 1825 when she died, her father and all but one of her seven brothers having already succumbed to tuberculosis. Like so much of the tuberculous poetry of the German *Lied*, her poems were steeped in longing – in looking at passing clouds, in listening to the rustle of the wind in autumnal trees, in death in youth, in faith and – forever – in hope.

> Reich mir die Hand, o Wolke,
> Heb mich zu dir empor!
> Dort stehen meine Brüder
> Am offnen Himmelstor.
>
> Sie sind's, obgleich im Leben
> Ich niemals sie gesehn,
> Ich seh' in ihrer Mitte
> Ja unsern Vater stehn!
>
> Sie schaun auf mich hernieder,
> Sie winken mir zu sich.
> O reich die Hand mir Wolke,
> Schnell, schnell, erhebe mich! [9]

In the existence of the tuberculous there were also times of exuberance, an intense enjoyment of life while it lasted; and this too found expression in Elisabeth Kulmann's simple lyrics:

> Wir sind ja, Kind, im Maie,
> Wirf Buch und Heft von Dir!
> Komm einmal hier ins Freie,
> Und sing ein Lied mit mir.
>
> Komm, singen fröhlich beide
> Mir einen Wettgesang,

---

[7] He died in 1856 aged forty-six, having spent his last years in a mental hospital.

[8] As did the present writer.

[9] "Reach me your hand, O cloud; / lift me up to you! / There stand my brothers / at the open gate of heaven. / There they are, although / in life I never saw them, / and I see our father too, / standing in their midst! / They look down on me / and beckon me to them./ O reach me your hand, cloud; / quickly, quickly, lift me up!"

Und wer da will, entscheide,
Wer von uns besser säng.[10]

The poet who more than any other expressed – though he also transcended – the spirit and disease of the age was Friedrich Leopold Freiherr von Hardenberg, better known as Novalis.[11] Born in 1772, his family were Protestant Saxon nobility but simple and pietistic – and riddled with tuberculosis. In 1790 he went to Jena where he was one of the group of students who took it in turn to look after the forever ailing but much-loved Herr Professor Schiller. He also met Johann Gottlieb Fichte, on the point of inventing German Romantic philosophy, and became immersed in the works of Kant and Friedrich von Schlegel. They helped him to evolve his own Magical Idealism. In 1796 he was appointed auditor to the Saxon state salt-works at Weissenfels, a nearly hereditary post of the von Hardenbergs; and he also had his first premonitory haemoptysis. By then he had already met the twelve-year-old Sophie von Kuhn and the two had fallen in love. They were betrothed in 1794, the year when she too developed the first signs of tuberculosis. She died three years later. During the next few years her memory inspired him to create his best work. *Blumenstaub* (Pollen) and *Glauben und Leben* (Faith and Living), published in 1798, were short poetic fragments and aphorisms, mystical and often a little obscure but exquisitely phrased. *Heinrich von Ofterdingen* was an unfinished novel, the blue flower in the story later becoming the symbol of Romantic and tuberculous pining, the mirage of ever elusive happiness.[12] With greatest intensity he wrote poetry, deeply religious but to some of his contemporaries shockingly unorthodox, mixing Evangelical piety and Marian mysticism, sexual allusion and spiritual frisson.

To the casual reader much of Novalis's verse may be impenetrable; but many tuberculous patients, including his fellow poet a hundred years later, Christian Morgenstern, recognised in it the truest reflection of their own destiny: moments of total despair alternating with almost schizophrenic (rather than religious) detachment. In the end love, in Novalis's case love

[10] "May has come, child; / throw aside your books! / Just come out into the open / and sing a song with me./ Come, let us both have / a cheerful song contest, and let who will, decide / which of us sang better!"

[11] The name was his own coinage, meaning roughly "one who is seeking new ways". This he certainly did, one reason perhaps why outside Germany his poems were not widely appreciated until the mid twentieth century. He was then discovered by English poets like Kathleen Raine and Jeremy Reed, some noting an affinity between him and the young T. S. Eliot. Among Novalis's many new verbal inventions was the use of the word genius in its modern sense.

[12] *The Blue Flower* is also the title of a fine biographical novel about the love of Novalis and Sophie by Penelope Fitzgerald.

for the dead Sophie, and the overwhelming prospect of mystical union after physical death, vanquishes all fear. But it is Schubert who dispels the last doubts. To have inspired some of his most solemn and deeply-felt songs Novalis's extraordinary outpourings must have been more than the ravings of a poetic but deranged mind. As the last vocal line in the chorale-like *Nachthymne*, "Ich fühle des Todes verjüngende Flut" ("I feel death's rejuvenating stream"), "vanishes into the stratospheres [in fact the top of the stave] and as the postlude climbs higher and higher on the keyboard, we feel that the Soul is on its way".[13] The poet was twenty-nine – to Schubert's thirty – when he died.

Even if it was the German *Lied* which most perfectly expressed the Romantic image of tuberculosis – or the tuberculous image of Romanticism – the image was not the product of one country or one particular genre. In *La chute des feuilles* the Frenchman Charles Hubert Millevoy, dying slowly of tuberculosis, saw the "mournful hues of autumn" mirroring his own doom. Lamartine was more fortunate, surviving by half a century the poems in which he took tearful leave of the world; but his beloved Julie, whom he met while recovering from his own illness near Lake Annecy, did succumb to tuberculosis at the age of twenty-two.[14] After her death the love she had inspired lived on in his melancholy verse in which the glowing, multicoloured foliage of autumn became the image of the passing of life and the mourning of nature. To Shelley too the colours, the crisp air and the pungent odours of the woods and fields of autumn evoked only

> the leaves dead
> Are driven, like ghosts from an enchanter fleeing,
> Yellow, and black, and pale, and hectic red,
> Pestilence-stricken multitudes ... [15]

And the restlessly wandering Hungarian poet, Michael Csokonay, apostrophised hope in his anguished ode as "a blind cruel mirage sent by the gods to tease and deceive us all".[16]

---

[13] From Graham Johnson's inspired notes to volume 29 of the Hyperion Schubert edition of the Complete Songs, CDJ 33029.

[14] She appears as Laurence in *Jocelyn*, Julie in *Raphael* and Elvire in *Méditations*. He died in 1869, aged seventy-nine.

[15] From "Ode to the West Wind" (1819). There were exceptions of course. Despite his illness, autumn to Keats remained a "season of mists and mellow fruitfulness": he was a much more robust character than suggested by some of his biographers.

[16] Csokonay was an itinerant scholar, student and soldier as well as a poet until his death in 1804 at the age thirty-two from tuberculosis. His wonderful ode "A reményhez" was set to music by Joseph Kossovits. (On record in Musica Hungarica, Qualiton, 1964.)

The sentiments became more sophisticated but no less intense as the nineteenth century advanced. Strolling in his garden under an autumnal sky in a fine drizzle, on an October day in 1852, the Swiss philosopher Henri Amiel saw the whole of nature reflecting his own "inexorably advancing disease": "Sky draped in gray ... mists trailing on the distant mountains: nature despairing, leaves falling on all sides like the lost illusions of youth under the tears of incurable grief ... The fir tree alone in its vigour remains green and stoical in the midst of this universal phthisis".[17] In the same year Thoreau wrote in his journal (in which he hardly ever mentioned his own disease by name) after seeing the first spotted maple leaves of autumn "with their greenish centre and crimson border": "Decay and disease are often beautiful like the hectic glow of consumption".

There was perhaps a grain of truth in the cynical view that Romantic attitudes and attitudinisings were as much a cause of the disease as its result. Because young men of fashion had developed or professed to have developed a passion for pale young women apparently dying of consumption, young women took to drinking lemon juice and vinegar to kill their appetites and make themselves look more alluring. Even in France for a decade or two the hallmark of a successful Romantic dinner was the apparent indifference of the participants to the food and drink on offer. The fashion was neither new nor did it last longer than such fashions generally do. In 1583 Montaigne had recorded with resigned horror that young women swallowed sand in order to ruin their stomach linings and acquire a pallid complexion. By 1840 Théophile Gautier lamented that "when I was young I could not have been accepted as a poet weighing more than ninety-nine pounds. Now that I have become thin, all men of genius must be fat".[18] Perhaps, while the fashion lasted, it contributed its small share to genuine consumption, just as the eating disorders of today can lead or predispose to life-threatening physical illnesses.

Fashions in dress reflected the trend. By 1800 the boisterous females of the Revolution dancing the carmagnole in the vivid colours of the tricolour had become languishing damsels dressed in vaporous white. Some doctors

---

[17] So he wrote in his famous *Journal intime* (translated into English by Mrs Humphrey Ward in 1885). It proved to be an overpessimistic forecast. Some years later he became professor of moral philosophy in Geneva and died in 1881, aged sixty.

[18] There was, according to Chateaubriand, a similar change of fashion in London. "When I came here in 1822", he wrote twenty years later, "the man of fashion had to present the appearance of an unhappy and sick man. Today it is different. His health must be perfect and his spirits overflowing." The Romantic image of tuberculosis in France is discussed in two books by L. Maigron: *Le Romanticisme et les moeurs* (Paris, 1910), and *Le Romanticisme et la mode* (Paris, 1910).

claimed that the wearing of such unsuitable attire in winter contributed to the vicious influenza epidemic of 1803 – *mal de mousseline* Dr Jules Potain was to call it – which in turn may have lowered patients' resistance to phthisis.

By the mid nineteenth century tuberculosis had pervaded literature even in far-off China. In *The Dream of the Red Chamber,* said to be the first realistic novel in the Chinese language, it is the symptoms of tuberculosis which symbolise the emotional crisis of the heroine, Black Jade.[19] In Europe tuberculosis became the natural manner in which to dispose of youthful lovers and characters without the horrors of disfigurement or character-destroying physical pain. In *The Bride of the Village* Washington Irving could let his young heroine pass away in slow and hopeless, but physically almost imperceptible, decline at the thought of her lover's unfaithfulness. In *David Copperfield* Dickens could allow Little Blossom to die gracefully almost without symptoms. If this was unrealistic, in *Nicholas Nickleby* he also drew what was perhaps the most truthful as well as the most stirring pen-portrait of the illness as it appeared to his contemporaries:

> There is a dread disease which so prepares its victim, as it were, for death; which so refines it of grosser aspects, and throws around it unearthly indications of the coming change – a dread disease in which the struggle between soul and body is so gradual, quiet and solemn, and the result so sure, that day by day and grain by grain the mortal part wastes and withers away, so that the spirit grows light and sanguine with its lightening load, and, feeling mortality at hand, deems it but a new term of mortal life; a disease in which death and life are so strangely blended that death takes the hue of life and life the gaunt and grisly form of death; a disease which medicine never cured, wealth never warded off or poverty could boast exemption from; which sometimes moves in giant strides and sometimes at a tardy sluggish pace, but, slow or quick, is ever sure and certain.[20]

Not surprisingly perhaps, writers surrounded by tuberculosis, tuberculous themselves or both made ample use of the disease in their plots. In *Wuthering Heights* several of Emily Brontë's characters die of consumption. When one of them, Frances Earnshaw, first appears in the book at the funeral of her husband's father, everything seems to delight her except the presence of the mourners. The mere sight of black triggers in her a strong emotional response.

> She felt so afraid of dying! But I imagined her as little likely to die as myself. She was rather thin but young and fresh-complexioned and her eyes sparkled as

---

[19] Tsao (Hsueh-Chin) began writing his novel in 1754. He died in 1763 having completed some eighty chapters and the general outline of the story. The book was completed by others after his death.

[20] Dickens, C., *Nicholas Nickleby* (London, 1838–39), chapter 6.

bright as diamonds. I did remark ... that mounting the stairs made her breathe very quick, that the least sudden noise set her all a quiver and that she coughed troublesomely sometimes; but I knew nothing of what these symptoms portended and had no impulse to sympathise with her.[21]

In June, after Frances has given birth to a boy, the doctor recognises the symptoms of consumption and thinks that she will die before the winter. A few days later, as she is telling her husband about her plans to get up the next day, she is seized by a small fit of coughing. He raises her in his arms and she puts her hands around his neck. Her face changes and she is dead.

The Goncourts in mid century Paris prided themselves on their unflinching realism and made a determined effort to get to grips with consumption as it really was. They spent some time at the Hôpital de la Charité to obtain material for their novel, *Soeur Philomène*, and saw their first death there, that of a "thirty-year-old phthisic, his mouth wide open as that of a man who had expired while trying to breathe but finding no air". A few days later they witnessed an older man "with bony and emaciated face and sunken eyes ... shaking like an old dead tree blown in the winter wind, begging for admission with a soft extinguished slow and humble voice". Unable to admit him and turning him out into the snow, the intern explained a little apologetically: "If we accepted phthisics ... we would not have any room left for other patients". When the brothers transformed their real – if limited – experience of the disease into literature even they romanticised it: Mme Gervaises's death became in *Renée Mauperin* a "strange and exciting seduction ... almost seraphic ... her progressive disembodiment carrying her ever more towards the saintly folly ..." It was but a step from here to generalising:

In contrast to the diseases of crude and baser kind which clog and soil the mind, the imagination and the humours of the sick, phthisis is an illness of the lofty and noble parts: it calls forth a state of elevation, tenderness and love, a new urge to see the good, the beautiful and the ideal in everything, a state of sublimity which seems almost not to be of this earth.[22]

On the other side of the Atlantic Edgar Allan Poe too revelled in "the terrible beauty of consumption". One evening in January 1842 he and his child-wife, Virginia, gave a party at their Fordham cottage. Dressed in white, "delicately, morbidly angelic", Virginia was singing and playing the harp in the glow of the lamplight. "Suddenly she stopped, clutched her throat and a wave of crimson blood ran down her breast ... It rendered her even more

---

[21] Brontë, Emily, *Wuthering Heights* (London, 1847), chapter 3.
[22] Goncourt, E. L. de and J. A. de, *Renée Mauperin* (Paris, 1864), chapter 13.

ethereal!" [23] Later, fascinated, he watched Fanny Osgood "dying of a cough by inches and there are not many inches left".

To some the disease gave a moment of Romantic fame which otherwise might have eluded them. Mrs Davidson of Plattsburg was a poetess and a consumptive. Her two daughters, Lucretia and Margaret, published poetry which was acclaimed both in America and in England. Lucretia wrote in a darkened room to the music of an Aeolian harp strange and wild poems about the Near East; Margaret composed on western themes. Both young women died of tuberculosis before they were twenty. Poe, Washington Irving and the Poet Laureate, Robert Southey, wrote of them as embodiments of poetic fire, their consumptive death a fitting climax to their genius.[24]

Tuberculosis was everywhere; but in one country it was more deeply embedded than anywhere else. Bohemia, a land of the mind, spirit and imagination (not the Czech Republic), has disappeared and still awaits its inspired historian; but, while it lasted, it was far more than what the current usage of the term Bohemian might suggest. It was born in the late 1820s in Paris on the Left Bank of the Seine; it could not have been born anywhere else at any other time. The France of the Bourbon Restoration had been bled white by the Revolutionary and Napoleonic wars. What remained were the unfit and the disillusioned, together with a section of the small bourgeoisie – mean, crafty, prudent, dull, moral, small-minded and ugly – who had not merely survived but had also profited from the political and economic catastrophes. By the time Louis-Philippe, Daumier's pear-faced king, supplanted the legitimate but addled Charles X on the throne,[25] they were the backbone of society, a class to which anything that smacked of unorthodoxy, let alone genuine creativity, was anathema. As the first crop of young men who had escaped the wastes of Russia and the killing fields of Leipzig and Waterloo reached manhood they faced a stark choice: they could conform to the precepts of their timorous but vengeful elders or they would be treated as outlaws.

The young Bohemians whom Henri Mürger was soon to portray with tearful gaiety were not of course criminals. They were poor, laughter-loving, irreverent, at times heroic, more often merely silly, always disorderly, sentimental, generous, careless of the law, inconsiderate of landlords and contemptuous of the stultifying virtues of the bourgeoisie. They were also,

[23] Poe married his cousin, Virginia Clemm, when she was fourteen (after making a false statement about her age) in 1836. She died at their cottage in Fordham near New York City ten years later.

[24] Dubos, R. and J., *The White Plague: Tuberculosis, Man and Society* (London, 1953), p. 204.

[25] After the July Revolution of 1830 immortalised by Delacroix.

as they flit across Mürger's pages, riddled with tuberculosis. The book, which the author later turned into a more successful but inferior play,[26] is now known mainly through Puccini's magical opera; and in the opera it is Mimi whose hands are frozen, whose terrible cough becomes so hard to bear, and who in the last scene dies in her lover's arms. In the book she is only one of many of the grisettes and midinettes whose lives intertwine with the lives of the Bohemians. Francine, another of Mürger's consumptive heroines, is, like Mimi, "pale like the angel of phthisis". When told of her disease and warned that she may die with the falling leaves she laughs. "Why should the falling leaves worry us? Let us spend our lives among pine trees whose leaves are always green." Autumn arrives and when weakness compels her to stay in bed in October her lover places a curtain over her window to hide the plane tree in the courtyard which is slowly losing its leaves. One day in November "a sharp wind opened the window and blew a yellow leaf torn from the tree. She hid it under her pillow. Then she quietly went to sleep from which she never awoke". The last of Mürger's victims was Mürger himself: he began to cough in his late twenties and soon he wrote to a friend: "Do you remember Schaunard, the musician, presenting himself to a prospective patron – I can't for my life remember his name – and telling the fat bourgeois that one of his lungs was gone? Of course it was a fib to arouse the patron's compassion. Well, I'm like Schaunard now, except it's not a fib and it's not one of my lungs which is gone but both." He died after a convivial evening with friends, aged thirty-eight.[27]

To the bourgeois of Mürger's generation the Bohemians were an ineffectual and transient nuisance, the noisy but fragile flower – or weed – of a post-catastrophe decade (like the flappers would be in the 1920s and the teddy boys in the early 1950s). But the bourgeois were wrong. Paris's infant Bohemia soon lost its innocence but it did not die. Distant outposts, each with its local character but sharing basic spiritual allegiances and sustaining hatreds, sprang up in Berlin, Munich, Vienna, Budapest, Copenhagen, Oslo, Odessa and Moscow. The split in society widened. On one side, the big battalions of the bourgeoisie went from strength to strength, firmly keeping their grip on the moneybags. On the other, Bohemia became not only more vicious but also tougher: soaked in absinthe and riddled with syphilis and tuberculosis, the life expectancy of her guerilla forces frighteningly short, but for nearly three generations much of what was new and important in the creative

---

[26] A little confusingly Mürger's original short stories were collected and published under the title *Scènes de la Bohème* (but called *Vie de Bohème* in the English translation), the play was called *La vie de Bohème* and Puccini's opera *La Bohème*.
[27] In 1861.

arts and literature was born in a territory occupied by them. It was into this country that Edvard Munch of Oslo (then still called Christiania), the sprig of a God-fearing middle-class family, plunged, first in his native city, then in Paris and finally in Berlin, the most depraved and the most brilliant of the Bohemias. His images of tuberculosis are haunting, not only *The Sick Girl* but also *Spring*, painted a few years later but more traditional in style and no less deeply felt.[28]

Munch was not the only Scandinavian obsessed with disease and death. By the turn of the century, tuberculosis was slowly retreating in most of western Europe, but it was still nearing its peak in northern Europe, one reason perhaps why it was northern artists who most memorably portrayed it. In Norway Christian Krogh, Munch's teacher, painted his tuberculous sister more than once, as did Hans Heyderdahl; in Sweden it was Ernst Josephson and in Denmark Michael Archer. The most harrowing and perhaps the most truthful representation of the illness in its final stage was the work of another Dane, Ejnar Nielsen.

Nielsen was a penniless student when he painted his masterpiece;[29] and most of the other artists were Bohemians in their youth, some never achieving the fame and affluence that in old age came to Nielsen and Munch.[30] But Bohemia eventually took its revenge. On 28 June 1914 it was two shots fired by a consumptive Bosnian student – the archetypal Bohemian – which brought the self-confident and seemingly indestructible bourgeois world crashing down.[31] Neither the bourgeois world nor Bohemia ever recovered.

London had a café society and Europe's toughest and most populous criminal underworld rather than a Bohemia – but for a few decades it had the Pre-Raphaelite Brotherhood. Elizabeth Siddal, who married Dante Gabriel Rossetti shortly before her death, was a pale, fragile beauty with abundant

---

[28] "My whole art", he later said, "was rooted in the contemplation of disease: without fear and illness my life would have been without a rudder." He painted *The Sick Girl* eight years after Sophie's death from memory. The mother had died (also from tuberculosis) some years before Sophie. See Hodin, J. P., *Munch* (London, 1977).

[29] In 1896 as a first-year student at the Academy of Fine Arts in Copenhagen.

[30] Nielsen was eighty-four when he died in 1954 and Munch seventy-nine when he died in 1944.

[31] Gavrilo Princip was born in Objaj in Bosnia in 1894 and studied in Belgrade. He was known to be tuberculous for some years before he became a member of a small band of patriotic Serb students resolved to assassinate a high-ranking Austrian official or member of the imperial family. He was arrested immediately after he shot Archduke Franz Ferdinand and his wife and sentenced to twenty years in prison, the maximum sentence allowed for those under twenty. He developed overt tuberculosis of the right elbow in prison and had his arm amputated. He died in the prison hospital a few days after the operation, two months before the collapse of Austria-Hungary in 1918.

red hair, the perfect model for the group.[32] Most famously she posed for John Everett Millais' *Ophelia* in a splendid old brocade dress with silver embroidery, drowning – for an hour at a time – in a bath filled with tepid water, not even protesting when the heating arrangement broke down.[33] Sad and quiet, perhaps she was composing in her mind one of her sentimental poems about tombstones and weeping willows. She had probably developed tuberculosis as a young girl: she was sickly throughout her short life. Her illness was never adequately diagnosed: curvature of the spine, pulmonary phthisis and "mental power long pent up and lately overtaxed" were the verdicts of three different doctors. Ruskin, who was fond of her, helped her financially to go in search of a cure first to the south of France and then to Algiers. It was of no avail: her health continued to deteriorate and her mood to darken. An overdose of laudanum, whether taken by accident or with suicidal intent, at last provided an escape.

Soon the Brotherhood grew rich, healthy, respectable and artistically even more deplorable than before; but others took up the tuberculous torch and brush. Kathleen Newton was the mistress of James Tissot, one of the most gifted chroniclers of the late Victorian social scene; and she enacted in her short life all the radiance and doom of the consumptive demimondaine. A convent-educated Irish beauty, she was born Kathleen Irene Ashburton Kelly, genteel but penniless. At the age of seventeen she was sent to India to marry Isaac Newton, a surgeon in the Indian Civil Service.[34] On board the *Empress of India* she was seduced by an Indian Army officer, a Captain Palliser, a *faux pas* which she confessed to Newton on their wedding night. Newton instantly shipped her back to England, instituting divorce proceedings at the same time. The action was undefended and the marriage was dissolved on the day she gave gave birth to Palliser's daughter.[35] In 1872 she met Tissot, who installed her in a stuccoed Italianate villa in St John's Wood near his own house. A year later she gave birth to his son. This was more or less as social conventions prescribed and it could have worked (as it did for many

[32] She was born in 1829 into a respectable lower middle-class family and worked in a milliner's shop in Leicester Square when she was discovered by the Brotherhood. She soon became Rossetti's exclusive possession and dominated his life and art until her death in 1862. See Doughty, O., *Dante Gabriel Rosetti: Victorian Romantic* (New Haven, 1919); Gaunt, W., *The Preraphaelite Tragedy* (London, 1943); March, J., *The Pre-Raphaelite Sisterhood* (London, 1985); Tate Gallery, *The Pre-Raphaelites*, exhibition catalogue (London, 1984).

[33] Her father threatened to take Millais to court to recover Lizzie's medical expenses (including two weeks' convalescence in Hastings). As befitted a future Baronet and President of the Royal Academy, John Everett Millais paid up without a murmur.

[34] Kathleen herself was the daughter of an Indian army officer. Nothing is known about the further career of the seducer. See Wood, C., *Tissot* (London, 1984).

[35] Violet by name: she later became a governess in Golders Green.

other fashionable Victorian and Edwardian artists) but for two unexpected developments. Soon after her move Kathleen began to cough, her illness making her (if Tissot's paintings of her are a true record and they surely are) more ethereally beautiful than ever; and Tissot fell deeply in love with her. He made her move into his own house; and the curious household of a French painter, an Irish divorcée and two illegitimate children put him beyond the pale. (To keep a mistress and her illegitimate offspring in a villa in St John's Wood was one thing; to live with her and flaunt the liaison in painting after painting was another. That the paintings were his best, and some of the best painted in England at the time, mattered not at all.) As happened to so many late Victorian mistresses living in the hothouse atmosphere of café society, she became melancholic and neurotic, especially when her illness began to destroy her; and he became tormented, impotently watching her slow but inexorable decline. Her death in 1879 also shattered his talent: he returned to France to devote the rest of his life to barely mediocre (though profitable) religious painting.[36]

Aubrey Beardsley was only seven at the time but already astonishing his teachers with his precocious skill at drawing and his knowledge of the classics. Twelve years later, after an unsettled childhood,[37] he shocked London society with his brilliantly erotic sketches but also realised that his lungs were "touched".[38] One of the few genuine prodigies in the history of the visual arts,[39] he became art editor of *The Yellow Book* at twenty-one and then editor of the *Savoy*. In his drawings he progressed as his health deteriorated from the still vaguely Pre-Raphaelite illustrations to *Morte d'Arthur* to the inimitably elegant series illustrating the *Rape of the Lock*, Wilde's *Salome* and *Mademoiselle de Maupin*. Until the day before he died in Menton on the Riviera at twenty-six he was working on the series of Volpone 3. He knew that he was dying and at times he was very frightened. A few great artists have been drawn on their deathbed by friends. Beardsley alone drew himself – as Pierrot (see frontispiece). The sheet shows the clown falling into his last sleep as dawn breaks. "Then, upon tip-toe, silently up the stairs, came the comedians Arlechino, Pantaleone, il Dottore and Columbina. With much

[36] He died in 1902 aged sixty-six.

[37] He had a precariously middle-class upbringing and education in various private establishments paid for by relatively affluent relatives. His father was a gambler and an alcoholic. See Weintraub, S., *Aubrey Beardsley: Imp of the Perverse* (Philadelphia, 1997).

[38] "Even his lungs are affected", Wilde is said to have quipped when Beardsley's tuberculosis became known; but it seems too cruel a joke for Oscar.

[39] Among Beardsley's near-contemporaries in England there was only Millais, who started brilliantly in his early teens but ended up a baronet, a millionaire and the painter of *Bubbles*, one of the sad losses of English art.

love they carried away upon their shoulders the white frocked boy of Bergamo whither we know not." A few weeks later he drew what could have been his own valediction, a wonderful illustration to Catullus's farewell to his brother, "Ave atque Vale".

Did Beardsley serve as a model for Shaw's Louis Dubedat in *The Doctor's Dilemma*? Shaw never said so; but the play captures the Edwardian artistic as well as the medical scene.[40] Both were dominated by tuberculosis, the illness from which the angelically handsome and plausible but amoral hero, the young artist Dubedat, is dying in the play. Around him are gathered a gallery of medical luminaries, caricatures but so real that they are instantly recognisable even today. There is Sir Ralph Bloomfield Bonnington, royal physician, ornament of the profession, full of optimism, compassion, reassurance, "his speech a perpetual anthem": also deeply ignorant and deeply ignorant of his own ignorance. There is Sir Patrick Cullen, a grumpy grand old man of the profession who has heard it all before and thinks little of new-fangled theories but is strong on common sense. There is Mr Cutler Walpole, the successful surgeon, convinced that all ill-health is the result of blood poisoning and that all blood-poisoning is caused by the nuciform sac, a useless but profitable anatomical appendage which he has discovered himself and which he specialises in removing. There is Dr "Loony" Schutzmacher, a fashionable and successful general practitioner, whose secret of success has been his motto: "cure guaranteed". There is his counterpart, poor old Blenkinsop, a down-at-heals doctor to the poor and himself tuberculous. There is Sir Colenso Ridgeon, a scientific whiz-kid and head of laboratory on his way to discovering the cure for tuberculosis, whose dilemma it is to choose between saving a divinely gifted scoundrel or a worthy but dim colleague. All are eclipsed by the tuberculous artist himself, dying but still putting the assembled company of medical eminences to shame for their hypocrisy and religiosity with an ease that shows Shaw at his disputatious best. If the death scenes of Mimi, Violetta and the Duke of Reichstadt are moving for sentiments beautifully expressed, Dubedat's is no less so for the sheer defiance of his last great speech and Bohemian creed – and for its truth:

> I'm perfectly happy. I'm not in pain. I've escaped from myself. I'm in heaven, immortal in the heart of my beautiful Jennifer ... I know that in an accidental sort of way, struggling through the unreal part of my life, I haven't always been able to live up to my ideal. But in my own real world I have never done anything wrong, never been untrue to my faith, never been untrue to myself. I've been threatened and blackmailed and insulted and starved. But I've ... fought the good

---

[40] It was first produced in 1905.

fight. And now its all over there is an an indescribable peace. I believe in Michael
Angelo, Velasquez and Rembrandt; in the might of design; in the mystery of
colour; in the redemption of all things by Beauty everlasting, and the message
of Art that has made these hands blessed. Amen.[41]

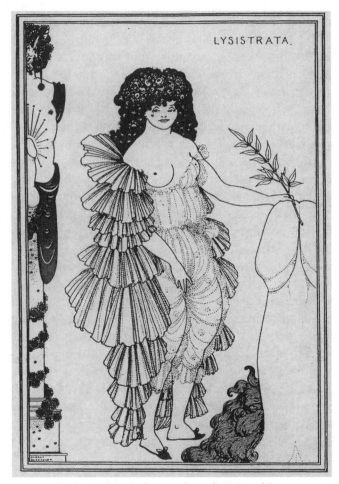

Lysistrata (1897), drawing by Aubrey Beardsley.

[41] Shaw, G. B., *The Doctor's Dilemma* (London, 1905), Act 4.

9

Staying at Home

The Reverend Patrick Brontë was born on Saint Patrick's Day in 1777 into a poor farming family in County Down, Ireland. It must have taken great tenacity against the odds to take him to Cambridge. He was ordained and became a curate in 1798. In 1812 he married Maria Branwell of Penzance in Cornwall. During the following seven years they had six children.[1] Mrs Brontë's health was already failing when the family moved to Haworth on the edge of the Yorkshire moors, where her husband had been offered a living. She died the following year, 1821, aged thirty-eight, of some vague ailment diagnosed as "internal cancer".

There is much that is obscure about the personality of Patrick Brontë. His rise from a poor farming background is testimony enough that he did not lack ability or an enterprising spirit. Mrs Gaskell thought well of him, though he does not emerge as a wholly credible character from her biography of Charlotte.[2] In Haworth he kept himself and his family aloof from the village folk, as if the humble social setting of the parish did not satisfy some never-revealed ambition. He professed and practised extreme austerity, believing, it seems, that his children should be brought up simply and hardily. There were no carpets in the parsonage (except in the parlour), despite the cold and damp of the stone floors and stairs: hardly any meat was served at the table; and the wearing of fanciful silk dresses "that might lead to vanity" was forbidden. Yet he was not without a certain vanity himself: at least his change of the family name from the Irish-sounding Brunty to Brontë suggests it; and he could on occasion present a front of great charm and even brilliance. Even in the hottest weather he wore an enormous white cravat to protect his throat, as he suffered from bronchitis. He took most of his meals alone because he also had digestive troubles; and he liked to go on long and

---

[1] None of the large Brontë literature dealing with single members of the family or the family as a whole has eclipsed Mrs Gaskell's *The Life of Charlotte Brontë*, ed. A. Shelston (London, 1975); but J. Barker's *The Brontës: A Life in Letters* (London, 1997), following on her massive family biography, *The Brontës* (London, 1994), is unlikely to be superseded for a long time.

[2] This is not perhaps altogether surprising since it was Patrick Brontë who commissioned – or at least invited – Mrs Gaskell to write a biography of Charlotte, "long or short ... just as you may deem expedient and proper".

always solitary walks. He doted on his son, Branwell, but took no visible interest in his five daughters: of their literary efforts he learnt only after their books had been published.

In this strange environment the six Brontë children grew up and developed as a close community of their own: they roamed their beloved moors, returning to play fantasy games or read aloud to each other in the tiny room that was allotted to them as their study. When the time came for the older girls to receive a more formal education, Maria, Elizabeth, Charlotte and Emily, aged between seven and eleven at the time, were sent to a semi-charitable boarding school at Cowan's Bridge founded some years earlier for the the daughters of indigent clergy. It was this ghastly institution – as awful in its different way as Dickens's workhouses – which later emerged from Charlotte's memory as Lowood School in *Jane Eyre*. She assured Mrs Gaskell that she had not invented or exaggerated the horrors of the place.

The boarders were always cold and hungry. The food was usually spoilt or burnt, the milk tainted, the supper nothing more than a thin oatcake and a drink of water taken from a common mug by all sharing a table. Some of the staff were clearly sadistic. At night the "pale thin girls slept two in a bed in tightly packed dormitories and during exercise time they went into the low damp garden. They herded together for warmth on the veranda ... and as the dense mist penetrated to their shivering frames I heard frequently the sound of a hollow cough".

During January, a few months after the arrival of the Brontë girls, a terrifying epidemic, referred to in *Jane Eyre* as "typhus", broke out among the pupils. But it does not, from the vivid account Charlotte gave to Mrs Gaskell, sound like typhus. The girls became "dull and unresponsive, heavy to understand remonstrances or to be roused by speech or spiritual exhortation ... sinking away into a dull stupor and half-unconscious listlessness ... All heavy eyed, flushed, indifferent and weary with pains in every limb ... they lay about resting on tables or on the floor". Although some forty girls developed the distemper, only one of them died in the acute phase; but within three months of the epidemic Maria and Elizabeth, twelve and eleven respectively, went into a decline with a persistent cough and loss of weight. They had to be sent home, where they died in the following May and June.

The three remaining girls and Branwell spent most of the next six years at Haworth, apparently happy and beginning to write poetry and fantasies. In 1831 Charlotte was sent as pupil to a girls' school, Roe Head House, and four years later she returned there as a teacher. Emily joined her as a pupil but soon became "literally ill with homesickness". "Every morning", wrote Charlotte, "the vision of home and the moors rushed on her and darkened and saddened her day. Her white face, attenuated form and failing strength threatened rapid decline. I felt in my heart that she would die if she could not go home." Soon after Emily returned to Haworth the youngest surviving sister, Anne, joined Charlotte at Roe Head House; but she too developed a cough with difficulty in breathing and pain in her side. Charlotte remembered the similar symptoms of Maria and Elizabeth and, frightened, took Anne home with her to Haworth.

During the next few years the three sisters left home only on a few occasions and for brief periods, to go school or to work as governesses, always with disastrous results to their health. "Only at Haworth", as Mrs Gaskell was to put it in her biography, "did their souls expand." When away they longed for each other's company and for their brother as much as for the austere beauty and freedom of the countryside. Between 1842 and 1844 Emily and Charlotte spent a year in Brussels – ostensibly learning French with a view of starting a small private school of their own. Nothing came of the plan, except Charlotte's later book *Villette* (her own favourite). Determinedly, at time feverishly, all three pursued their literary ambitions and under various male pseudonyms soon succeeded in having their first works published. But their poetry and novels remained almost unnoticed until the appearance and success of Charlotte's *Jane Eyre.* Emily's *Wuthering Heights* achieved recognition only after her death.

In any case it was Branwell with his poetry and his painting on whom the hopes of the family centred. The sparkle of his conversation was the pride of the local pub and those who met him casually were charmed by his wit. Despite his gifts, his attempts at any occupation ended in failure: during his brief spell as a private tutor he fell in love with the mother of his charges and was sent home in disgrace. He was undoubtedly developing consumption and one reason at least for his addiction to laudanum and alcohol was to relieve his cough and chest pain and the torments of sleepless nights. He never allowed himself to be confined to bed or to be sent away for con-valescence, ending his increasingly dissipated life in the village. Dissipated or not, tuberculosis has always inspired poetry as no other disease. Visiting Haworth churchyard thirty years later Matthew Arnold wrote some memorable lines about Branwell:

> A Brother – sleeps he here? –
> Of all his gifted race
> Not the least-gifted; young
> Unhappy, beautiful; the cause
> Of many hopes, of many tears.
> O Boy, if here though sleep'st, sleep well!
> On thee too did the Muse

Bright in thy cradle smile:
But some dark Shadow came
(I know not what) and interpos'd.[3]

That same dark Shadow (if Arnold meant tuberculosis rather than opium and alcohol) was to strike at Emily next. As the family followed Branwell's coffin to the grave, in September 1848, the sharp autumn wind started her coughing. It was quickly followed by the by now familiar symptoms – painful breathing, hectic fever, almost visible loss of weight. She refused to see a doctor and went about her household tasks with "catching rattling breath and a glazed eye". She died three months after Branwell, aged twenty-nine.

Less than two weeks later Dr Crawner, the local doctor, diagnosed Anne, "gentle ... a very sincere and practical Christian whose tinge of religious melancholy communicated a sad shade to her brief life ...", as suffering from advanced consumption. Full of anxiety, Charlotte sent a detailed account of her symptoms to Dr Forbes, the eminent London physician who twenty years earlier had translated Laënnec's work on auscultation into English. Forbes replied kindly but gave little hope of a cure and endorsed Dr Crawner's prescription of cod-liver oil. In desperation Charlotte took her sister to Scarborough to see if the sea air might help. It did not: four days after their arrival Anne died. She was twenty-seven.

Charlotte returned alone to the ghost-filled parsonage. In her letters – with increasing frequency over the next few years – she mentions her cough, the pain between her shoulders, the frequent bouts of fever, her poor appetite and her troublesome thirst; but she continued to write her novels, including *Villette*. Fame did not overcome her timidity, and though she was now invited into literary circles, she felt unhappy away from Haworth. In 1854 she married Arthur Bell Nicholls, her father's curate, a kindly man though not one to encourage her writing. Soon she was expecting a baby. But early in her pregnancy she developed what seemed like a cold but was quickly diagnosed as consumption, the family disease, and a few months later at the age of thirty-nine she too died.

The Reverend Patrick Brontë survived his wife and six children, struggling on against his bronchitis and digestive ailments till his death in 1866 aged eighty-nine.

---

[3] Arnold, M., "Haworth Churchyard", published in 1855.

10

Seeking the Sun

The Brontës stayed at home; but escape from illness by moving to another place – to almost any other place – is probably as ancient as hope. In 86 BC Cicero fell gravely ill: he was coughing, spitting blood and "became thin like a pole". He was sent on a long sea voyage to Greece and Egypt and returned fully recovered.[1] It was this kind of lore as much as medical evidence which inspired later migrations. And fear. The Black Death of the late middle ages saw the wandering of desperate people from north to south, from south to north, from east to west and from west to east. Only slightly more rational was the exodus of people from cities during later epidemics of plague and cholera. Tuberculosis, an epidemic as devastating as the plague but wholly unlike it, gave the seeking of life under more gentle skies a new meaning.[2]

The pilgrimage of consumptives from northern fog to southern skies had begun long before Keats's doomed voyage to Rome or Shelley's flight to Venice, Florence and eventually Pisa. Among their literary forebears Tobias Smollett (1721–1771), a not notably successful medical practitioner in Edinburgh but one of the creators of the English novel, travelled to France and Italy in search of his vanished health and wrote one of the most tetchy, xenophobic and delightful travel journals of his age.[3] He and his wife spent altogether a year and a half in Nice in 1763 and found a small English-speaking consumptive colony already established there. (Most, he discovered, had originally set out to consult the famous Professor Fizès of the University of Montpellier; and, for what Smollett regarded as an outrageous fee payable in advance, all had received exactly the same elaborate written prescription and the advice to seek better health in Nice.) Nice itself had a population of about 12,000 at the time and was "nothing to write home about"; but the countryside around it was "most pleasing, resembling a garden with fruit and olive trees and every kind of flower but especially carnations".[4] The only feature the travellers missed was bird-song: "scarce a sparrow, redbreast or

---

[1] Schuckburgh, E. C, introduction to *Cicero's Letters* (London, 1900), p. 8.
[2] R. L. Stevenson's phrase.
[3] Smollett, T., *Travels Through France and Italy*, ed. F. Felsenstein (Oxford, 1979), p. 192.
[4] Ibid., p. 212.

tomtit can escape the guns and snares of these indefatigable and greedy fowlers".[5]

Smollett's health was not improved by his travels. "I am returned to England", he wrote to John Hunter, "after an absence of two years ... I have brought back no more than the skeleton of what I was, but with proper care that skeleton may hang together for some years yet."[6] It did, for another six. He went to Scotland and then to Bath where "I must have lapsed into some 'coma vigil' and expected to die".[7] But he recovered and left England again for Italy. His last home, where he "rusticated on the side of a mountain overlooking the sea", was a villa on the slopes of Monte Nero near Livorno (Leghorn). It was there, slowly fading away, too weak to walk, that he wrote *Humphrey Clinker*, to Hazlitt "the most pleasant gossiping novel that was ever written".[8]

Seventy years later, in 1838, Frédéric Chopin (1810–1849) travelled to Majorca accompanied by George Sand in search of the sun. He had been delicate since his teens: it was at Bad Reinerz, a Silesian spa where he had been sent to recover from a "cold in the chest" at the age of sixteen, that he gave his first solo recital.[9] He carried with him the memory of his older sister, Emilia, who died from galloping phthisis after repeated blood-lettings, purges and cuppings. They had undoubtedly hastened her end; he would never allow his doctors to perform any of these cruelties on himself. He was not aware of the seriousness of his own illness until after his arrival in Paris in the autumn of 1831: nor, it seems, was anybody else. A year earlier, during his stay in Vienna, he was a frequent visitor in the house of the court physician, Malfatti,[10] and there is no mention in Malfatti's correspondence that their divinely gifted and yet charmingly modest guest was ailing. Even in Paris his worries about his cough and occasional feelings of faintness were pushed into the background by his success in the world, and a ceaseless flow of musical inspiration. He was admired as a pianist and as a composer, and

[5] Quoted by Spillane, J., *Medical Travellers* (Oxford, 1984), p. 126. A hundred and seventy years later D. H. Lawrence, on the Riviera on the same hopeless quest as Smollett, made the same comment.

[6] Ibid., p. 128.

[7] Ibid., p. 129.

[8] Ibid., p. 134.

[9] He was born in Zelazowa Wola near Warsaw, the son of a French father (who migrated to Poland under Napoleon) and a Polish mother. He always regarded himself as a Pole. A. Zamoyski's biography, *Chopin* (London, 1979), is both sympathetic and informative. Medical aspects of Chopin's illness are discussed by E. R. Long in *A History of the Therapy of Tuberculosis: Chopin's Illness* (Kansas, 1956).

[10] Who had attended not only the Duke of Reichstadt and other Austrian royalty but also Beethoven.

cherished as a person, by a dazzling circle of artists and musicians – the young Liszt, Berlioz, Mendelssohn, Bellini, Hiller, Delacroix, Heine, the famous cellist Franchomme, a particularly close friend, and the piano-maker Camille Pleyel among them – and patronised and later lionised by fashionable and aristocratic hostesses. His naturally elegant manners, fastidiousness and sensitivity made him a favourite both as a recitalist and as the private teacher to the delicate and highborn. His pupils adored him. He also became to many the epitome of the Romantic artist, pale, almost transparent, but alight with the flame of creative genius. As indeed he was.[11]

The year 1835 was a memorable one for him: there was a brief and happy reunion with his parents in Karlsbad (today's Karlovy Vary) and then a visit to Polish friends, the Wodzinkis, in Dresden. There he fell in love with the sixteen-year-old daughter of the house, Marie, and she with him, but his illness once again surfaced and caused heartbreak. Though attached to the young man, Mme Wodzinska was too worried by his precarious health to allow the marriage plans to proceed. After his return to Paris and the dispatch to Mademoiselle Marie of the waltz, *L'adieu*, the lovers were encouraged to drift apart.

Chopin's illness did not deter the provocative, free-thinking, free-living and free-speaking novelist Aurore Dupin, formerly Mme Dudevant, alias George Sand; nor were his naive moral scruples and dislike of gossip allowed to stand in the way of a liaison.[12] But his hectic life in Paris was proving too much for his fragile frame: after a bad attack of influenza he had several bouts of severe haemoptysis. They jointly consulted the fashionable physician Alphonse Gaubert. Gaubert declared to Aurore that Monsieur Chopin was not "actually tuberculous" but only "extremely delicate" and that he could be saved by "sunshine, rest and loving care".[13]

Their visit to Majorca tested and proved her love but was otherwise a disaster. During their first winter, with the weather wet and cold, Chopin had a succession of "respiratory exacerbations". They called in the three leading physicians of the island, "one more asinine than the other". As Chopin described their visit in letter to his agent in Paris, Julius Fontanal:

[11] Chopin belonged to the first generation of famous artists who were caught (in their last years) by the photographic camera; but it is Delacroix's wonderful portrait of him – though only the severed half of a double portrait of Chopin and George Sand – which seems to catch on canvas not just a likeness but also the creative genius of the greatest tuberculous composer.

[12] She was six years older than him and the liaison as distinct from the friendship probably did not last for longer than a year or two. She had two children from her marriage, Maurice, whose delicate health was one reason for their journey to Majorca, and Solange. Chopin was very fond of both and his feelings were reciprocated. ·

[13] Quoted by Zamoyski, *Chopin*, p. 192. Chopin had been coughing up blood intermittently for several years by then; but (partly following Laënnec's teaching) haemoptysis in France was not regarded as pathognomonic of tuberculosis and certainly not of advanced tuberculosis.

One sniffed at what I spat out, the second tapped where I spit it from, the third poked about and listened how I spat it. One said that I was going to die, the second that I was dying and the third that I was dead ... I can scarcely keep them from bleeding me. All this has affected the Preludes and God knows when you will get them.[14]

Worse than the doctors' ministrations was their gossiping. Their tales, as George Sand was to describe in *Un hiver en Majorque* many years later, stirred up great terror.

Phthisis is scarce in these climates and is regarded as contagious! ... The owner of our small house threw us out immediately and started a suit to compel us to replaster his wretched house which we had contaminated. We then went to take up residence in the uninhabited monastery of Valdemosa ... but could not secure any servants or any help of any kind from the local peasantry, as not even the poorest wretch wants to work for a phthisic ... We begged for a last service, to be given a carriage to take us back to Palma, but even this was refused ... So we had to go three leagues on neglected, deserted side roads in a *birlocho*, that is a wheel-barrow. When we arrived in Palma Chopin had a terrifying haemorrhage. We had to leave at once; but the only boat that would give us room was one transporting pigs to Barcelona. Even there our presence had to kept a secret: so we spent the journey in the the smelly, stifling hold among the cargo.[15]

On the journey Chopin had another bleed, coughing up "basins of blood". In Barcelona, Sand secured the help of the French consul who in turn summoned the ship's doctor of a brig-of-war in the harbour. The doctor managed to stop the bleeding – presumably by rest and plentiful sedatives – "but the inn-keeper later insisted on us paying for the bed which the police had given him orders to burn".[16]

In Marseille, under the gentle care of Dr Cauvières,[17] Chopin's health improved: "I am beginning to play, eat, walk and speak again almost like other men!" [18] But he was far from cured: in the winter of 1839, back in Paris, he still suffered greatly. "Feeble, pale, coughing much [one of his pupils,

---

[14] Chopin, F, *Selected Correspondence*, edited and translated by A. Hedle (London, 1963), p. 98. Chopin had a gentle self-deprecatory wit; but in fairness to the Mallorcan physicians, inspection of the sputum was a recognised medical aid and if the other two were percussing and auscultating his chest they were following up-to-date practice.

[15] Sand, George, *Un hiver en Majorque* (Paris, 1852).

[16] Ibid., p. 196.

[17] Little is known about this physician except that he clearly practised the art of medicine well, if not its science. "This worthy and amiable man", George Sand wrote about him, "the most charming and most devoted friend, is the kind providence occasionally sends to sufferers." He assured Chopin that the composer could by no means be classified as a consumptive with any certainty, certainly not an advanced one.

[18] Chopin, *Selected Correspondence*, p. 185.

Frederike Müller, wrote], he often took drops of opium on sugar and gum water, rubbed his perspiring forehead with *eau de Cologne* – and nevertheless taught with great patience, perseverence and zeal." [19] Fortunately, he could spend the summers of the next six years in Nohant, George Sand's beautiful country estate, about 200 miles south of the capital. He was not temperamentally a country person (unlike Aurore); but he loved the trees and the roses in the park and he wrote some of his loveliest music there – the Fantaisie in F minor, the Polonaise Fantaisie, the Ballades in A flat Major and F minor and the Sonata in F minor among others.[20]

The winters in Paris saw a steady deterioration of his health, aggravated by the annual epidemic of *la grippe* which regularly decimated the city's population.[21] He saw most of the leading physicians of the day, including the pioneer homeopath Mollin: they tended to reassure him in a rather perfunctory way, perhaps realising that his case was hopeless. His personal doctor and boyhood friend, Matuszynski, started to have haemoptyses a year or two after him and died in 1845.[22] Chopin felt the loss keenly. Also, sadly for both Chopin and Sand, their relationship grew strained: both were proud and self-willed and missed more than one chance at a reconciliation. The final rift came in 1848.[23]

Chopin's last two years, fleeing from revolutionary Paris in 1848, as a guest in aristocratic houses in Scotland and feted in London, were a constant struggle against an illness which was sapping the last of his physical strength – though not his inspiration. Some of the last compositions to survive are among his loveliest – but much of what he created during those months was probably never written down. Like many consumptives, he was often too weak to do anything during the day but rallied in the evening; and at small gatherings in Scottish baronial halls or in his rooms in London he would improvise at the piano till dawn, "transporting us to regions none of us had known before and none of us would revisit again". Jane Stirling, one of his

---

[19] Zamoyski, *Chopin*, p. 184.

[20] Dr Gustave Papet, George Sand's friend and physician in Nohant, stated in 1843 that Chopin no longer showed any evidence of pulmonary disease and suffered merely from chronic laryngeal infection.

[21] It continued to do so – skipping a few years now and again – for the best part of a century. Like the London smog, it killed mainly those who were already suffering from heart or lung disease, including many tuberculous.

[22] Another contemporary whom Chopin mourned was the virtuoso violinist Artot. "This boy", Chopin wrote, "so strong and robust, with such broad shoulders … died of consumption. Nobody could have guessed, seeing both of us, that he would die first and also of phthisis." But he did, in 1845.

[23] She survived him by twenty-seven years.

most devoted pupils and friends, wrote later that these were his greatest works.

He was too sensitive to continue indefinitely to accept hospitality which he knew he could not reciprocate;[24] and in 1849 he returned to Paris. There, living on the secret charity of friends, he spent most of his last months in a room in the then quiet suburb of Chaillot. He was seen by some of the leading physicians in the city: Pierre Charles Alexandre Louis, the author of the standard French textbook, *Recherches sur la phthisie*,[25] Blache, a famous paediatrician,[26] and Jean Cruveilhier, professor of pathology and still a revered name in morbid anatomy.[27] They discussed whether or not to send him to rest in the south of France. "Rest?", Chopin whispered, overhearing them, "I'll have plenty of that soon enough." In October he was moved back to the Place Vendôme to be in easy reach of his many friends, both Polish and French.[28] A piano was installed in the room and the Polish beauty, Delphine Potocka, perhaps his one-time mistress, sang for him.[29] He listened and nodded but he could no longer speak. Some biographers have ascribed this to tuberculous laryngitis; but the cause was probably the accumulation of sputum in his larynx which he was too weak to cough up. Now forgotten, it was the commonest terminal event in pulmonary tuberculosis. Before he

[24] He was also haunted by the ghost of another tuberculous composer whom he much admired and who died seeking his fortune in London. Carl Maria von Weber was the already famous creator of two operas, *Der Freischütz* and *Euryanthe*, when in 1824 he accepted an invitation by the Covent Garden Opera House to write and conduct an opera for London. Suffering from advanced tuberculosis, he was strongly advised by his doctor in Dresden not to undertake the arduous journey; but he was a family man and always in financial straits and the London offer was too good to refuse. The new opera, *Oberon*, was much acclaimed and he conducted eleven performances of it, each occasion costing him an almost superhuman effort. In the morning following the eleventh performance he was found dead in his room in a pool of blood. He was thirty-nine. There were no funds to transport his body back to Germany until Wagner raised the cost by public subscription forty years later.

[25] He was a sane and conservative doctor, at loggerheads with the Broussais school of therapy (then at its height) which was letting off untold gallons of blood in most Paris hospitals. For Chopin, Louis prescribed an infusion of moss, syrup of gum and opium.

[26] On the staff of the Hôpital Cochin, he was also acknowledged as an expert on the treatment of tuberculosis. When Chopin was told that he had been called in he remarked: "Good. There has always been something of a child in me."

[27] For more than a hundred years his *Pathological Atlas* remained the most beautifully illustrated medical book on the market; but he was also a practising doctor, physician to Talleyrand and Chateaubriand.

[28] They included his much-loved sister, Ludwika, who arrived from Poland to nurse him, Princess Marcellina Czartoryska, Mme Matuszevska, Solange Clésinger (George Sand's daughter), Franchomme and his faithful servant, Daniel.

[29] She travelled to Paris from Nice where she was nursing her own lungs.

died – in the early hours of 17 October 1849 – he asked for Mozart's *Requiem* to be played at his own requiem.[30]

After George Sand had made Majorca notorious, it was Nice which was to be the goal of the sun-seekers. (Menton or Mentone, a few miles down the coast, caught up with it around the turn of the century.) Here Niccolò Paganini came in 1839 to spend his last winter, shaken by fits of coughing, reduced to a shadow of his former self, his face cadaverous.[31] Although consumptive from early youth, he had lived a life both strenuous and disorderly; his "diabolical feats" on the violin being reputedly matched by his amorous and gambling exploits. During his last years he was so thin that "as he bowed to acknowledge the applause of his audience they feared that that his frame would fall apart in a heap of bones". His voice was also stilled, probably by tuberculosis of the larynx. "Was that a man on the point of death who wishes with his convulsions to delight his audience in the arena of art like a dying gladiator … or a dead man risen from his grave, a vampire with a violin who would suck the blood from our hearts?" Heine asked. On the night before his death, and already completely mute, he played an improvisation from his bed, his double-stopping as heart-stopping as ever, the roundness and beauty of tone of his famous Guarneri undimmed. He did not receive the last rites of the Catholic Church and his body was refused burial in consecrated grounds, despite his son's protestation to the Bishop of Nice. "My father was a devout if grievously sinful believer but, as commonly happens in phthisis, he never thought that his end was approaching." The last statement was probably true and young Paganini's predicament was to trouble many a bereaved family throughout the century.

Less than a year after Paganini's death came the incomparable Rachel "to beg of the Mediterranean sun a last ray of hope". Born Elisa Rachel Felix, the daughter of an itinerant Jewish pedlar, she was uneducated, mean and uniformly unfaithful to her lovers – but she transformed French classical theatre.[32] How far this was calculated art and how far she followed the dictates

[30] He was laid to rest in the Père Lachaise cemetery under soil enriched with a few clods brought from Poland. His funeral march was not played on that occasion; but it *was* played and repeated over and over again for six hours on Radio Warsaw on 23 September 1939, after the announcement that German troops were in possession of most of the city and would soon be entering the radio station. This was signalled by the interruption of the Chopin record, a brief pause, and then the Blue Danube Waltz.

[31] He was born in 1784 and was probably syphilitic as well as tuberculous. See Pulver, J., *Paganini: The Romantic Virtuoso* (London, 1936).

[32] She was born in 1821. James Agate wrote a splendid biography of her, *Rachel* (London, 1928).

of her illness is uncertain; but instead of ringing declamations and loud outbursts of grief or joy she uttered the alexandrines of Racine and Corneille with a hoarse intensity and concentrated passion that kept her audience spellbound. "She stood", Charlotte Brontë wrote about her Medea,

> not dressed but draped in pale antique folds, long, regular and white like alabaster sculpture … or rather like death. Wicked she is, yes. but also strong … disclosing power like a deep swollen winter river thundering in a cataract and bearing the soul like a leaf in the steep and stately sweep of her descent.[33]

In 1855 she had been playing *Les Horaces* with her French troupe in New York when she collapsed and the curtain fell on her prostrate figure. She fainted again a few days later in Philadelphia. Ordered to a milder climate, she appeared in public for the last time in Charleston. Back in Paris she realised that she was now a shadow of her former self: "you who knew her in the brilliance of her splendour would not believe that the gaunt spectre who wearily drags herself over the world is Rachel". In Nice she lingered for only a few weeks and died murmuring verses from Racine and calling for her sister, Rebecca, who had died of tuberculosis a few years earlier.

Only a few hundred yards from where Rachel spent her last weeks the Tsarevitch Nicholas, heir presumptive to the Russian throne and one of several tuberculous Romanovs, lingered a little longer. In 1865 his father, Alexander II, came to listen to his last words and then to order the frigate *Alexander Nevski* to convey his body to be buried in the soil of Holy Russia.

By the mid 1860s steam trains and wagons-lit had made the previously long and hazardous journey to the south of France fast, comfortable and – above all – affordable for people less exalted than stars of the concert hall or the theatre or heirs to imperial thrones; and what had been a trickle became a sad, slow, steady stream. One of those who came, Marie Bashkirchev, had been born in Russia in 1860 but had settled in Paris with her mother to study art. She began in childhood to write a diary which was published after her death first in French and then in English under the title *The Journal of a Young Artist*. Queen Victoria found it "a most affecting little tale" and the stern Mr Gladstone described it as "a book without parallel".[34] Marie loved clothes, society and love itself and yearned for glamour, and although sickly and fragile she had seemingly unbounded energy. At first she wanted to become a singer but tuberculous laryngitis put a stop to that. Instead she became a painter.

---

[33] Dubos, R. and J., *The White Plague* (London, 1953), p. 21.

[34] Bashkirtseva, M. K., *The Journal of a Young Artist*, translated by Mary J. Serrano (New York, 1926). Gladstone himself had lost his much-loved elder sister, Anne, to a long drawn out wasting disease, probably tuberculosis.

There was much tuberculosis in Marie's family and household. Her governess was a sorrowful-looking creature with consumption. Her father was pale, delicate in health and the son of a sickly mother who had died young. She told the doctor who diagnosed her disease that one of her grandfathers, two of his sisters, a great-grandfather and two great-aunts had died of consumption. Coughing, ailing much of the time, often in pain, she was seen by the most eminent physicians of her day; but, suspecting that they were concealing the truth from her, she dressed in her maid's clothes and went to a charity clinic in one of the poor districts of Paris. There she learnt that both her lungs were severely affected. In Nice she enjoyed the beauty of the scenery and consciously added to its poetic charm walking along the Promenade "silent as a white shadow". In the evening she attended the opera, one of the "beautifully dressed and lavishly bejewelled young women but so pale beneath their curls that their faces appeared to be powdered with scrapings of bone".[35] (It seemed to one visitor as if the cemeteries were not closed at night but allowed the dead to escape.) She was twenty-two when she joined the dead, leaving behind not a masterpiece but one of the enduring literary memorials to tuberculosis.

The English by and large continued to prefer Italy to the south of France. The Brownings and Fanny Trollope, Anthony's mother, went to Florence for the sake of consumptive members of their families and became the nucleus of a wide literary circle. They also welcomed Americans, among them the Reverend David Home from Connecticut who had been compelled by tuberculosis to give up the ministry and devoted himself to spiritualism instead. His seances were followed with intense excitement by Elizabeth Browning.

Inevitably the migration spawned a voluminous literature of guidebooks, much in the vein of today's travel guides but concentrating on the vagaries of an ill-understood and unpredictable illness rather than on cuisine, shopping, opera, antiquities, gambling or sex. The most widely read and the most peremptory was Mrs Carleton's *Brief Advice to Travellers to Italy, Addressed to Persons who Travel for the Purpose of Health, Economy or Education*. She warned that, despite its "soft, balmy air", the climate of Palermo was deceptive and "unfavourable to diseased lungs, being of an exciting nature though to a lesser degree than the treacherous breeze of Naples which may be described as positively irritating to the throat". Nice, she felt, was

> agreeable but not always safe as it caused some complaints to shift from one part
> of the body to another ... A person whose system has been too much lowered at
> Rome will recover through a short sojourn in Amalfi, one coming from Switzerland

---

[35] Cahuet, A., *Moussai: ou la vie et mort de Marie Bashkirtseff* (Paris, 1926).

or Germany will find the nervous action let down to the right point in Rome, while those coming from the East Indies ...[36]

The length of time a person should spend in any one place was of the utmost importance. "One who arrives with a good reserve of nervous excitement in Florence may feel well for several years; but then some functions will become torpid, the liver may become clogged and a journey further south may become necessary." [37] Pages and pages of such drivel rise at times to the surrealistic inanities of today's holiday brochures.

Trains and steam-boats also made travel to more distant lands more accessible to many. For a decade or two boat trips around the world were particularly recommended by fashionable physicians in London and Edinburgh; and tours were specially designed to be undertaken in sailing boats to prolong the cure but supported by steam power in case the weather turned inclement.[38] Funerals at sea were not uncommon: a clergyman on board was one of the amenities advertised by the tour operators.

Egypt was another favourite destination – especially recommended by doctors in Germany and Austria. One of those dispatched there was the exasperatingly clever son of rich German Jewish parents, a chemist when his parents would have preferred him to have become a doctor. Paul Ehrlich was ten years younger than Koch who became (replacing more orthodox deities) his god; and he was probably the first person actually to see tubercle bacilli under the microscope – though without realising at the time what the micro-apparition was. What is not in doubt is that he was the first person to diagnose tuberculosis in himself by looking for and finding the organism in his own sputum. According to his diary, his elation – "positively a warm glow" – at this diagnostic triumph quite eclipsed any dismay he might have felt at its implications. Perhaps his optimism was justified (or his diagnostic acumen not quite so sharp as he supposed): after a year in Egypt he returned apparently cured. Apart from becoming the founder of clinical chemistry – his reagents are still used in the laboratory diagnosis of jaundice – he was to discover the arsenical Compound 606, the first effective cure of syphilis and arguably the first usable chemotherapeutic agent.[39]

In terms of time and distance the tuberculous traveller who surpassed

---

[36] Carleton, Mrs, *Brief Advice to Travellers to Italy: Addressed to Persons who Travel for the Purpose of Health, Economy or Education* (London, 1856), p. 68.

[37] Ibid., p. 128.

[38] Some physicians (like Sir Timothy Benninson of Harley Street) suggested that the benign influence of sea travel resided in being seasick and for those who could not afford such a journey he recommended using a swing. Erasmus Darwin had earlier suggested that results "as good as seasickness" could be obtained by the rotary motions of a chair thirty times a day.

[39] He died in 1915, aged sixty-two.

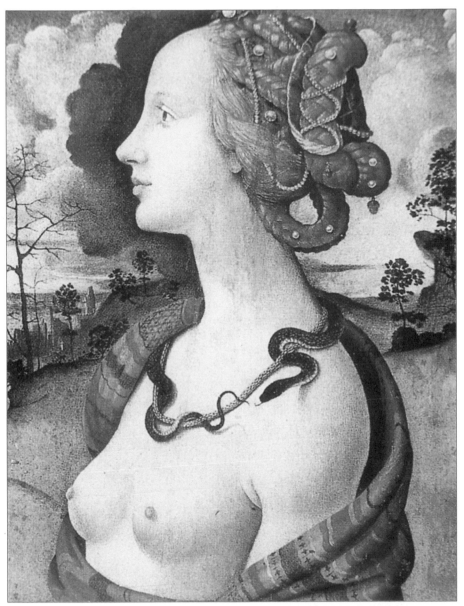

1. Was it tuberculosis which killed Simonetta Vespucci, the model for Botticelli's Venus, at the age of twenty-three? The serpent round her neck represents the disease. Painted by Piero di Cosimo after Simonetta's death.

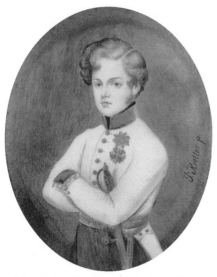

2. The Duke of Reichstadt, in his white Austrian uniform. Miniature by P. Kretter. (*National Gallery, Budapest*)

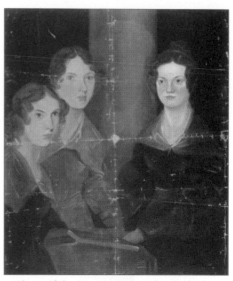

3. Three of the Brontë sisters who died of tuberculosis by Branwell Brontë who himself died of the illness. (*National Portrait Gallery*)

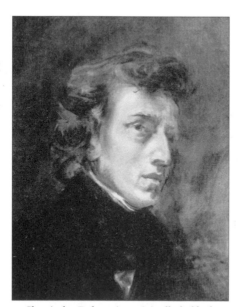

4. Chopin by Delacroix; originally half of a double portrait with George Sand. (*Louvre*)

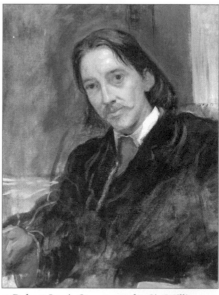

5. Robert Louis Stevenson, by Sir William Blake Richmond, 1885. (*National Portrait Gallery*)

6. *The Sick Child* by Edvard Munch, 1885–86. One of Munch's many paintings and etchings inspired by the memory of his sister Sophie, who died of tuberculosis aged sixteen. (*Tate Gallery, London*)

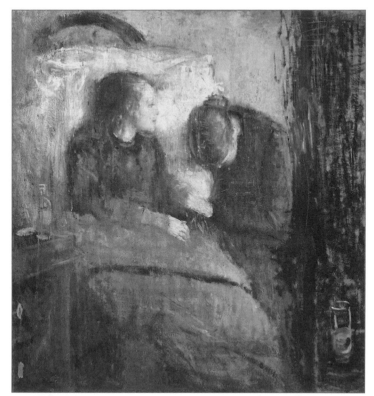

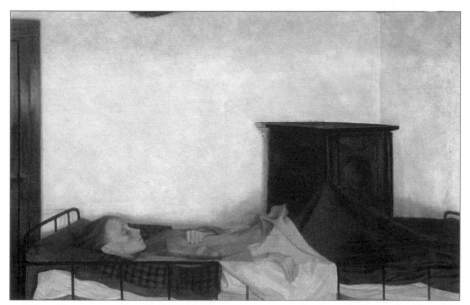

7. *Sick Girl* by Ejnar Nielsen. Nielsen was twenty-four when he painted this masterpiece, the image of a young girl near the end of her illness. (*Statens Museum for Kunst, Copenhagen*)

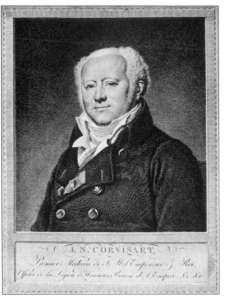

8. Jean Nicholas Corvisart (1755–1820).
Napoleon said "I don't believe in medicine
but I believe in Corvisart".

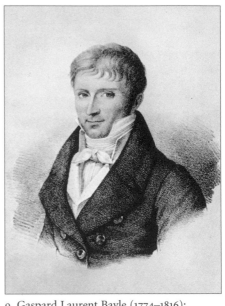

9. Gaspard Laurent Bayle (1774–1816);
pathologist, friend of Laënnec and victim of
tuberculosis.

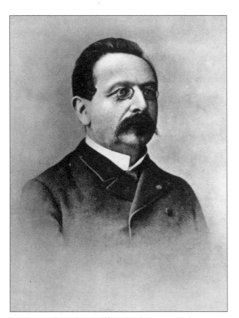

10. Jean-Antoine Villemin (1827–1892),
Koch's grudgingly acknowledged
forerunner.

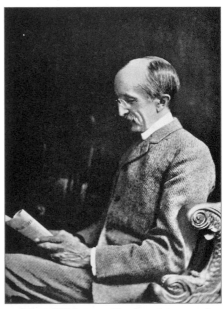

11. Edward Livingston Trudeau (1845–1915),
the founder of Saranac Lake.

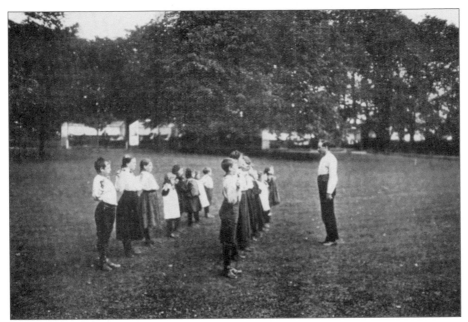

12. Respiratory drill for young patients at the Royal Victoria Hospital, *c.* 1910.

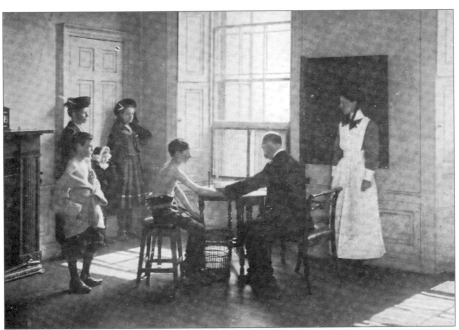

13. "March Past" of the family of a newly diagnosed tuberculous patient, *c.* 1910. Dr Robert Philip's invention, aimed at detecting "early cases" among the patient's contacts.

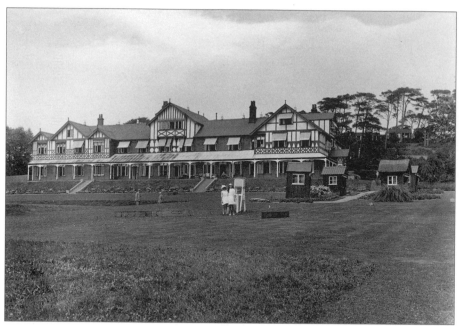

14. Mundesley Sanatorium, Norfolk. The only sanatorium in Britain with its own golf course. (*County Record Office, Norwich*)

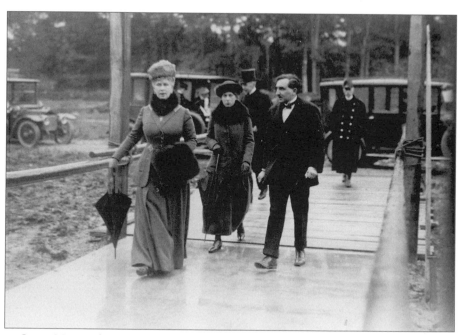

15. Queen Mary and Princess Mary, visiting Papworth Hospital in 1918; accompanied by Dr Pendrill Varrier-Jones, the Medical Director (*County Record Office, Cambridge*)

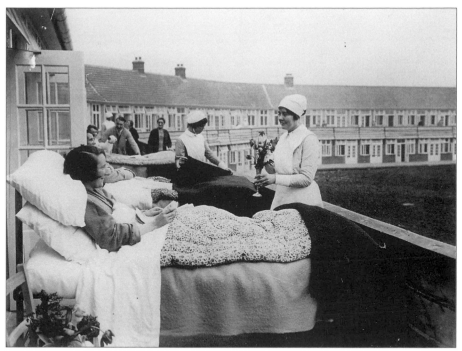

16. On the balcony, Papworth Hospital. (*County Record Office, Cambridge*)

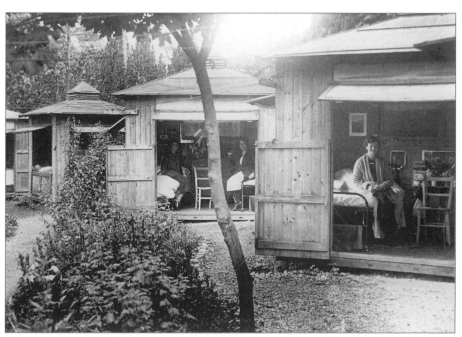

17. Chalets at Papworth Hospital. (*County Record Office, Cambridge*)

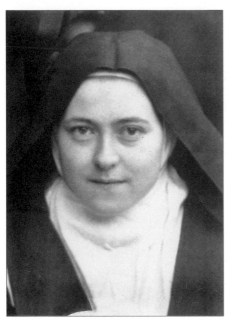

18. St Thérèse of Lisieux (1872–1897).

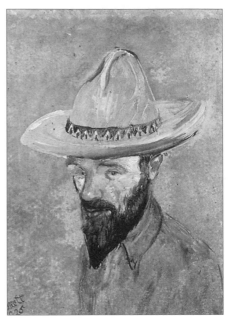

19. D. H. Lawrence (1885–1930). (*National Portrait Gallery*)

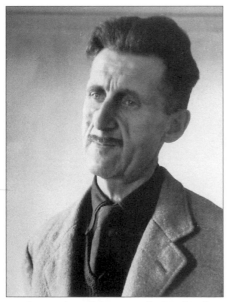

20. George Orwell (1903–1950). (*National Portrait Gallery*)

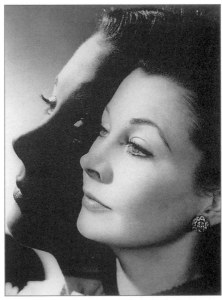

21. Vivien Leigh (1913–1967). Photo by Angus McBean. (*National Portrait Gallery*)

them all was the only son of a Scottish civil engineer and his English wife, Robert Louis Balfour Stevenson. He probably contracted tuberculosis quite young: he was certainly a sickly child whose attendance at Edinburgh Academy and other schools was fitful. He was also a kindly but determined rebel who decided early to devote himself to writing rather than to the family profession of engineering or to the law. By the age of twenty-five his lungs were sufficiently far gone to persuade his parents to send him to the Riviera, the beginning of his life-long travels.

> Crack goes the whip and off we go;
> The trees and houses smaller grow;
> Last, round the woody turn we swing;
> Good-bye, good-bye to everything! [40]

On his many visits to France – the country became almost a second home – he wrote some of his most delightful travel books.[41] He also befriended some of France's best painters,[42] and became a life-long admirer of the still struggling Rodin.[43] In 1876 he met Fanny Vandegrift Osbourne, an American woman separated but not yet divorced from her husband, and the two fell in love. The horror of his parents was only temporarily assuaged when Fanny decided to return to California: soon their son was on his way to join her there.

After a journey that would have taxed even a fit person (and most of the time Stevenson was coughing up blood and suffering from disabling "asthma"), he arrived penniless and in desperate physical straits in California. Fanny had by then obtained a divorce and the two got married. A telegram from Robert's relenting father offered much-needed financial help. They returned to Scotland; and *Treasure Island* (started as a game with his stepson, Lloyd Osbourne) was begun in Pitlochry.

Then Robert's ill-health forced him and his family to leave once again and they spent two spells in Davos in Switzerland and a happy year in Hyères in the south of France. The threat of cholera sent them hurrying back to England; but the climate even of balmy Bournemouth proved too severe. Between or even during bouts of incapacity he finished *Dr Jekyll and Mr Hyde*, *Kidnapped* and the lovely poems of *A Child's Garden of Verses*.

In 1887, still in search of health, he set out for America again, this time

---

[40] Stevenson, R. L., "Farewell to the Fawn", from *A Child's Garden of Verses* (London, 1885). The tuberculosis imagery in these poems was of course unconscious – or possibly prophetic.

[41] Among them *An Inland Voyage* (1878) and *Travels with a Donkey in the Cévennes* (1879).

[42] He was particularly close to the artists working in Barbizon like Millet and Diaz whom he visited regularly.

[43] With W. E. Henley, he was largely responsible for introducing Rodin to England and England to Rodin, probably the sculptor's longest-lasting love affair.

with his wife, mother and stepson. He was now famous and was offered lucrative contracts in New York; but New York was ruinous to his lungs and he took refuge in the Adirondack Mountains. It was at Saranac Lake that he began *The Master of Ballantrae*. But:

> I have a little shadow that goes in and out with me
> And what can be the use of him is more than I can see.[44]

To escape that shadow, after a few months he and the family set sail from San Francisco. They originally planned a short health-giving cruise of the South Seas. It proved to be the last stage of his long wanderings. They toured many of the islands – the Marquesas, the Gilberts, Tahiti, then Hawaii – and he produced some of his most evocative travel pieces. Eventually they settled in Vailimi in Samoa, which he loved and where he felt better than he had felt anywhere for years. "It is like a fairy story that I should have at last recovered liberty and strength and should be able to go round among my fellow men again, boating, riding, bathing, toiling hard with a woodknife in the forest." [45] It could not last: he died in 1894, aged forty-four, probably from a cerebral haemorrhage.

---

[44] Stevenson, R. L., "My Shadow", from *A Child's Garden of Verses*.

[45] Balfour, G., *The Life of Robert Louis Stevenson* (New York, 1915), p. 352. The events are also described in an excellent more recent biography by McLynn, F., *Robert Louis Stevenson* (London, 1993).

11

Going West

As in Europe so in the New World "lungers" living under northern skies looked for milder climates for their salvation. A few who were wealthy and enterprising enough to brave the journey crossed the Atlantic to the Mediterranean; and at least one, Washington Irving, returned not only healthy but also famous. Many more travelled to Florida or to the Caribbean: in 1852 when Franklin Pierce was elected President his new Vice President was in Cuba unsuccessfully trying to cure his consumption and his Secretary of State was in mourning for his son who had just died there. (The President's reclusive and sickly wife, Jane, was also rumoured to be suffering from the disease.)

But for most consumptive Americans salvation lay not to the south but in the west. George Weeks, whose autobiography, *California Copy*, was to inspire tens of thousands, was born in 1851 on a small subsistence farm in New York State.[1] His mother died from tuberculosis when he was five and the rest of his childhood was one of poverty and physical abuse. He eventually found a steady job as a typesetter for the *New York World*, married and had several children; but at the age of twenty-four he began to suffer from "violent and prolonged fits of coughing, pains in his side and profuse night sweats". He consulted the famous Dr Austin Flint who told him bluntly that, if he cared to live for more than another five or six months, he should go west. To avoid the hardships of a transcontinental train ride in winter he booked a passage on a ship to Panama, then crossed the isthmus by train and finally boarded a steamer bound for San Francisco. By the time he set sail his health had deteriorated further and by the time the steamer docked in San Francisco, several months later, he had barely strength to visit a booking agency and arrange lodging for himself on a ranch in a sparsely settled region in the San Bernardino Mountains. Although utterly exhausted on the final leg of his journey – he had had to go to Los Angeles first and then travel on a dilapidated stagecoach for four days – the first sights and smells of the orchards which lined the end of the road convinced him that he had entered Paradise. "The perfumed life-laden air was so grateful to my weakened lungs,

[1] Weeks, G., *California Copy* (Washington, 1928).

rasped and worn by the harsh winds of the Atlantic coast and the unsanitary atmosphere of the composing room that there was no opportunity for weariness."

Within a month Weeks was strong enough to begin exploring the region; and on one excursion he met a rancher and beekeeper who needed an assistant. He became a "choreman", collecting honey, and "commenced [his] outdoor life under health giving conditions". After a few months and a steady gain in strength, he secured a claim to an abandoned vineyard, planted more vines and started to cultivate bees himself. Soon he had accumulated enough health and wealth to send for his family. Many years later he accidentally met a Mr Van Tassell who had been a fellow passenger on the boat which had taken him to California. Apparently Weeks had then looked so ill that his fellow passengers had placed bets on whether he would just about survive the journey or die at sea. When he realised that the giant of a man bursting with vigour was the same Weeks he had known on board ship, Van Tassell was incredulous. "'How did you do it?', Van Tassell asked to which I replied 'That's easy. Life in the open air, hard work, plain food and plenty of sleep.'"

Just how many health-seekers like Weeks found a cure in the west will never be known. As usual with shrines and health resorts, the narratives of successes were so dramatic that they eclipsed the failures; and by the 1880s the migration of the sick began to rival that of those who came to seek their fortune. Many came for both and some even found them: "They came to cough", as the saying went, "and stayed to spray." [2]

It was a masculine world and a masculine myth but women came too. Catherine Haun, originally from Boston, recalled many years later her journey in 1849 as one of a female caravan of covered wagons:

> My health was not good: I was at the end of my strength. My four sisters had already died of consumption and I had reason to be apprehensive on that score. The physician advised an entire change of climate [and] finally approved of our contemplated trip across the plains in a "prairie scooter" ... In my case as in

---

[2] S. M. Rothman, *Living in the Shadow of Death* (Baltimore, Maryland, 1995), gives an excellent account of the migration. While practically every state west of the Mississippi had communities founded and developed by health-seekers, Colorado, Southern California, Texas, New Mexico and Arizona, all situated on the dry and arid plateau of the south west, received the largest influx. More than half of the residents of Pasadena (California), Silver City, Colorado Springs and Denver (Colorado), El Paso (Texas), Albuquerque (New Mexico) and Tucson (Arizona) reported in a 1913 health survey that they or one of their parents or grandparents had migrated there for health reasons. Other works covering the migration of both people and of diseases like tuberculosis include Bailyn, B., *Voyages to the West: A Passage in the Peopling of America on the Eve of the Revolution* (New York, 1986); Baur, J. E., *Health-Seekers of Southern California, 1870–1900* (San Marino, California, 1959); Long, E. R., "Weak Lungs on the Santa Fe Trail", *Bulletin of the History of Medicine*, 8 (1940), 1041.

that of many others, my health was restored long before the end of the journey. Had I stayed I would never have lived this long.[3]

The personal accounts – and fantasies – of health-seekers were reinforced by a flood of medical books. The most influential, Daniel Drake's *Systemic Treatise, Historical, Aetiological and Practical, on the Principal Diseases of the Interior Valley of North America*, was published in 1850 and gave a distinctive New World stamp to the practice of medicine.[4] It was strikingly different in tone from medical publications in Europe and had no difficulty in dealing with consumption. Drake mingled seemingly objective data on climate – hours of sunshine, number of cures – with popular anecdotes and semi-legends (the dying coming to life in California) and expressed a burning conviction that a natural life style, that is the life of the frontier, regenerated consumptive bodies even as it purified their souls. Drake himself had become by the 1840s Cincinnati's leading physician and was, according to Harriet Martineau, "the complete and splendid specimen of a westerner", apparently indistinguishable from any farmer on his way to the market place. "His sentences", Harriet reported, "take whatever form fate may determine but they bear the rich burden of truth hard won by experience."[5]

The "hard won" was undoubtedly true. The doctor had been raised in a log cabin in Kentucky, educated locally and sporadically, his medical training best described as empirical. (He later attended lectures at the Medical College of Philadelphia and obtained a diploma many years after he had begun to practise.) Yet he did not see his lack of formal education or his reliance on experience as in any way a handicap. His faith in the right environment and way of life to cure almost every ailment was unshakeable. Conceding that "some of these journeys over the deserts to the Rocky Mountains would abound with fatigues and in privations", without them "they would scarcely be more efficacious than the expensive and fashionable trips to Europe we hear so much about".

Failure did not exist for Drake and his like (as it still does not for their professional progeny), despite the evidence of the hundreds of solitary graves

---

[3] Rothman, *Living in the Shadow of Death*, p. 84. The autobiographical accounts of the first health-seekers became bestsellers in the east. Josiah Gregg's *Commerce of the Prairies*, published in 1844, was one of many relating his near-miraculous cure in New Mexico. George Ruxton, an Englishman, was similarly bowled over by the curative properties of Colorado. Of course it was not just the climate but also the natural open-air way of life – riding a horse all day, the buffalo meat roasted over an open fire, sleeping under the stars – which contributed to the miracle cures: the imagery is still potent.

[4] Schapiro, H. D., Miller, Z. L., *Physician of the West: Selected Writings of Daniel Drake on Science and Society* (Lexington, Kentucky, 1970).

[5] Martineau, H., *Retrospect of Western Travel* (London, 1838), p. 225.

along the routes across the prairies. "A short distance from our place of encampment", Henry Jones wrote in *Health-Seekers in the South West*, "I observed a newly made grave ... and on examining the wooden headboard I found it to be the resting place of George W. Tindal ... who died here from consumption." Such finds were not admissible as evidence. When a resident at Mackinac Island, a favourite stopping place of the health-seekers and gateway to the west, told Drake that consumption was common there and introduced two of the sufferers to Drake, the doctor insisted that their ailment was chronic bronchitis. Perhaps it was.

As in Europe with the south, the railway companies did not invent the myth of the health-giving west but they did not object to profiting from it; and, as in the case of the Riviera, after the 1870s the trickle of health-seekers turned into a flood. "Go West and Breathe Again!" was one company's slogan and it was heeded by tens of thousands. The benefits derived by those who did go west were often more subtle than the advertised "new lungs". What many of the early health-seekers appreciated most was the sympathy they encountered among the fit. Here there was no stigma yet attached to them as there was in the east. "Several consumptives have come here totally unfit ...", the *Colorado Springs Gazette* stated in 1873. "They are drowning men clutching at straws and are worthy of our sincerest sympathy." Such charitable sentiments survived into the early 1890s and encouraged openness. "They don't hesitate to inform you that they are consumptive and that they wish to live through the winter to give the climate a chance to do them some good." But charity and tolerance in human societies have their limits; soon there was greed and exploitation as well. While brochures which reached the East Coast depicted well-designed and spacious resort hotels with well-ventilated rooms, porches and extensive grounds, the reality was often wooden shacks in remote, barren regions. But so potent was the lure of the west, and so terrible the prospect of a lingering death in a more rigorous climate, that many patients could not be bothered to investigate the claims in advance. Their disappointment was all the more bitter because it was the first hint that the promise of cure might prove no less deceptive.

Often, for men with limited financial resources, "a regimen of outdoor living" consisted of working as hired men in jobs well beyond their physical capacity. Unlike Weeks, many lacked the capacity to cultivate bees or care even for a small place with a cow, a horse, a chicken coop and a strawberry bed interspersed with a few lemon and orange trees. It sounded idyllic from a distance and might have been for the healthy; but it could be too much for those with hardly any lungs left. "Often", one health-seeker reported, "I had to stop for fifteen, or twenty minutes coughing and gasping for breath every half hour, every bone in my body aflame. Eventually I caved in and

sold the farm for a pittance." Many partially planted vineyards were, as
George Weeks observed, a memorial to "those who had waited too long
before coming to this Land of the New Lungs".

As sooner or later happens to all refugee populations, everywhere in the
west the health-seekers were put off by the army of their fellow consumptives.
"Oh what a lot of coughing suffering mortals are coming here!", D. M. Berry,
one of the founders of Pasadena wrote to his sister. "And many come too
late, much too late! One man died in sight of the harbour." The army of
breathless, hawking invalids became a living testimony against the myth of a
miracle cure. "At every street corner", a health-seeker wrote from Los Angeles,
"I meet a poor fellow croaking like myself . . . Wherever I go I meet men with
broken lungs who speak of nothing else but their ailment. 'Well, how do you
feel today? Did you have a good night? . . . Did you cough much after breakfast?
Any blood in the spit?'" The view from the writer's window was of "men
muffled in shawls on the porch, parchment faces and sunken eyes and cough,
cough, cough; leaning over the handrail another fellow with spindle legs and
shrunken form; another joins them, and still another, feebly walking to and
fro to save the funeral expenses". Pasadena was no different. Indeed, "we see
more health-seekers here", Jenny Collier wrote home, "of every possible shade
of ghostliness than can be found anywhere else. They shuffle about the streets
with aimless unsteadiness which says plainer than words that hope has died".
She found her visits to the post office particularly unnerving. "Those poor
wanderers driven from home by failing health congregate here about the
doors or sit coughing upon the steps or lean exhausted against the wall with
eager anxious faces waiting, hoping for letters from home."

Yet the myth lived on, fuelled by the occasional cure but more by propaganda and most of all by hope. Mark Twain gave *spes phthisica* the ultimate
accolade of parody in *Roughing It*: "Three months of camp life in Lake Tahoe
would restore an Egyptian mummy to its pristine vigour. The air up there
in the clouds is pure, fine, bracing and delicious: and why shouldn't it be?
It's the same the angels breathe."

By the turn of the century the old attitudes of hospitality and compassion
were almost completely gone: they were replaced by a terrible fear of the
vast encroaching contagion. In *Chasing the Cure in Colorado* Thomas Gal-
braith described his odyssey, moving like a fugitive or a leper from one
boarding house to another because of objections of the neighbours or fellow
boarders. Yet most of them were consumptives themselves.

> As I entered the dining room for the first time [at his second place of residence]
> I was introduced by the landlady to the assembled boarders as the gentleman whom
> she had told them about – the one who came to Denver for his *rheumatism* . . . It

was surprising the number of diseases I found represented in that house. But it was more surprising that everyone coughed – dyspeptics, rheumatics, nervous wrecks, heart patients, kidney patients, ear patients, Keely cure patients – all coughed. For fear of being called consumptives, no one exercised any of the simplest sanitary precautions … In the business world, the consumptive isn't wanted except when he buys and gives cash in return. Want "ads" specify, "No invalids need apply".[6]

In 1902 the young physician John Bruce MacCallum came to Denver seeking to regain his failing health. "There are 600 doctors in Denver already", he wrote, a ratio of 1 to 250.

I was never so horribly impressed with the struggle for existence as I have been here … It is a city of people … fighting against almost impossible odds of sickness and poverty. Although it is bright and sunny, there is something horribly depressing about it all … No one belongs here – everybody is moving on or dying.[7]

Flight from consumption took some victims to exotic places and changed their lives and even perhaps the course of history. While studying in Oxford, Cecil Rhodes's health broke down at the age of sixteen. The diagnosis was early consumption and he was sent to join his elder brother who was farming in Natal.[8] It happened to be the year when diamonds were discovered in the Kimberley fields and he found in South Africa not only renewed vigour but also an immense fortune. He also decided that, for the benefit of mankind and of all races, the British should rule the Dark Continent. Back in Oxford he became sick again in 1873 and was told that one of his lungs was completely gone and the other partially gone and that he had less than six months to live. He returned to South Africa and his health was once again restored. He visited Oxford for the last time five years later but did not stay. On the outbreak of the Boer War in 1899 he returned to Kimberley and died there in 1902, at the age of forty-nine.[9]

---

[6] Quoted by F. R. Rogers in "The Rise and Decline of Altitude Therapy of Tuberculosis", *Bulletin of the History of Medicine*, 43 (1969), p. 1.

[7] Malloch, A., *Short Years: The Life and Letters of John Bruce McCallum, M.D., 1876–1906* (Chicago, 1938), p. 192.

[8] Thomas, A., *Rhodes: The Race for Africa* (London, 1997), is a recent addition to the Rhodes literature, a good biography written for an unsuccessful television series.

[9] Rhodes's illness remains something of a mystery. Pulmonary tuberculosis was the diagnosis of the family doctor, Dr John Morris, who was trusted by the Rev. Francis Rhodes, Cecil's father. There had been several cases of consumption in the family. The diagnosis was the reason – at least the main reason – for Cecil's departure from England. It is true that he rarely referred to his ill-health later in life; but it was at times incapacitating even in South Africa. He had several spells of haemoptysis; and cough and attacks of "asthma" troubled him for most of his life. Subject to the perennial question of the "successor diseases" (discussed in Chapter 33 below), tuberculosis seems to the present writer to have been the likeliest cause, more probable than a congenital cardiac abnormality, atrial septal defect (suggested in the

Rhodes himself and some eminent physicians believed that hot dry air could save consumptives and perhaps it did save some. The Reverend John Hamilton, of Christ Church, Oxford, pointed out that the Old Testament, a mine of recondite medical clues, mentions nothing that could reasonably be interpreted as phthisis; and for a decade or two health-seekers joined religious pilgrims and over-the-top Pre-Raphaelites in trips to the arid deserts of the Holy Land.

In addition to tracking south or west – to deserts, to the Veldt, to the Riviera, to Colorado or to Polynesia – there was one other direction in which consumptives could travel: upward. Since the brothers Joseph and Etienne Montgolfier sent up live animals in a balloon and recovered them live (to receive the plaudits of France and their reward from the hands of royalty) in 1783,[10] and the ascent in a captive balloon of Pilâtre de Rozier four months later, ballooning for scientific and for military purposes (and, of course, for fun) advanced by fits and starts. Sixty-six balloons defeated the Prussian blockade during the Siege of Paris of 1870–71,[11] and by the 1880s most western countries had at least one well-equipped ballooning corps. In peacetime the workshops tried to keep in business by finding civilian uses for their products; and prominent among these was altitude therapy for tuberculosis.

This was respectable medicine, not a branch of quackery. The eminent French physician, Christian Beck, reported in 1907 to the Académie des Sciences in Paris on the incalculable benefits of the treatment to selected patients: breathing a pure atmosphere free from germs and dust even for a few hours virtually guaranteed improvement and sometimes a rapid cure. The respective merits of various regimes were hotly debated in the light of ample but somewhat contradictory scientific evidence, ranging from daily ascents to 4–500 metres for up to eight hours to once- or twice-weekly ascents to a greater altitude (up to 1200 metres) for one or two hours. The treatment was not of course for the indigent poor, since the more frail had to be accompanied by at least one nurse and a doctor (in addition to the navigator

1960s by some biographers). The final event was probably acute or chronic pulmonary oedema. The doubt about tuberculosis arose from the fact that no reference to a tuberculous lesion was made in the report on the necropsy performed at Muizenberg; but the examination seems to have been surprisingly perfunctory and the report does not inspire much confidence.

[10] The Montgolfiers were no scientists – they believed that it was the smoke rather than the heat which lifted off their balloon – but theirs was probably the prettiest balloon ever built and modern ballooning is generally dated from their experiments.

[11] They mostly carried post and messages but famously one balloon helped Léon Gambetta to escape in order to inspire resistance and organise the relief of Paris. The mission failed but historically this was the golden moment of ballooning.

and his mate or mates); but it was cheaper than travelling to Egypt or to the South Seas. Among Beck's patients was one Grand Duchess who was virtually restored to health after twenty eight-hour ascents, as well as the wife of a prominent diplomatist whose single excursion enabled her to take her place among the President of the Republic's New Year guests at the Elysée. Despite such triumphs, the treatment did not catch on widely outside France and the First World War put an end to it as it did to so many other expensive pleasures.

So what was – and is – the importance of climate, air and altitude in tuberculosis? Despite weighty monographs which filled bookcases in university and hospital libraries and the proceedings over several decades of learned societies dedicated to the subject, nobody knew then and nobody knows now. Rudolf Virchow, impatient of all crazes and unscientific fads (other than those which buzzed under his own capacious top hat) made great play of the fact that the healthy inhabitants of Nubia were said to have become tuberculous and succumbed to the disease when they moved to Egypt, in Virchow's day one of the places of pilgrimage for German consumptives. In a famous textbook Augustus Hirsch, another would-be iconoclast, argued against mountain resorts, pointing out that many people moving from lower to higher altitudes almost predictably developed scrofula. Such observations were often factually correct but the interpretation put on them was usually dubious. Egypt has many different climates and could be expected to affect fit Nubian warriors differently from the way it affected the ailing sons of German industrialists from the Ruhr. The actual move from low to high altitudes – or the reverse – could expose sufferers to other trying conditions, probably far more important than height.

Even in the golden age of medical climatology unprejudiced observers recognised that climate was multifactorial and tuberculosis variable. A dry but dust-free atmosphere usually benefited patients with infections of the larynx. Sunshine was good in some cases of bone and joint tuberculosis. The smog of big cities – London leading the way – was a killer. But it was always difficult to formulate general rules. In the late 1940s, the last time before effective chemotherapy made it impossible to evaluate natural aetiological factors, the mortality rate from tuberculosis was highest among the Innuits of the frozen Canadian North, the Bantu of dry sunny Africa, the inhabitants of the most humid regions of India and the people of Cyprus. Yet a change in climatic conditions could undoubtedly have an effect on the course of the disease – not always for the better. Guinea-pigs from the high Andes transported to animal houses at sea level were not only more susceptible to tuberculosis than breeds native to the plain: they could also be rendered more resistant by being maintained at a reduced atmospheric pressure.

Faith in such matters was (and is) always more important than statistics. The firm of Göbel of Gmunden in Austria was founded in 1865 and did not go out of business until the early 1930s. Its sole product was bottled air, collected, compressed and preserved (so the firm's brochure informed prospective customers) from every famous spa in Europe. Its best-selling line before the First World War was *Luft von Ischl* (Ischl Air). It was especially recommended for those with consumption unable to travel and forced to live in a dusty atmosphere. Its unique properties were endorsed on the label by more than one *Professor Ordinarius* and extolled by a Royal and Imperial Highness, two Princes, a Countess and a Rothschild. It had received numerous gold medals and diplomas of honour at international exhibitions. It hardly needed such recommendations. Ischl was a charming Alpine spa near Salzburg, celebrated for its pine forest, its lake, its almost continuous rain, its incomparable Ischler cakes, but above all, for being the the summer residence of the Emperor, Franz Josef.[12] The bottles of Göbel's *Luft von Ischl* were prettily shaped, not unlike those of the "pure, natural and health-giving" spring waters which are sold by the billion today. In loyal middle-class households of the Dual Monarchy a bottle would be solemnly opened in the master bedroom (and in any sick-room in the house) every evening an hour before master and mistress retired for the night. A faint but pleasing scent of pine forests soon wafted from its direction, carried by the same air which gave the Emperor and Apostolic King, the father of his people, his legendary wisdom and vigour.

With the rise of sanatoria faith in travelling as such began to wane. Fewer and fewer geographical locations were recognised as safe. By 1900 tuberculosis was killing young men and women as surely in San Francisco, Cape Town and Melbourne as it was in Paris, Edinburgh and Moscow; and it was as rife among Polynesian Islanders as it was among the people of Old and New England.

---

[12] It was also Brahms's favourite resort toward the end of his life.

The Cause

Landmarks in art and literature can usually be dated and attributed with reasonable certainty to an individual artist or author. In science (outside old biographical films in which the swell of a heavenly choir often marked the event) this is rarely possible. But there can be no doubt that the first person actually to see microbes was the Dutchman, Antony Leeuwenhoek (1632–1723), and that the event occurred some time in 1660 in Delft. Leeuwenhoek was descended from a long line of respectable burghers, mostly brewers and basket-weavers, and for most of his long life he himself was a respected draper. Respected but (even in the proverbially tolerant Netherlands) probably regarded as a little cracked. He spent most of his time grinding lenses – a craft at which he was not to be surpassed for at least two centuries – and constructing dozens of what were in effect the first microscopes. Peering through these a fantastic world was revealed to him – minuscule creatures of a staggering variety which populated everything from rain water to scrapings from teeth and skin. Leeuwenhoek spoke only Dutch and probably his main if not his only reading matter was the Bible; but, at the prompting of and through the mediation of a famous local scientist, Régnier de Graaf, he eventually communicated his findings in long and discursive letters to London's Royal Society. The original debating club had recently been raised to that status by Charles II and it counted Robert Boyle, Isaac Newton and Christopher Wren among its Fellows. They rewarded him with a medal and a diploma; and microbiology was born.[1]

It did not at first advance very fast. Good microscopes were difficult to make and it was not immediately clear where Leeuwenhoek's tiny animalcules came from, what purpose they served, if any, and what, if anything, should be done about them. Leeuwenhoek himself was so fascinated by what he saw (who can blame him? The wonder of it is still sometimes recaptured when a schoolchild peers down a microscope for the first time) that he gave little thought to anything other than to describing them. For almost a hundred years the subject was also befogged by the Vegetative Force, the misty brainchild of an English Catholic priest, the Reverend John Turberville

[1] Dobell, C., *Antony van Leeuwenhoek and his Little Animalcules* (London, 1932).

Needham, who saw "with his own eyes" living creatures emerging from pure incubated mutton gravy.[2] The idea was vigorously promoted by the great French naturalist, Georges Louis, Comte de Buffon, and accepted by advanced scientific opinion in most of Europe.[3] Though "spontaneous generation" was contested and eventually demolished by the Abbé Lazzaro Spallanzani (1729–1799), a flamboyant Italian polymath and one of the biological sciences' great experimenters, this left both the provenance and the significance of Leeuwenhoek's animalcules unaccounted for. The man who almost single-handedly transformed a diverting pastime of a few *dilettanti* into a scientific discipline was Louis Pasteur (1822–1895).[4]

Pasteur, like many other pioneers whose discoveries changed the course of medicine, was not a doctor. Born into a farming family in Dôle in the Jura he studied first mathematics and then chemistry, his work on isometric tartrates landing him the chair of chemistry in the University of Strasbourg at the age of thirty. There he married Mlle Marie Laurent, among the longest-suffering and most supportive of scientist's wives, and his attention gradually turned to fermentation. In 1854 he was appointed professor at Lille, where he was persuaded (perhaps against his inclinations) to try to rescue the city's ailing brewing industry. He did so by demonstrating that microorganisms, much like the ones described by Leeuwenhoek 200 years earlier, were responsible both for normal and for abnormal fermentation. (Ironically for a non-drinker, he remained involved with the brewing and wine-growing industry for most of his life.) Almost incidentally his discovery inspired Joseph Lister of Edinburgh (later Lord Lister) to develop antisepsis, the most important single surgical advance of the past 200 years.[5] But if Pasteur's interest in microbiology was kindled nearly by accident, once kindled there was no stopping him.

There is always an element of luck in scientific discoveries and favourable circumstances are often more important than individual talent and dedication; but it is impossible seriously to question Pasteur's genius. Yet

[2] He was a man of integrity and a Fellow of the Royal Society; one wonders what he did see. He died in 1781 aged sixty-nine.

[3] Buffon was an outstanding representative of the French Enlightenment, wrong on almost every biological question he addressed but the first to treat biology as a science in its own right, independent of theology. Darwin revered him as his intellectual forerunner. He died in 1788, aged eighty-one.

[4] Unlike most great scientists, Pasteur has had several good biographers. Outstanding among them is the work of his son-in-law, R. Pasteur-Valéry-Radot, *Pasteur* (Paris, 1924).

[5] Lister never failed to acknowledge his debt and remained a great admirer of Pasteur. (The esteem was reciprocated: to Pasteur Lister was "le vrai gentleman Anglais", which, despite Lister's faults and allowing for the all-inclusiveness of *Anglais* for all Britons to Frenchmen, was a fair judgement.)

he was in many ways not only a monster but also a persistent offender against the rules of sound scientific research. In private he was arrogant, vain, impatient, bigoted, a chauvinist (both French and male). He was not above vulgar abuse and thought nothing of vilifying the work of Claude Bernard as soon as the great physiologist was in his grave; or of physically assaulting the venerable surgeon Jules Guérin (past eighty) in the Académie when the latter dared to question some of Pasteur's assertions. He worked his assistants like a slave-driver but never appropriated their ideas and he was intensely loyal to them. Professionally he always preferred to circumvent, ignore or bypass difficulties on the way to some distantly glimpsed goal rather than to solve them. He knew what he wanted to prove rather than eliciting answers with an open mind; he was often wrong in his guesses, illogical in his arguments and even slapdash in his experiments; and there was a wholly unscientific, mystical element to his approach to scientific problems which often disconcerted more hard-bitten colleagues. With such deficiencies it would be possible to explain one or even two major discoveries by invoking good luck or the concatenation of happy circumstances; but Pasteur's career was a succession of scientific triumphs, both improbable and imaginative, quite as inexplicable by accident as are the symphonies of Mozart or the plays of Shakespeare.[6] Not only was his own work ground-breaking in half a dozen fields but it also inspired others, as clever or almost as clever as he was himself. In the rare first category was the German general practitioner turned scientist, Robert Koch (1843–1910).[7]

Koch was born in Clausthal in the Harz Mountains, the most northern mountain range in Germany, the third of thirteen children of a mining engineer. He graduated in medicine with honours at the University of Göttingen, a leading medical school at the time. He was a slightly built, studious, near-sighted young man with a well-concealed Romantic streak. As resident physician in a lunatic asylum in Hamburg he met Emmy Fraatz, who agreed to marry him on condition that he jettisoned his secret ambitions of exploring the South Sea Islands and winning the Iron Cross in battle in favour of the more humdrum prospect of rural general practice. For several years, based in the small and rather drab Prussian town of Wollstein, he did his rounds on horseback to back of beyond hamlets and villages to attend farmers, farmer's wives, their babies and often their dogs and cats as well. Apart from

---

[6] By demonstrating that the cell-free extracts of yeast cells could catalyse fermentation as readily as intact cells he became the founder of modern biochemistry. Since the catalyst was contained in yeast, that is ἐν ζύμῃ, he called it enzyme.

[7] Brock, T. D., *Robert Koch: A Life in Medicine and Bacteriology* (New York, 1958); Robinson, V., *Robert Koch* (New York, 1932).

reading the *Deutsche medizinische Wochenschrift* once a week, he was completely cut off from developments in medicine or science. But on his
twenty-eighth birthday Frau Emmy surprised him with a present that was
to change their lives. She gave him a microscope of quite a modest capacity,
the kind that is bought today for bright ten-year-olds to awaken their minds
to the wonders of of the natural world.

Koch's first microbiological interest (or obsession; all his interests became
obsessional) was one which had also excited Pasteur some years earlier:
anthrax. The disease was a savage, seemingly capricious and ill-understood
killer of sheep and occasionally of man, and had many characteristics which
suggested microbial transmission. Koch had to teach himself the very rudi-
ments of microbiological research; and he had to fit his studies into the time
left over by a busy and exacting practice. He also had to make almost every
implement he needed himself, prepare sharpened slivers of wood for injections, build his own cages and look after his menagerie of experimental
animals. Often he had to improvise techniques; and some of his early improvisations, like the hanging drop preparation, are still in use.[8] He was in
many respects the antithesis of Pasteur, meticulous to a fault, wary of jumping
to conclusions, critical of his own results, determinedly avoiding short cuts
which might lead him astray, but he had the same total dedication. It is not
known how well he looked after his cases of whooping cough, diarrhoea and
obstructed labour (which must have taken up what others might have
regarded as a full day's and often night's work); but it is impossible to imagine
him careless in any professional capacity. Outside his practice his priorities
were the same as Pasteur's: the guinea-pigs came first; family, friends and
private life nowhere.

It took Koch six years in the wilderness before he was sufficiently satisfied
with his results to emerge from isolation and to take his notes, microscope
and microscopic preparations to the University of Breslau (now Wroclaw).
Here he struck gold. Two professors, Cohn and Cohnheim,[9] recognised the

---

[8] The ingenious simplicity of the device was typical of Koch. A drop on the underside of
a microscopic cover-slip which fitted into a hollowed-out space on the slide itself allowed the
examination of the contents of the fluid in depth.

[9] Both were products of the Jewish emancipation in German academic life. (Jews had been
barred from studying medicine or holding chairs in the University of Berlin until 1870 and
in many other prestigious seats of learning for much longer: hence the flowering of previously
insignificant schools like Breslau which could not afford to be choosy.) Ferdinand Cohn
(1828–1898) was a founder of modern plant physiology who made no pretence of knowing
much about human diseases; but he immediately grasped the significance of Koch's work.
He called in his colleague, Julius Cohnheim (1839–1884), head of the pathology department
and already famous for his *Lectures on General Pathology*, a classic text setting forth the basic
events of acute inflammation (and many other pathological phenomena). Though Cohnheim

importance of his work and set the wheels in motion to find him a place where he could continue his researches without distraction. Seven years earlier Pasteur had a little flamboyantly predicted that science would soon be ready to eliminate all parasitic, meaning microbial, diseases. Koch's work on anthrax had added a new element of reality to this prospect. Not only did he establish that the disease was caused by a specific and identifiable bacillus and by nothing else; he also demonstrated how anthrax spores could remain dormant under extreme adverse conditions – in dead and buried carcasses for example – only to revive and to start to multiply when transferred to new living hosts and kill again.[10]

There was still a wait of two years before Koch's Breslau patrons and his own growing reputation secured for him a proper laboratory in the Imperial Health Office in Berlin. His transfer gave him scope for working on essential technical problems, including ways of growing homogeneous colonies from single organisms. Pre-echoing Fleming's discovery of penicillin thirty years later (but no more accidentally), the solution stemmed from a boiled potato cut in half and left uneaten on the laboratory bench by a careless – or, more likely in Koch's department, desperately overworked – assistant. Next morning Koch noticed the beadlike growths on the cut surfaces, and his prepared mind conceived the notion that each colony could represent the multiplication of a single bacillus. This in fact proved to be the case; and Pasteur himself hailed it as a great advance. Despite the more salubrious surroundings than the garden shed in Wollstein, Koch still had much to contend with. Rudolf Virchow, revered by the whole of the German and much of the European medical establishment and by Koch himself as the fount of all wisdom, found the chase for microbes more than a little ludicrous.[11] When

was a pupil of Virchow's, he had an open and well-ventilated mind and was quickly convinced by Koch's demonstration and converted to what was still the revolutionary concept of microbial diseases.

[10] The term "spore" (meaning seed) was ancient but Koch's demonstration of anthrax spores was the first time that their nature and importance was established in modern microbiology.

[11] Virchow still gets a bad press in relation to tuberculosis which he had studied for many years before Koch's emergence. In fact he was a classic case of the young rebel who cannot later accept any modification to his beautifully worked out and comprehensive new system. He was born into a poor family in 1821 in East Prussia and advanced by highly competitive state scholarships; he graduated from the University of Berlin in 1843. His most important book, *Cellular Pathology*, was published while he was a youthful professor at Würzburg: it went through twenty-eight editions in his lifetime (growing in bulk each time) and established the cell – rather than humours, organs or tissues – as the basic unit of pathology. In 1856 he was invited to head the department of pathology at La Charité Hospital in Berlin and also entered the *Reichstag*. An effective social reformer, he introduced useful public-health measures, including the best medical statistical recording system in Europe. He was one of the few academic politicians whom Bismarck respected, almost feared, despite their political

Koch explained the advantages of isolating individual organisms in pure culture Virchow expressed the fear that now a new institute would now have to be built for every *verfluchte Mikrobe*: the whole business was getting out of hand, as expensive and silly as Germany's new African colonies. (His sarcasm was not entirely misplaced.) Undismayed, with his assistants, Löffler and Gaffky,[12] and with a thoroughness which some of Pasteur's more mercurial team regarded as hopelessly plodding and indeed typically teutonic, Koch pressed on in pursuit of what all agreed was the most problematic but also potentially the most glittering prize, the organism – if it was an organism – causing tuberculosis.

General opinion about this had shifted slightly since the frosty reception given to Budd and Villemin. "While admitting the apparent specificity of the infection resulting in animals from the inoculation of tuberculous material", wrote the *Lancet* in 1867 in an unsigned editorial, " ... and impressed with the fact that two independent observers (M. Villemin and Dr Budd) from two different and perfectly independent points of view, have arrived at a zymotic theory of tuberculosis, we cannot but confess to the excessive difficulty of reconciling with this theory clinical facts ... as well as daily experience about the origin of phthisis." Powerfully persuasive though still entirely indirect evidence supporting contagion continued to accumulate. In 1868 Jean-Baptiste Auguste Chauveau of Lyon,[13] reported to the Académie des Sciences that he had succeeded in producing tuberculosis in three healthy heifers by feeding them tuberculous products; and in 1872 Luigi Armani inoculated the centre of the cornea of guinea-pigs with a needle dipped into a watery suspension of caseous material from the tuberculous lesion of a recently dead patient and watched, some weeks later, tubercles develop in the inoculated animals while the controls remained clear. Cohnheim and Salomonsen performed similar experiments a few years later, inoculating the anterior chamber of rabbits' eyes. In a spectacular series of demonstrations (repeated in several laboratories), H. Tappeiner produced tuberculosis in every dog enclosed in kennels sprayed with a dilute solution of tuberculous

---

differences. ("To the Herr Professor politics is only an extension of public health", the Iron Chancellor once remarked.) He also wrote fiction and historical and anthropological works of some distinction. He died aged eighty-one in 1902, eponymously commemorated in several branches of medicine.

[12] Both became successful microbe hunters in their own right. George Gaffky (1850–1918) succeeded Koch as director of the institute named after the master and was the first to culture the typhoid bacillus in pure culture. Friedrich Löffler (1852–1913) was the first to culture the diphtheria bacillus (first described by Edwin Klebs). He was also the first to provide evidence of the existence of pathogenic filterable viruses.

[13] The Virchow and Koch rolled into one of veterinary medicine.

sputum. Respectable opinion still remained on the fence: in 1881, almost at the eleventh hour, Austin Flint and W. H. Welch, in the fifth edition of their magisterial textbook *The Principles and Practice of Medicine*, committed themselves to the statement that "the doctrine of the contagiousness of the disease ... has its advocates but general belief supported by the weightiest of evidence is in its non-communicability".

Koch's original material came from the body of a thirty-two-year-old labourer, Heinrich Günther by name, strong and fit until three weeks earlier when he started to cough, little pains began to shoot through his chest and his body seemed to melt away. Four days after admission to hospital he died, post-mortem examination revealing almost every organ in his body to be riddled with tubercles. Koch began by injecting this material first into guinea-pigs and then into rabbits, using a procedure developed by Cohnheim some years earlier. Within a few months he and Löffler caught their first glimpse of the small, slender and seemingly fragile rods that they suspected of being the cause of tuberculosis. After a year's further work there was no doubt left in their minds; nor could there be in the mind in any objective observer. This was not enough for Koch. He had by then laid down three criteria which in his opinion had to be fulfilled before a cause and effect relationship between a germ and a disease could be accepted as proven. These, "Koch's Postulates", soon to become famous, were:

1. The organism must be found in every lesion.

2. It should be capable of being cultivated pure outside the body for several generations.

3. After pure culture for a sufficient length of time and for several generations, it should be able to reproduce the original illness in laboratory animals.

What ensured the fame – or notoriety – of these seemingly simple criteria was not so much their content as their style. Though doctor literally means a learned man, and though the title had been bestowed on those qualified to practice medicine for centuries, learning let alone scientific rigour was not recognised in Koch's day as hallmarks of successful doctoring. To say that science was held in contempt would be an exaggeration. It was simply not essential for the pursuit of that particular profession. Even those engaged in teaching and research usually based their claim to be described as learned on their practical skills, their familiarity with hallowed texts, their long experience, their understanding of the vagaries of human nature, their intuition and sometimes merely on their common sense. The functioning of the human body, let alone its malfunctioning, was viewed, not only by the Sir Ralph Bloomfield Bonningtons but also by such academic eminences as

Rudolf Virchow, as far too complex a mechanism to be encapsulated in postulates. Koch's whole approach smacked of the rigid laws of physics, mathematics or astronomy, even of theological doctrine, leaving no room for inspiration or the hunch, the very essence of traditional medicine. Nor was it just a question of tradition versus the new. The traditional view was endorsed even – or most of all – by the leaders of the new disciplines. Pasteur's papers would be rejected with more or less polite expressions of horror today by the editor of any reputable medical or scientific journal for lack of solid experimental evidence and proof of statistical significance. Not Koch's. His was unashamedly a different approach; and, in the face of much blustering, as well as a certain amount of reasoned argument, his postulates established the science of medicine as the equal of the art of medicine. For better or for worse, once established it could never be dislodged.

The tuberculosis bacillus was and remains one of the most difficult organisms to culture; and it is doubtful if many scientists would have had the mulish tenacity of Koch in persevering in order to satisfy his own postulates. But on 24 March 1882, a cold and cheerless evening, he reported his findings to the Berlin Physiological Society gathered in the Reading Room of the Physiological Institute under the chairmanship of Professor du Bois-Reymond. The audience was small, only thirty-six in all. Among them was Helmholz, Ehrlich and Löffler; but the pathologists, including the great Virchow and the leading clinicians of Berlin, were notable absentees.[14] It did not matter much. There was an initial slightly disparaging reference to Villemin's work – dislike of the French was never far below the surface in Prussia and was heartily reciprocated – but, apart from this blemish, Koch's communication was a model of what a scientific paper should be: brief, clear and irrefutable.

The news travelled more quickly perhaps than it would today. Koch's paper was published in the *Berliner klinische Wochenschrift* on 10 April and a copy of it landed on the same day on the desk of the eminent British scientist, John Tyndall, in London. Realising its importance, he summarised its main findings in a letter to *The Times* which published it on 22 April. Next day, a Sunday, the *New York World* carried a brief cable dispatch announcing the discovery; and two days later both the *New York Times* and the *New York Tribune* published Tyndall's letter in full. Newspaper readers in Paris, both lay and medical, did not learn the news for another six months,

---

[14] Contrary to what was shown in a famous and frequently revived German film of 1938, now a classic despite its Nazi provenance. In the film Virchow (played by Werner Krauss) is present during the meeting and every eye is fixed on him after Koch (played by Emil Jannings) has finished his incontrovertible demonstration. After a dramatic silence Virchow gets up, puts on his top hat and walks out without saying a word. Consternation – but followed by a happy ending.

when it appeared in *L'écho* hedged in with doubts and reservations; but surprisingly perhaps – or not – it was at once endorsed as an important discovery by both Pasteur and his medical colleague and right-hand man, Emile Roux.[15]

To many, perhaps to most practising doctors outside Mediterranean countries, it remained a difficult concept to swallow. At the annual meeting of the British Medical Association in Worcester in August 1882, Dr C. Theodore Williams, physician to the Brompton Hospital, gave voice to the concern of what was still almost certainly the majority. "The chief difficulty", Williams said,

> is that many of the most potent causes of phthisis – dampness of the soil, bad ventilation and deficient food – are also the conditions which would promote the multiplication of low organisms; and, on the other hand, heredity which is the source of a large amount of phthisis cannot be reconciled with the bacillus theory... How can we account for cases where the parents having died of consumption, their children are attacked at the same age as the parents had been? And I know of several instances where children who happened to be scattered in various parts of the world were yet attacked and succumbed to the fell disease at about the same age.[16]

Williams was particularly concerned about the possible implications of Koch's discovery for his own famous hospital. "The evidence of large institutions for the treatment of consumption directly contradicts any idea of consumption being an infective disease like a zymotic fever. In the rare and in my opinion still doubtful instances of contagion through inhalation I would put the prime blame on improper ventilation rather than on close intimacy." Others continued to pursue their own favourite ideas. Only a few years earlier Henry F. Formad of Philadelphia had constructed an ingenious hypothesis attributing tuberculosis to certain to him clearly defined inborn tissue changes in individuals predisposed to the disease; and he was not easily shaken.[17]

Many claimed to have repeated Koch's experiments but, having observed his "so-called bacilli", clearly recognised them as artefacts. In the United States Dr Bertram Smith dismissed them as "fatty globules soluble in boiling water"; and, a little more kindly, Dr Rollin Grigg scouted them as "quite obviously fibrin filaments of no pathological importance whatever".[18] In Vienna Professor Franz Skaunditz had seen bodies with his own eyes "indistinguishable from Herr Professor Koch's so-called bacilli in many normal

---

[15] Pasteur's anti-German sentiments did not go so far as to deny the importance of a scientific advance if he regarded it as important.

[16] Williams, C. T., *British Medical Journal* (1882), no. 1, 618.

[17] Landis, H. R. M., *Annals of Medical History*, new series, 4 (1932), 531.

[18] Ibid., 535.

joints".[19] More seriously, Watson Cheyne of King's College Hospital, London, reported that he had vainly tried to repeat Koch's experiments over a period of almost a year.[20] Latin countries took to the concept more readily: indeed, Vittorio of Turin wrote (though he phrased it more politely) that his countrymen did not need a German professor to tell them that phthisis was catching.

Some of the resistance to Koch's ideas was fuelled by humane considerations. The eminent advocate of the dry climate therapy, Dr Henry Bennett, argued that acceptance of Koch's ideas would "increase a hundredfold the miseries and sufferings of patients and their families ... phthisics would have to be treated like medieval lepers, separated from their beloved, isolated, shut up, refused admission to hospitals". (Some of these dire prognostications would prove to be well founded.) He took comfort from his belief that Koch could not possibly be right and that his own favourite aetiology, rebreathed air, was the only correct one.

The unbelievers were fighting a losing battle. In 1883 Babesiu of Bucharest and Rosenstein of Munich independently demonstrated the bacillus in the urine of patients with genitourinary tuberculosis, both stressing the diagnostic value of the finding.[21] In the same year Hoadley Garb of Hastings cultured the organism from caseous material recovered from cervical lymph-nodes.[22] In New York Austin Flint instituted regular sputum examinations at Bellevue Hospital immediately on learning of Koch's discovery and published an

[19] Skaunditz, F., *Wiener medizinische Wochenschrift*, 38 (1883), 132.

[20] He later visited Koch's laboratory, saw his methods, brought back the appropriate dyes and fully confirmed Koch's findings.

W. (later Sir William) Watson Cheyne was the nearest to a pioneer bacteriologist Britain produced during the heroic age of the new science (other than Ronald Ross, who was not really a bacteriologist). The son of a sea captain, he was born at sea off the coast of Tasmania in 1852 and brought up by his grandfather, a clergyman in the Shetland Islands. He graduated from Edinburgh University and, having inherited £150, decided to follow his inclinations and study laboratory medicine in Germany. He returned fired with enthusiasm for microbiology and spent two years complementing Lister's surgical researches with bacteriological studies carried out in a "little blind passage behind the operating theatre of the Edinburgh Infirmary with no benches, no incubators, no staining facilities and only one rickety microscope abandoned by the histologists". When his money ran out he was on the point of entering general practice, when Lister, about to move to London, offered him the post of house surgeon. His surgical career advanced steadily – professor in 1880, baronet in 1908 – but, though he continued laboratory work for some years, he was lost to microbiology. Many clever physicians and surgeons (such as Shaw's friend, Clifford Allbutt, the model for Sir Colenso Ridgeon) dabbled in microbiology over the next twenty years; but no specialist consultant microbiologists were appointed to British hospitals until the 1920s.

[21] *Lancet* (1883), no. 1, 464.

[22] Hoadley Garb, D., *British Medical Journal* (1883), no. 2, 1190.

appendix to the next reprint of the fifth edition of his and Welch's *Principles and Practice of Medicine*, strongly advocating the investigation to provide conclusive diagnosis in all patients in whom the symptoms and signs were equivocal. Ironically, it was a French pathologist and an initial unbeliever, Henri Vignal, who showed in 1885 that bacilli in sputa could be ground under foot, dried, moistened, dried again and remoistened eight times and could still kill a guinea-pig. The next year, 1886, saw France enacting the first legislation of any country prohibiting spitting in public places; and on 5 March 1887, after prolonged and careful deliberation, the Council of the Brompton Hospital decreed that spittoons in the wards should be emptied and disinfected at least once a week.

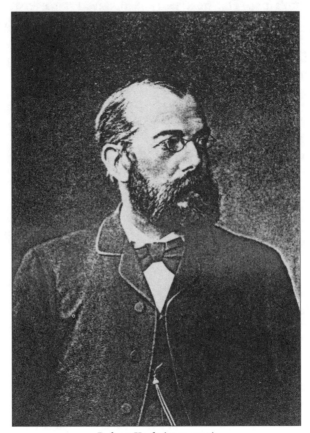

Robert Koch (1843–1910)

13

Tuberculin

After his triumph of 1882 Koch was occupied for a time with the investigation of cholera in Egypt and India, but in 1894 he published a second paper on tuberculosis, more exhaustive than the first, in which he gave credit to the work of others (including Villemin) as well as giving details of his own investigations. It was a staggering record. He had studied in careful detail ninety-eight cases of human and 334 cases of animal tuberculosis; he had inoculated 496 experimental animals and had recovered 143 pure bacillary cultures and had tested their virulence in 234 animals. He described his techniques of preparing suitable culture media and his incubation and staining methods in meticulous detail. The paper contained little that was new but it confirmed Koch's reputation as an obsessively factual investigator. This makes subsequent events even more puzzling.[1]

Although after 1884 Koch retired behind a barrier of silence on the subject of tuberculosis, as the century drew to a close rumours began to circulate that another advance, even more momentous than the isolation of the causative organism, was in the offing. The bombshell exploded at the Tenth International Congress of Medicine in Berlin in 1900 when Koch announced that he had discovered a substance that could "in some cases" protect against tuberculosis and even "under certain circumstances" cure the disease.

Such tantalising announcements, however guarded, were quite out of keeping with Koch's character and reputation. Pasteur, his forerunner and later rival, had often been accused of rushing into print with insufficient evidence, or, even more often, of staging dramatic and slightly preposterous public announcements; and it had often been predicted by his rivals that sooner or later his overconfidence would lend him in trouble. By the grace of God, or because of his uncannily accurate hunches, it never did. In contrast, if Koch had a fault it was to be too circumspect, almost pedantic; he had never spoken before until the truth of his message had been tested and established beyond reasonable doubt. The question therefore remains as to what prompted him to make an announcement that, despite its

---

[1] Webb, G. B., *Annals of Medical History*, new series, 4 (1932), 509; Flick, L. F., *Developments of our Knowledge of Tuberculosis* (Philadelphia, 1925), 71.

apparently cautious wording, was bound to trigger off an explosion of interest and upsurge of hope.

Koch was never to provide a completely satisfactory answer – and indeed the whole truth is still not known with certainty – but an unsigned editorial in the *Lancet* a few months after the original announcement hinted at a likely scenario. "Professor Koch has never yet rushed into print with a discovery until he has been sure of his facts, and all who are in any way acquainted with the circumstances know that he was practically compelled by his government superiors and his colleagues to make a premature statement ..." Having made this accusation – it would be a grave one even today – the leader writer added a little quaintly that "everybody will sympathise most deeply with Dr Koch that he was compelled to break through his usual reticence".[2] Compelled by whom? Wilhelmine Germany was a swaggering sycophancy but not a regime that could or probably even wished to dispatch uncooperative scientists to a Gulag or a concentration camp.[3]

This is to anticipate. The immediate effect of Koch's announcement was electrifying. The *Lancet* welcomed it in an editorial as "glad tidings of great joy"; no less enthusiastically the *British Medical Journal* reprinted Koch's paper in full;[4] and the *Review of Reviews* devoted its entire December issue to it. "Europe witnessed a strange spectacle last month", its editor wrote. "In the Middle Ages the discovery of a new wonder-working shrine often led to a rush of the sick and the lame to God's chosen spot. It was a similar rush which took place over the last two months to Berlin ... The consumptive patients of the Continent have been stampeding for dear life to the capital of Germany."[5] On the Riviera, the last ditch of the consumptive, the news that a German scientist had discovered a cure "sounded as the advent of Jesus must have sounded in the villages of Judea". It flashed through the region like lightning and the newspapers announced that all sleeping-car accommodation from Nice "to the inclement latitudes of Berlin" had been booked for months ahead. The Grand Duke Sergei Nikolaievitch had no

[2] *Lancet* (1890), no 2, 118.

[3] After Bismarck's dismissal in 1890 Wilhelm II announced: "The ship's course remains the same. Full steam ahead is the order of the day." The first statement was a blatant lie, the second became the guiding motto of his reign. The only question was "full steam ahead where?" Most obviously ahead of all other nations in every field of human endeavour, in the sciences and medicine as much as in military power. The acceptance of the objective did not in fact require coercion: with comparatively few exceptions (like Virchow, now retired, who hated swagger of any kind) most German scientists and doctors responded with enthusiasm. Whether or not Koch was among them is uncertain.

[4] Dubos, R. and J., *The White Plague: Tuberculosis, Man and Society* (London, 1953), p. 104.

[5] *Review of Reviews* (1890), p. 557.

such problems: though nearly dying, a special train was to convey him and his entourage from his villa on the Corniche to Germany.

Not inappropriately perhaps, the first of the international medical contingent to arrive in Berlin was Arthur Conan Doyle, already celebrated as a writer but not yet a knight and still in medical practice. The details of his visit, as reported in the *Review of Reviews*, reveals the atmosphere of adulation that had built up around Koch, "a veiled prophet ... unseen to any eyes save those of his immediate co-workers", but also the slightly more sceptical attitude of the creator of Sherlock Holmes. "Koch has never claimed", Doyle reported, "that his fluid kills the tubercle bacillus. On the contrary, it has no effect on it, but it destroys the low form of tissue in the meshes of which the bacillus lurks. Should this tissue be then sloughed off in the case of lupus or be expelled as sputum in the case of phthisis then it might be possible to hope for a complete cure." Even in the first flush of general enthusiasm Doyle thought that this was unlikely.

Although such caution was to prove sadly justified, nobody listened during the heady autumn of 1884. Doctors, patients and entrepreneurs of every degree of disrepute and from every corner of the world jostled for access to Koch's laboratory and competed for samples of his magic fluid. Fabulous fortunes and more exotic inducements, including it was rumoured a princely title, were being offered for a course of treatment. Clinics and hospitals were besieged by newspaper reporters. Sir Joseph Lister was among the early luminaries who arrived to be convinced, and immediately nominated his own tuberculous niece for treatment.[6] By then Koch was frantically insisting – but in vain – that his statement had been no more than a preliminary communication and that much more work was necessary before his "tuberculin" could be released for general use. It is still uncertain whether he was trying to withhold the material (or the formula how to prepare it) because of belated scientific scruples or because his employers wanted the process of manufacture, promoted to a kind of national trophy, to become a monopoly of the Fatherland.

There have been several but only modestly successful attempts to cast a veil over the episode and to explain away the publicity or at least to exonerate Koch. Against this, there is no doubt that on 22 November his colleagues publicly claimed to have cured fourteen cases of lupus, three of scrofula and eighteen of joint, bone and laryngeal infections, and that they insisted that the effect of the vaccine on lung cases had been less dramatic but encouraging: the patients had lost their cough and expectoration after a course of injections (though sometimes only after a significant increase of the initial dose), their

---

[6] Lister's endorsement was reported in the *Lancet* on 12 November 1890.

sputa had become clearer, their bacillus count had diminished, their night sweats had ceased, and they had started to gain weight. After four to six weeks early-stage patients could be regarded as cured. Somebody was fantasising and perhaps deliberately lying and Koch did not disown the report.

Yet he had tried the remedy on himself and it is now known that it produced a "horrid reaction with a rise in temperature, vomiting and lassitude lasting several days". He was probably suffering from a severe positive reaction to what was almost certainly a widely variable preparation. This was not made public and Koch went on record or at least signed an official statement that his vaccine could be given in large and increasing doses, beginning perhaps with two to eight milligramme (the dose he had injected into himself) but rising if necessary to 500 milligrammes.

After several months of stonewalling, and mounting indignation in the world press, both lay and medical, over the secrecy, it was officially revealed that "Koch's Lymph" (subsequently called "Old Tuberculin") contained proteins from killed bacteria originally harvested from infected guinea-pigs: the extract was concentrated in a filtrate of the ox bile and glycerine medium in which the bacilli had been cultured. Doctors could now hurry to their selected patients with samples to test the efficacy of the preparation and the way was open for the manufacture of alternative and cheaper vaccines.

The response to the belated disclosure was variable. Led by Professor Voisin of the Académie de Médecine French medical leaders refused even to test the material. In a sudden volte-face the Royal College of Physicians of London advised extreme caution. Soon it was reported that eight patients at the City of London Chest Hospital had shown no improvement in response to Dr Koch's Lymph injections and eleven subjects at King's College Hospital had responded variably.[7] Many, it was whispered, had shown alarming side-effects. Going as usual from one extreme to the other, nobody suggested that the trial period might have been been too short or that the vaccine might have been too old to be effective; but for once longer and better controlled trials confirmed the negative results. Watson Cheyne (who had been beaten by Koch in the vaccine race) experimented with a range of dosages between two to eight milligrammes and up to three injections a day. In many patients the injections caused severe inflammation and soreness which could last for up to three weeks. After six weeks' treatment thirty-eight cases of lupus and of bone and joint tuberculosis "had improved and the improvement had been maintained for up to three months; but none was cured".[8]

[7] *Lancet* (1890), no. 2, 1173.
[8] Watson Cheyne, W. W., *Proceedings of the Royal Society of Medicine* (1910), no. 5, part 3, 129.

Characteristically, Watson Cheyne emphasised that his trials – by far the most thorough since Koch's original announcement – were not entirely conclusive; but after a few months he had already encountered some of the incidental drawbacks of the new therapy. Prolonged (let alone continuous) treatment was, as one doctor complained to the meeting of the British Medical Association in Bristol, debarred by cost alone. There were others. Once they realised that the injections were not a miracle cure, patients refused or evaded it because of the pain, fever, headaches and general depression which the treatment induced. Those who did not lost weight and were pulled down during the first week or two of the course: they also seemed abnormally vulnerable to the influenza epidemic which swept over Europe in 1901 and to another in 1904. At the Brompton Hospital even submissive patients refused to participate in trials after reading "alarmist reports" in the newspapers.

A few doctors held out against the tide and their isolation made them pugnacious. Among the more eminent R. W. (later Sir Robert) Philip of Edinburgh and W. Canac Wilkinson of London continued to use the vaccine in "early" cases in sufficiently high doses to horrify even well-disposed colleagues. It is possible that the treatment did contain local lesions; but both Philip and Wilkinson refused to publish results. In any case, tuberculosis was so diverse and so unpredictable, and its assessment still so subjective, that a controlled trial would have been conclusive only if the benefits had been dramatic (as they were later with streptomycin). Yet the treatment, promoted by small charities and well-meaning believers, took a long time to fizzle out: for more than three decades it continued to cause suffering and distress to thousands and was almost certainly responsible for deaths.[9] At last, in 1932, Dr F. G. Chandler in his opening address to the annual meeting of the British Medical Association (in the presence of both Sir Robert Philip and Canac Wilkinson) publicly dismissed it as "one of the ingenious errors of the human mind like the mythical antiphlogistones".[10] After that standard textbooks began to change their message: from commending tuberculin as a form of therapy they moved rapidly to a mere mention and eventually to advising strongly against it.

The tuberculin debacle had a few beneficial side-effects. In his paper announcing his ill-starred cure Koch also described the different responses of normal and of previously infected animals to the injection of dead tuberculous materials, the beginning of the study of tuberculosis as an immunological phenomenon.[11] Indeed, Conan Doyle, with a percipience

---

[9] Smith, F. B., *The People's Health, 1830–1910* (London, 1939), p. 82.
[10] Chandler, F. G., *British Medical Journal* (1932), no. 2, 262.
[11] See below, Chapter 18.

worthy of his creation, suggested within a few days of the announcement from Berlin of Koch's vaccine that the material might prove more useful in diagnosis than in treatment. His forecast became reality when, ten years later, it set off Clemens von Pirquet on his search for a diagnostic skin test.

At the personal level, for a time Koch's reputation hung in the balance. Rumours circulated that he had accepted a bribe of a million marks from the government anxious to bask in his reflected glory and to trumpet around the world Germany's pre-eminence in science (as in everything else). Nobody who knew him believed it; but upheavals in his private life gave the calumny a veneer of credibility. He had fallen love with a pretty and gifted art student, Hedwig Freiberg, thirty-two years his junior, and the liaison could not be kept a secret.[12] Eventually he obtained a divorce from Emmy, his wife of twenty-eight years, and set out on a round-the-world honeymoon with his new bride.[13] Despite his reputation as a great scientist, the scandal could have ruined him; but it was ruthlessly and effectively suppressed by the imperial government. On his return the Kaiser personally decorated him with the Order of the Crown and Star: he became director of the Institute of Infectious Diseases (soon to be named after him) and travelled to Africa and India, making useful contributions to the aetiology of cholera, typhoid and sleeping sickness. By the early years of the new century he was once again among the most revered international medical figures, the recipient of countless academic and state accolades, including a prize and medal instituted in his honour and named after him by the Pasteur Institute of Paris. In 1905, a little belatedly perhaps, he received the Nobel Prize. He died of a heart attack in Baden-Baden on 27 May 1910, aged sixty-seven.

As if to balance the tuberculin fiasco, its unfolding coincided with another leap forward, a genuine one this time. On the night of 8 November 1895, Wilhelm Conrad Röntgen (1845–1923),[14] professor of physics in the University of Würzburg in Bavaria, was completing a routine investigation into

[12] Hedwig was seventeen when they first met, five years younger than Trudy, Koch's daughter, who had by then married and had left home. One of his letters to Hedwig from Egypt fell into the hands of a newspaper and blackmail was attempted. The details are still obscure and should perhaps remain so.

[13] Koch had purchased the Koch family house in Clausthal a few years earlier: this now went to his wife in their divorce settlement. After Koch's death, Hedwig took a great interest in oriental religions and lived in Japan for a time. She died in 1945.

[14] He was born in the small provincial town of Lennep in the Ruhr. An allegorical statue erected in his memory now stands in front of the house. For a biography, see Glasser, O., *W. C. Röntgen* (Springfield, Illinois, 1945).

phenomena accompanying the passage of an electric current through a vacuum tube. The laboratory was in darkness and the tube was enveloped in black cardboard. Since this was supposed to make it impervious to light, Röntgen was surprised to notice that a few crystals left by accident on the bench some distance away became brilliantly illuminated. He placed them at a greater distance and still they fluoresced. Then he placed materials of varying density between his vacuum tube and the crystals. First he used a book, then a piece of timber, then glass, then various metal objects; and he found that to a lesser or greater degree all were transparent to the newly discovered rays. Finally he placed his own hand into their path and became the first person to see outlined the bones belonging to a living human skeleton.

Röntgen christened the new rays "X-rays" and announced his discovery to the Würzburg Medical Society on 28 December 1895. Within a few months his paper was translated into several languages and, in contrast to most important laboratory discoveries, was immediately hailed as revolutionary. Indeed it created a sensation among the lay public as much as it did in medical circles:[15] a London clothing firm soon advertised "X-ray-proof underclothing for ladies" and Miss Marie Lloyd immortally sang:

> I'm full of daze
> Shock and amaze
> For nowadays
> I hear they'll gaze
> Through cloak and gown and even stays
> Those naughty, naughty Roentgen rays.

Chest X-rays and their lineal successors were to transform the diagnosis of tuberculosis; and the mass X-ray was to become the first and arguably

[15] The *Frankfurter allgemeine Zeitung* carried a front-page report of the Würzburg meeting the following morning; and students organised a torchlight procession in the evening.

[16] He also accepted (though he never used) the ennobling "von" from the King of Bavaria and several honorary doctorates of medicine. On a more sombre note, a Mr Hawkes, demonstrator at the popular roentgenology counter at Bloomingdale Brothers department store in New York reported painful burns – or what seemed like painful burns – on his hands in 1896 after a particularly busy pre-Christmas week. His nails stopped growing and he developed skin scaling. He was transferred to another department and his injuries eventually cleared – at least no more was heard about them – but others were not so lucky. To Röntgen's distress reports of similar and more serious damage from exposure to X-rays began to be published in both the lay and the medical press; and by the first years of the century heavy lead aprons, head-gear and gloves were becoming compulsory among workers with X-rays. Even so several hundred cases of cancer of the skin developed during the first twenty years of radiology, the majority ending fatally. The subject seems never to have been fully explored.

still the most successful screening programme in preventative medicine. Röntgen, an unassuming man, repeatedly refused to patent his discovery (letting others make their millions) but accepted the first Nobel Prize for Physics in 1901.[16]

14

Rest and Fresh Air

No comprehensive monograph chronicles one of the strangest episodes in the history of medicine: the rise, dominance and fall of the tuberculosis sanatoria. Perhaps the subject is too diffuse. Sanatoria varied not only from one country to the other but also from establishment to establishment. Many prided themselves on being unique. Yet they shared more than the name.[1] They subscribed to the same therapeutic approach. They cultivated a common and distinct ethos. The name itself carried a message entirely different from that of hospital, infirmary or convalescent home. Their basic assumptions were identical in the same way as the basic doctrines governing the great houses of different religious orders in the middle ages were identical.

The roots of the movement reached back into Antiquity. Most Greek and Roman shrines catered for short-stay pilgrims. The oracles of Delphi and Dodona were no more prolix (or more informative) than most modern hospital consultants. They would not therefore have qualified as sanatoria in the nineteenth century. A few, however, were equipped to cope with health-seekers for periods of many months. Aretaeus the Cappadocian in particular recommended that those "weak in the lungs" should try a prolonged sojourn in the blessed cypress groves of Apollo's temple of Aquinum (somewhere on the south coast of Anatolia), where the Sun God himself would both comfort them and look after their diseased organs.[2]

In England too there were forerunners. George Bodington's blunt turn of speech antagonised his colleagues; and in his own time the influence of his ideas about fresh air, exercise and wholesome food was therefore slight.[3] More successful and even earlier was the fashionable Quaker physician John

---

[1] Strictly (or pedantically) two names. "Sanatorium" and "sanitarium" were often used interchangeably but their derivation is slightly different, the first from *sanare*, to cure, and the second from *sanitas*, health. The German founding fathers preferred the former, implying that active medical intervention was involved, whereas many early American writers (though not Trudeau), expressing their faith in healthy living rather than in medical skill, often used the latter.

[2] Many inmates in nineteenth- and twentieth-century sanatoria might have suggested that from Sun God to Medical Superintendent was but a small step.

[3] See above, Chapter 5.

Cockley Lettsom, founder of the Royal Sea Bathing Infirmary for Scrofula in Margate. Like many good practical measures, his action was based on a mistaken idea. He was persuaded by a colleague and fellow Quaker, Jonathan Fox Russell, that fishermen never developed scrofula and that scrofulous children sent to the seaside returned to their families after a season of sea-bathing "the tumours of their necks cured and their countenances healthy".[4] Lettsom was already in the habit of dispatching his wealthier clientele to the seaside, and his philanthropic instincts could not bear the thought that what was good for the rich was not available to the poor. (Of the latter he had seen plenty while acting as a voluntary medical attendant to the the Port of London Dispensary.) He chose Margate for his venture, because of the clemency of its climate and its proximity to the city, and established a thirty-six-bedded infirmary (later enlarged to eighty-six beds) in 1791.[5] The building was so designed that patients could sleep on open but protected balconies and could spend most of the day resting or in gentle exercise on the beach. Actual bathing in the sea was encouraged but not compulsory: indeed, the considerable freedom enjoyed by the patients – that is the lack of medical discipline – was probably one reason why the venture got no more than a lukewarm reception.[6]

Sanatoria in the modern sense did not take off till the second half of the nineteenth century; but once launched sanatorium care (as perceived both by the public and the medical profession) became the bedrock of the treatment of tuberculosis. With ups and downs and local variations, it remained unchallenged for nearly a hundred years. It was in some respects a characteristic product of the bourgeois century; but sanatoria survived most other bourgeois certainties, as well as such developments as the discovery of the tubercle bacillus and the devastations of two world wars. Then, after a period of decline lasting barely a decade, they disappeared, their previously unquestioned tenets going under with the buildings and the sales talk. Today their

---

[4] The link between scrofula and consumption was not yet generally recognised.

[5] Lettsom, who founded the Medical Society of London when he was twenty-eight, was also one of the first to come out in support of Jenner's vaccination. Despite his many achievements and admirable character, he is perhaps best remembered for the ditty: "When any sick to me apply, / I physics, bleeds and sweats 'em. / If after that they choose to die, / Why verily – I Lettsom."

[6] Charles Lamb in *The Old Margate Hoy* describes a poor lad on his way to the Infirmary for Sea-Bathing at Margate. "His disease was scrofula which appeared to have eaten all over him. He expressed great hopes for a cure." The journey by foot from London took two days; but it was possible to catch a steamer from Westminster or the Tower of London which did the journey in about six hours. Margate was Turner's favourite resort, as it was that of the Sailor King William IV.

world seems as remote as that of medieval leprosaria or Tibetan lamaseries, and few with dim recollections of their sway have a good word to say in their memory. This is unfair. Of the two guiding principles of sanatorium treatment one at least was a real advance and its total loss today may be a real loss.

Although consumption was, in Bunyan's much-quoted (and much-misquoted) phrase, the Captain of the Men of Death,[7] it was always recognised that occasionally the Captain's advance could be halted: the Captain could even go into reverse. Intelligent pathologists and astute clinicians of the late eighteenth century were familiar with the often fine balance between the active destructive process on the one hand and the forces of natural defence and repair on the other. To quote Bayle's characteristic insight: "While the advance of phthisis is usually inexorable and is in the end almost always fatal, the body's protective mechanisms often seem to lose only by a hair's breadth".[8] The most perceptive of the next generation also realised that, while medical and non-medical miracle workers were never backward in claiming credit for the occasional cure, the credit almost always belonged to the patient's natural resistance, the recuperative power of nature. What the sanatorium ideal proclaimed was that, while medicine could do little on its own, it could help and promote this power by wholesome rest and graduated exercise. At the very least it could ensure that the working of the power was not impeded. It sounded and still sounds obvious. Most great truths do after being recognised. It was profound.

The second principle may have lacked the profundity of the first but it made the first acceptable. Although it was the patient's own body which could and usually did put up a vigorous defence against tuberculosis (as against many other chronic ailments) – far more effective than drugs, bloodletting, purgation and procedures even more drastic – the benefits of rest and graduated exercise were attainable only under strict medical supervision. With hindsight it is questionable how essential or even beneficial this condition was, but there can be no doubt about its political value. It could be argued that the first principle of sanatorium treatment was no more – and no less – than common sense. The second transformed it into medical wisdom. Both were necessary for the idea to prevail.

Even with the medical gloss, the sanatorium movement needed the usual

---

[7] Until comparatively recently no book or review of tuberculosis was complete without it. In *The Life and Death of Mr Badman* John Bunyan wrote: "The captain of all these men of death that came against him to take him away was the Consumption, for it was that that brought him down to the grave." It could have been tuberculosis but it could also have been a dozen other wasting diseases from cancer to pernicious anaemia.

[8] In *Researches on Pulmonary Phthisis*, translated by W. Barrow (Liverpool, 1810).

misapprehensions to get started. Several German and Austrian physicians in
the 1830s and 1840s had suggested that phthisis was caused by the failure of
a small and weak heart to pump the blood forcefully enough to prevent the
deposition of tubercles in the patient's body. Though totally without foundation, the hypothesis made a deep impression on a single-minded medical
student, Hermann Brehmer. Born in Silesia in 1826 (a day after Laënnec's
death),[9] he had been sent by his poor schoolmaster father to study mathematics in Berlin with a view to becoming a teacher himself; but, coming
under the spell of the great physiologist Johannes Müller, he soon switched
to the longer and more arduous study of medicine. In 1853 he devoted his
doctoral dissertation, *The Laws concerning the Beginning and Progress of
Tuberculosis of the Lungs*,[10] to the proposition that at its onset pulmonary
tuberculosis is always and inherently curable. He argued that the smallness
and weakness of the heart of phthisics (of which he claimed to have seen
many examples at post-mortem dissection) could be compensated for by
living above sea level: there the reduced atmospheric pressure would ease
the pumping action of the heart muscle and this in turn would improve the
body's general metabolism, including its capacity to overcome diseases. He
was encouraged in this series of mistaken beliefs not only by his teacher,
Johan Lukas Schönlein (who liked both Brehmer and mountains), but also
by the distinguished explorer Alexander von Humboldt, who assured him
(also mistakenly) that the disease did not exist in mountainous countries.
Most powerful perhaps – if never admitted in later medical texts and scientific
books – was the close, almost mystical association of spiritual and physical
renewal with the mountains. This was one of the most pervasive images to
which German Romanticism had given birth: and it lingered on longer than
most of the movement's other accoutrements. It also spread (though never
with the same force) to other European countries. Popular acclaim for a
medical or scientific concept entirely devoid of experimental basis or empirical proof is always difficult to explain; but Brehmer's extraordinary
success probably owed more to the lyric poetry of Goethe,[11] the songs of

[9] The peasant house where he was born in the small village of Kurtsch still stands and is
now a museum.

[10] *De legibus ab initium atque progressum tuberculosis pulmonum spectatibus.* It was published
in book form in 1857 but was for many years totally ignored. By the time the second edition
was published in 1869, the fame of his settlement at Göbersdorf had spread by word of mouth
and the book remained a best-seller for decades.

[11] Most poignantly perhaps in *Der Wanderer's Nachtlied*, said to have been scratched on
the window pane of a mountain hut by the poet near the end of his life : "Über allen Gipfeln
ist Ruh / In allen Wipfeln spürest du / Kaum einen Hauch./ Die Vöglein schweigen im Walde,
Warte nur balde / Ruhest du auch." It was set to music by Schubert, Schumann, Wolf and
Liszt, among others.

Schubert and the vision of moonlit forests and snow-capped mountain peaks by Caspar David Friedrich than to scientific mumbo-jumbo about metabolic purification.

It certainly owed nothing to official support from the Prussian government, the less inclined to offer help since Brehmer had a sharp tongue and had voiced vaguely democratic sentiments. Fortunately, he also had powerful friends in medical and academic circles; and with their support in 1854 he set up in the village of Göbersdorf in the Bavarian Alps the first sanatorium dedicated to the treatment of pulmonary tuberculosis. The establishment was in fact for some years no more than a group of makeshift wooden chalets; but those admitted followed an elaborate regime of carefully mapped out walks in the forest, monitored daily by Brehmer (or, later, by one of his assistants), coupled with lengthy and measured periods of rest and a simple but nutritious diet based on the fresh spring water of the region.[12]

None of Brehmer's ideas were startlingly new; but while he lacked literary polish, he had (like Freud) a gift for encapsulating the commonplace in an incisive phrase or memorable metaphor. "The two great causes of death in phthisis have nothing to do with the disease itself", he proclaimed: "they are the indiscipline of patients and the carelessness of doctors." He also had a brilliantly inventive mind for seemingly insignificant but captivating details. To make it easier for patients to complete their prescribed walks – not a inch more, not an inch less – he had weatherproof wooden benches fixed into the ground at regular intervals along the forest paths, a bold innovation that was to survive the age of sanatoria and from Yalta to Hampstead Heath and from Kyoto to New York's Central Park still commemorates his obdurate faith.[13]

Like all effective innovators Brehmer was a gifted proselytiser; and it was one of his ex-patients and converts, Dr Peter Dettweiler, who carried his message a stage further. In Dettweiler's sanatorium in Falkenstein in the Rheinland measured periods of rest in sheltered open *Liegehallen* (covered balconies) were added to the carefully graded open-air walks and other forms of exercise. The small heart was now happily forgotten; but, unlike Brehmer, Dettweiler published his results in prestigious medical journals and became a popular speaker at medical conferences. Over a ten-year period starting in 1886 he claimed that, out of 1022 patients who had come and stayed at his sanatorium for more than a month, all of them "confirmed phthisics",

[12] Knopf, S. A., "Hermann Brehmer", *New York State Medical Journal*, 1 (1904), 98.

[13] Ornamental marble benches had of course been a feature of princely gardens since the Renaissance; but their purpose was entirely different from the simple wooden structures along forest paths provided for tired walkers and young lovers free of charge the world over today. The latter benches are Brehmer's legacy.

232 had departed "completely cured" and 310 "cured".[14] It is not clear from
the published works what the difference between the two groups was; nor
did Dettweiler give details of the eighty-nine "relapses" after departure or
of an unstated number who were dead at the time of counting.

The institution which made the deepest impression outside Germany was
Dr Otto Walther's sanatorium in Nordrach in the Black Forest. (By 1910
there were many sanatoria in other countries which had adopted not only
its methods but also its name: Nordrach-in-Wales and Nordrach-on-Mendip
were among them.) This "abode of Spartans" 1500 feet above sea level was
exposed to every wind: the *Liegehallen* were open day and night, summer
and winter, to "dissipate the impure air expired by patients and to allow
them to inhale nature's clean air". Exposure developed the appetite. Walther
was a firm believer in building bodily resistance by overfeeding: each patient
every day had to consume several pints of milk, together with an abundance
of cheese, meat, potatoes, butter, bread, sweets and fruit. "It is amazing",
rejoiced an English convert, "the amount one can eat when forced to." The
three gargantuan main meals of the day were consumed in teams and were
both preceded and followed by one hour's compulsory and complete
rest.[15] Drugs (except morphine for the seriously ill) were forbidden: they
were unnatural and upset the stomach. Patients who were improving were
allowed carefully graduated walks; but otherwise rest was the key to the cure.
Mental exertion was deemed to be potentially as harmful as physical stress:
the Oxford don Jeremiah Prescott asked for a set of Plato's Dialogues to be
sent to him but "could the volume be rebound in a manner suggestive of
light romance?" It might otherwise be summarily confiscated. Walther was
too much of a music-lover – a great admirer of Brahms both as a person
and and as a composer – to forbid the occasional chamber-music concert
or piano recital. Music therefore became a beneficial because soothing part
of the therapeutic regime; but visiting artists, even Rachmaninov (who came
twice), were asked to take their final bow after an hour and a half. The lights
went out at nine, after which the rooms were patrolled by nurses. "The four
highlights of the day", one patient later wrote, "were the times when every
patient took his or her own rectal temperature, a manoeuvre requiring some
skill and practice – too many breakages could lead to mercury poisoning –
and entered the result on an elaborate chart." [16] Dr Walther studied the charts

---

[14] Dettweiler, P., *Lancet* (1886), no. 2, 124.

[15] Today such a diet would be regarded as a crude provocation of the coronary and cerebral
arteries; modern physicians might want to know how many of Walther's cured tuberculous
patients subsequently succumbed to a myocardial infraction or a stroke. Probably none.
Conversely, the idea of jogging would have horrified Walther.

[16] From mercury from broken thermometers readily absorbed through the rectal mucosa.

at length. He spoke to every patient every day: he was even known to listen. He proceeded to a full, unhurried physical examination once every month. Sputa were also regularly cultured.[17]

Nordrach housed a maximum of fifty patients (half of whom were usually English), the most in Walther's opinion who could be adequately supervised by one person. It was extremely expensive and a hundred days of treatment had to be paid for in advance. It never published detailed results and even disdained the then popular booklet of printed testimonials by ex-patients, yet it was always oversubscribed with a waiting list rarely less than a year long. What was its secret? As with most successful sanatoria the question is almost impossible to answer after a lapse of hundred years and the disappearance of its charismatic medical founder, but according to the somewhat acid comment of one inmate the institution provided "a haven for affluent consumptives obsessed with their misfortunes and infatuated with tracing the diurnal variations in their ailment while seeking, through the regime, punishment for having fallen ill".

Although healing establishments of the German type soon sprung up everywhere in Europe,[18] the German model was soon challenged by a country whose very name became (at least to upper- and middle-class tuberculous patients, their families, their friends and their doctors) virtually synonymous with sanatoria. The mountain resorts of Switzerland offered a regime infinitely more benign than those of Germany. Davos in the Grisons led the field and became something of a prototype. A local practitioner, Dr Walter Spengler, first recommended the rather dingy and sunless little village for the treatment of consumptives in the mid 1860s; and for some reason now impossible to fathom German, Dutch, Russian and American patients began to come almost at once. Then came the British, among them the Conan Doyles, Robert Louis Stevenson and John Addington Symonds (to give the place literary glamour),[19] and a sprinkling of minor royalty. Such an invasion of rich or at least comfortably off foreigners launched a building boom of inns, pensions and hotels, many now styling themselves sanatoria. By 1887 the original population of about one hundred had swelled to 3000. Even the small establishments

---

[17] Gibson, J. A., *The Nordrach Treatment* (London, 1901).

[18] Küss in Agincourt and Dumarest in Hauteville pioneered sanatoria in France. Mesnalian and Velefjord in Norway and the sanatoria on the Semmering in Austria all opened around 1900.

[19] Conan Doyle brought his consumptive wife, who stayed for a year. John Addington Symonds later wrote that tuberculosis had given him "a wonderful Indian summer of experience". His vivid account of Davos was first published in the *Pall-Mall Gazette* and partly reprinted in the *British Medical Journal*, 1882, no. 2, 89. Stevenson stayed only for a few months and did not like the place.

had double glazing and central heating but few had resident physicians or strict medical supervision; "the health-giving resinous aroma of the incomparable pine forests, ample and wholesome food, a glass or two of tannin-impregnated wines" but above all the "patients' own wisdom, restraint and self-denial" were expected to do the trick.[20] Four new sanatoria *de grand comfort* – the Angleterre, the Belvedere, the Victoria and the Buol – more or less targeted the British and were in all but name luxury hotels with armies of chambermaids, porters, messenger boys and chasseurs, a staff-guest ratio of about fifteen to one. Even guests like Lady Emily Anderson, used to the gargantuan breakfasts of Edwardian country house parties, found the five main repasts at the Angleterre "almost uplifting in their quality and abundance". The Swiss themselves came as hoteliers, cooks, waiters, teachers, doctors, mountain guides and shopkeepers – but stayed away as patients.

Inevitably and quickly Davos spawned other sanatorium resorts in nearby valleys and villages. St Moritz, formerly an unfashionable spa catering for elderly Swiss dyspeptics, started to develop in the 1880s. Samaden, "very windy but brisk", and Pontresina, "calm and cold because protected by mountains", began by taking the overflow from Davos but soon took off in their own right.[21] Arosa, another formerly poor mountain village with less than one hundred inhabitants, started an open-air school and began to employ English teachers (almost all consumptive) to attract the consumptive children of rich parents: it was sunnier than the rest and acquired the reputation of being more raffish.[22]

Davos nevertheless held its pre-eminence until the First World War: Thomas Mann took his tuberculous wife there as a matter of course and transformed it into the Magic Mountain. (In the public perception the book, a pulpit for philosophical ruminations, remains a monument to Davos in its sanatorium heyday; but few former inmates ever recognised in its pages the atmosphere of the place.)[23] By then the municipality, sensing competition, had canalised the small river which meandered through Davos Dorf;[24]

[20] *Davos Year Book* (1905).

[21] These had been some of the most backward villages of Switzerland (well portrayed in John Knittel's best-selling novel of the 1930s, *Via Mala*), where, until the compulsory addition of iodine to table salt, almost every person had a goitre and cretinism was rife.

[22] Among those seeking a cure there was the German poet, and master of *Galgenhumor*, Christian Morgenstern. His poetry and letters to Margarete Gosebruch von Liechtenstern remain eloquent and moving documents of the tuberculous life. He died in 1914.

[23] The book was written in the early 1920s and it has been suggested that it is emblematic of post-war Europe; but it was supposed to portray Davos in about 1912, the time of Mann's visit.

[24] It improved but did not entirely eliminate the choking mists which in October and November tended to descend on the village. The more expensive sanatoria were built above Davos Dorf, in what came to be called Davos Platz.

hoteliers were ordered to instal proper sewage systems; and, most importantly, a new mountain railway from Landquart eliminated the seven-hour
trip by diligence which had killed many a wan phthisic before they could
even reach the mountain top. Despite its cultivated reputation for liveliness
and luxury, by the turn of the century the graveyards as well as the hotels
were filling up.

Patients who arrived in the Swiss resorts expected to find the clean, still,
cold altitude exhilarating and healing without too much medical meddling;
and many had their expectations fulfilled. John Lowe, medical officer of
health for Wokingham, whose career had seemingly ended at thirty-five with
a massive haemorrhage from the lungs, had tried several English resorts but
continued to lose weight and strength. In 1887 two eminent London colleagues, Dr C. Theodore Williams and Dr Clifford Allbutt, advised him to
try Davos. Within days of his arrival he found that his sleep and appetite
began to improve and his anxiety to abate. Thereafter he gained a pound in
weight each week. After eleven weeks of careful self-management he could
walk sixteen miles a day. He returned to England after nine months with all
the signs of phthisis gone "except for dullness in both lungs". He was lucky,
he believed, partly because he was an early case and partly because he had
held aloof from the dissipations Davos had to offer. The latter were beginning
to detract from – or add to – Davos's allure: "some patients, especially
hopeless cases, were tempted to plunge into a round of parties, drinking,
gambling and worse!", Lowe wrote. "I had witnessed some terrible scenes in
the winter." [25]

Of course none of this came cheap, even though clusters of cheaper chalets
were mushrooming on the slopes behind the luxury establishments. Around
the turn of the century the minimum outlay at a reputable chalet for a
twelve-month stay was the equivalent of two to three thousand pounds. The
bigger sanatoria cost much more. Glossy advertisements emphasised the
quality and abundance of their tables (with sample menus in full) rather
than details of the therapeutic regimes or cure rates. Extras were numerous
and expensive, ranging from meals in one's room and private bathrooms to
regular specialist consultations. Periodic disinfection of one's room was also
an extra. Most of the senior medical staff were owners or co-owners, assisted
by underpaid and almost invariably tuberculous juniors; and competition
between the leading sanatoria was intense. The high cost had its advantages:

[25] Lowe, J., *Lancet* (1888), no. 2, 513. Not everybody among London's top tuberculosis doctors
approved of Swiss mountain resorts. Sir William Jenner advised John Addington Symonds to
spend his winters on the Nile, after passing no more than a few weeks in the Alps as a
preliminary tonic. When Symonds decided to stay in the mountains, Jenner wrote to him: "If
you like to leave your vile body to the Davos doctors, that is your affair. I have warned you."

as Countess Anny Andrássy reported back to her parents in Hungary "one meets a good class of people here, quite unlike those in the sanatoria at home or in the Tatra: even a few maharajas".[26]

In addition to being of good class, the sanatorium population in Davos and Arosa were also for the most part young and ambulant (at least on arrival: hoteliers and the doctors did not like admitting bedridden patients). They were isolated at the top of the world – "*bei uns oben*" – with nothing to do except have daily but perfunctory medical checks and temperature readings, shop in the expensive shops, consume delicious cream cakes, organise concerts and amateur theatricals, go for long walks or sleigh-rides, collect stamps, play cards, flirt, gossip, quarrel and make up. Mammoth jig-saw puzzles were popular.[27]

The First World War cut the British ties and these were never fully restored. (Germans became the dominant national group after the war and remained so until the end of the Second World War.) During the Depression the Swiss resorts were beyond the means of all but the most affluent or successfully criminal; and British physicians obliged with deeply scientific reasons for staying at home. Dr John Bain spoke for many of his colleagues in the British Medical Association when he asserted that the weather in Davos, even in the summer, was worse than the weather in Inverness; and that Britons, delicate Britons especially, did better in the climate to which they were accustomed: his own patients, for example, did very well in South Shields.[28]

By the late 1920s – but especially after the New York stockmarket crash of 1929 – commercial interests behind the sanatorium industry began to sense that the pre-eminence of Switzerland in the field of nursing and burying the tuberculous rich might not last forever. Increasing effort and capital was then invested into developing and selling the old healing resorts as unrivalled venues for winter sports and related junketings. Despite the economic gloom and political uncertainty the transformation was, like most Swiss commercial ventures, conducted with unobtrusive efficiency: soon the perils and delights of the Parsenn and the Suvrettabahn became as famous among the Orient-Express set as the cleansing properties of the air had been to the generation

---

[26] Unpublished letter to Countess Geraldine Andrássy, 1905.

[27] A guide book compiled by Dr J. Weber, published in Davos in 1880, expressed the view that "Consumption has always been too timorously, too leniently, too indulgently dealt with. Parents and doctors united to soothe the patient at Rome, and when the last stage was drawing nigh, sent him to end his or her sadly useless life, fittingly in some remote region. Davos demands qualities the very opposite of resigned sentimentalism ... Here is no place for weak and despairing resignation ... here you are not pusillanimously helped to die." Many died nevertheless.

[28] Bain, L., *British Medical Journal* (1922), no. 2, 875.

before them. Nor were the medical facilities wasted: in an increasingly competitive field the uniquely efficient casualty departments for dealing with fractured skulls, hips and spines remained among the special draws of the Swiss skiing resorts.

There was another strand to the Swiss sanatorium culture aimed at a cosmopolitan and wealthy clientele which survived longer and which had its origin not in Switzerland but in Denmark. Niels Ryberg Finsen (1860–1904) was a lecturer in anatomy in the University of Copenhagen when he developed an interest in the effects of light on diseases of the skin. That sunlight could have a dramatically healing action on skin lesions had been known to Arab physicians and probably earlier; but in Europe the effect was feared rather than sought: indeed, until well into the twentieth century, the danger of exposing white skin to direct sunlight was one of the most deeply embedded medical notions of the European middle and upper classes. Finsen realised that "sunlight" was an omnibus term which covered a wide spectrum of radiations and that under certain conditions and carefully controlled some forms might be useful as well as dangerous. His researches soon led him to the ultraviolet end of the spectrum. To study its action he constructed a special lamp, subsequently known by his name, which both concentrated and cooled the rays. His first interest was in the natural history of smallpox pustules but inevitably – tuberculosis had killed several of his own family – he then turned to lupus vulgaris, tuberculosis of the skin. In some forms of this comparatively rare but destructive disease ultraviolet irradiation proved extraordinarily effective, the first successful specific treatment of any kind of tuberculosis.[29] For his discovery he was awarded the Nobel Prize two years before he died; and an institute dedicated to tuberculosis research in Copenhagen was named in his memory.[30]

A less immediate consequence of Finsen's researches was the development of heliotherapy, the treatment not only of skin but also of other

[29] Henri Vignal, who demonstrated the extraordinary resistance of the tubercle bacillus to drying, cold and mechanical crushing, also showed that the organism was quickly and irreversibly destroyed by exposure to sunlight.

[30] He died of constrictive pericarditis, a painful condition in which the heart is progressively constricted by a thickening pericardium. Many, perhaps most, cases in his day were of tuberculous origin. Water and salt retention with oedema were a feature and, throughout his illness, Finsen kept a meticulous record about his water and salt balance. Published after his death it became a valuable guide in the development of intravenous fluid replacement therapy.

Both heliotherapy and phototherapy have now virtually disappeared from the medical repertory; but Finsen's researches stimulated much later and still relevant work on the effects of radiation on cells and bacteria. The institute named after him is now dedicated to medical, rather than specifically to tuberculosis, research.

non-pulmonary forms of tuberculosis, mainly tuberculosis of the bones and joints, by exposure to sunlight. Its apostle was a Swiss, Auguste Rollier, a gifted publicist and entrepreneur as well as a doctor who probably believed in what he preached and who certainly succeeded in communicating his faith to some of his patients. To put his ideas into practice in a country already dotted with fiercely competing mountain *Kurorte*,[31] he chose a plateau above the upper Rhone at a level considerably higher than had been recommended in the past for tuberculosis and exposed to more and more intense sunlight than any other mountain resort. Arriving in Leysin by funicular from Aigle was indeed an awesome experience for anyone not familiar with the combination of brilliant sunshine and glittering snow, the air pure, the silence almost palpable. Here under Rollier's aegis row upon row of sanatoria dedicated to sun worship sprang up, their white clifflike simplicity hardly disturbing the starkness and stillness of the landscape. They catered for every purse – that is every purse above a substantial minimum – but all had open balconies facing south and there patients, clad in loin cloths or short shifts, spent most of the day. A high proportion of them were seriously ill, neither capable of nor perhaps wanting to indulge in the social whirl of Davos or Arosa; shops and restaurants were few.

Although Rollier never published statistics, he had devoted followers among eminent doctors both in Switzerland and abroad, especially in eastern Europe. Until the end of the 1940s, even during the war years, his sanatoria were always full. (Leysin was never regarded as ideal for winter sports.) Unlike the grand hotels for the tuberculous in Davos, they were equipped with the latest in X-ray and laboratory facilities, they had pioneering physiotherapy departments, and they were well staffed with nurses and doctors. They also accepted non-tuberculous patients suffering from chronic debilitating conditions.[32] One drawback (or the reverse) of the high altitude was that once patients were acclimatised they found returning to anywhere near sea-level difficult, even impossible. By the 1930s there was a cluster of chalets, as well as several churches and a school, behind the sanatoria for those fit enough to abandon sanatorium care, or unable to bear the cost, but incapable of descending from the mountains.

It was from Leysin that the young Rumanian pianist, Dinu Lipatti, dying from leukemia as well as tuberculosis,[33] descended for his last public concert

[31] There were 325 registered sanatoria in Switzerland in 1946.

[32] Rollier, A., *The Healer: How to Fight Tuberculosis*, translated by A. E. Glogue and M. Yearsley (London, 1925).

[33] Tuberculosis often developed as an opportunistic infection in patients suffering from some other debilitating illness such as leukemia, pernicious anaemia or, most commonly, diabetes mellitus (see below, Chapter 21). Lipatti was also on cortisone for his leukemia, now

in nearby Besançon in September 1950. After the concert he was rushed back to Aigle and a special funicular took him gasping for breath back to Leysin in the early hours of the morning.[34]

(but not then) a recognised cause for the flare-up and rapid dissemination of previously quiescent tuberculosis.

[34] The Bensançon concert was recorded and is now one of the classics of the gramophone. Lipatti, who was then thirty-three, gave one more recital in the sanatorium for fellow inmates, a few visitors who happened to be about and nurses and doctors: to many of them it would remain one of life's enduring memories. After finishing the last item, the Mozart Sonata in A minor, K 310, he looked totally exhausted and was about to rise when he heard the sound of sobbing from the audience. He immediately sat down again and, turning to the keyboard, launched into rousing medley of Gershwin and the Charleston, ending with a free fantasia on the *Rhapsody in Blue*. Everybody began to laugh and clap. He died five days later on 2 December 1950.

15

Under English Skies

After visiting a clutch of German cousins in their *Schloss* the Duke of Cambridge, Commander in Chief of the British Army,[1] and his travelling companion and personal physician, Dr Archie Munro, decided on an unscheduled visit to a newly established colony in the Black Forest, a kind of cranky spa, dedicated to the open-air treatment of tuberculosis. They arrived in Nordrach, on 9 June 1889, and were welcomed by the director, Dr Walther. "It was one of those perfect days of early summer, the crystalline air heavy with the scent of pine forests, the merest haze in the distance enfolding blue mountains", Dr Munro later recorded. They were treated to a "substantial but not too heavy breakfast" and then taken on a leisurely but invigorating tour of the cottages. "There, on open porches and verandahs patients reposed in peace and quiet, soaking up the sun on comfortable *Liegestühle*, some dozing, some reading, some merely admiring the incomparable view."

> Dr Walther knew them all by name, exchanged a few words with those not dozing, carefully checked their medical charts and gave us, where appropriate, a brief medical history. We then followed one of the winding path ... on a circular tour, meeting more patients as they made their unhurried rounds in one direction or the other or sat on wooden benches installed at intervals along the footpaths. Permeating the establishment was a kind of tranquillity that was by no means languorous or effete but rather full of vitality and optimism ... "A capital place this!" the Duke exclaimed as soon as we had bade our farewells to the ebullient Dr Walther and I could not but agree that it was capital ... at least much superior to any establishment for consumptives I have seen in Britain or even in Germany. "We should have such sanatoria in England", the Duke said, "and even in Scotland !" A quick learner and no mean linguist and classical scholar he had already familiarised himself with the name. I agreed and undertook to alert my colleagues to the development.[2]

It is difficult to say how far the Duke of Cambridge or Dr Munro were personally responsible for the sanatorium idea catching on in Britain; but catch on it did. The Royal Victoria Hospital of Edinburgh for the open-air

---

[1] He was Queen Victoria's second cousin and took a lively interest in the medical welfare of the troops. The military hospital in Aldershot was named after him.

[2] Munro, Sir H., *Memoirs of a Doctor* (Edinburgh, 1898), p. 98.

treatment of pulmonary tuberculosis opened in 1894; the National Hospital for Consumption in Newcastle, County Wicklow, in 1896; and a Glasgow philanthropist, William Quarrier, became the moving spirit behind the Consumption Sanatorium of Scotland at Bridge of Weir, Renfrewshire, in 1897. The institution which attracted most attention, however, and which under its first superintendent, Dr Marcus Paterson, gave the sanatorium movement in England a characteristic English flavour, was the outdoor extension of the Brompton Hospital at Frimley, Surrey.[3]

Soon after his appointment in 1903 Paterson came to the conclusion that many patients who had been employed in heavy manual labour until shortly before their admission had remained in remarkably good general health. From this he argued that if patients "under adverse circumstances and without the benefit of medical guidance could act thus without apparent injury they might, under ideal conditions and with their work graduated according to their physical state, be able to undertake useful labours". Instead of the leisurely walks of the German pioneers, he proposed that

> manual work should be of great advantage to patients undergoing treatment in a sanatorium, as, first, it would do much to meet the objections that members of the working class are liable to have their energy sapped and to acquire lazy habits; second, it would make them more resistant to the disease by improving their physical condition; and third, it would enable them by its effect on their muscles to return to their work immediately after their discharge.[4]

This was of course relevant mainly to the non-paying patients, 75 per cent of the projected total, who were to be referred to Frimley by the staff of the Brompton Hospital; but it might also appeal to some of those admitted privately at the very reasonable fee of twenty-five shillings a week.

With this in mind, Paterson devised a complex system of grades of work from carrying baskets of mould for the sanatorium lawns to the wielding of a pickaxe for felling trees. Soon another rationale behind this regime took shape. This was a reversal of the usual order of things. In medicine mistaken observations often lead to practical measures which for the wrong reasons prove beneficial. In Paterson's case a correct observation helped to germinate a practical course wholly devoid of merit. What Paterson noted was that many patients developed a temperature and began to relapse when put to work. To explain this he conceived the hare-brained idea that physical work led to "self-inoculation with the patients' own tuberculin". Instead of being interpreted as a warning sign, the rise in temperature then became evidence

---

[3] Paterson, M. S., *Lancet* (1908), no. 1 , 216; Bignall, J. R., *Frimley: The Biography of a Sanatorium* (London, 1979).

[4] Paterson, M. S., *Lancet* (1908), no. 1, 216.

of this self-inoculation. Most importantly, as a result of self-inoculation the patients' "recovery and progress after being put back to bed was more rapid than usual".[5] "Recovery no, progress yes: but progress to the grave", the eminent London cardiologist Dr Jenner Hoskin commented – but *sotto voce* and long after autoinoculation was safely buried. At the time Paterson was hailed as an endearingly eccentric genius, England's answer to Koch.

To achieve a cure Paterson's regime required "absolute obedience to medical orders regulating the amount of work to be done".[6] Walks were prescribed to the yard up to ten miles a day: patients were instructed to carry pebbles in their pockets to help them count the rounds. From walks men graduated to breaking stones with light hammers, from hoeing with light hoes to digging with large spades, from carrying bundles of sticks to manhandling logs. The final grades were intended to be physically more demanding than anything the patients might afterwards encounter while earning their living.

Rebellion was not encouraged: "obdurate cases were sent to the superintendent's office where they waited in fear and trepidation expecting instant dismissal".[7] Paterson noted with surprise that more women rebelled and were dismissed than men, the more remarkable since, as a matter of policy, Frimley reserved two-thirds of its places for men. This was "partly because bread-winners needed the cure more than wives and partly because they were more single-minded in striving for it".[8] The policy did not significantly unbalance the waiting list: woman applicants were always fewer. They were, the governors stated, "apparently more reluctant to leave their children and husbands and more antagonistic to sanatorium life". Women were also "notoriously more prone not only to disobey regulations but also to suddenly discharge themselves regardless of their health when they learnt even of trifling upsets at home, like a child breaking a leg or playing truant at school".[9] While Paterson made little effort to detain them – he would have preferred to run an all-male establishment – he was unforgiving to men who, against his advice, insisted on taking their own discharge. "Tell your widow to stay in touch with us", was his parting instruction to one such delinquent, "We need the details of your death for our records." The sexes were of course strictly segregated, taking their meals, exercises and Sunday devotions separately.

As in other sanatoria catering for the lower orders, alcohol was totally if not always successfully banned. Also like other sanatoria, Frimley was

---

[5] Paterson, M. S., *Autoinoculation in Pulmonary Tuberculosis* (London, 1920).

[6] Ibid., p. 248. After 1920 the concept was quietly allowed to wither away.

[7] Paterson, M. S., *The Shibboleths of Tuberculosis* (London, 1920), p. 52.

[8] Worthington T., ed., *Brompton Hospital Report, 1905-1910* (London, 1911), p. 82.

[9] Ibid., p. 122.

continually battling against the tendency of patients to wander outside the beautiful but difficult to guard grounds. This was worrying not for fear that harm might befall them but because it hardened local hostility to the establishment. Most villages near sanatoria feared the "lungers", especially when they tried to visit pubs and left their lip-prints on the glasses.[10] Frimley patients could leave the grounds only on producing a signed pass (not easily obtained) which read:

> I beg to ask permission to go for a walk outside the Sanatorium grounds on ... from ... to ... (state exact times). If granted this privilege I promise to carefully observe all the rules and directions of the medical staff. I also promise not to enter a public house. I understand that in the event of my breaking this rule I may be dismissed at once from the Sanatorium.[11]

Inside the sanatorium daily life was "admirably regulated for the benefit of all". Each patient was allocated his or her numbered eating utensils and told to use those alone. He or she was responsible for washing them after each meal with his or her numbered tea towel. This was perhaps less than arduous since the meals were frugal. Handkerchiefs too were numbered and allotted individually, though, in common with other English sanatoria, the management did not provide – or impose – uniforms.

> In practice this meant that the poorer patients – the majority – continued to wear their one good serge suit or worsted dress and the pair of pyjamas or nightgowns they brought with them ... Since the outdoor life was mandatory they soon began to look frowsy, their clothes always damp and muddy, the women's hair straggly from being blown and wet ... Their breath stank; their bodies were slimy from the night sweats. Bored, tired, strictly non-responsible for themselves most of them "felt TB" – "Totally Bitched".[12]

Because Frimley was relatively well funded, it could provide adequate nursing for difficult or febrile patients, or for those who coughed up much blood and were therefore judged to be in need of complete immobilisation. The objective of this regime was to "reduce lung activity": patients lay on their sides and were forbidden to move, read, wash themselves, go to the lavatory, talk, indulge in "unnecessary coughing" or receive visitors who might "evoke argument, crying or even laughter". Their food was cut up and fed to them or sucked through a straw. Cocaine sprays were used to ease the swallowing. Such periods were supposed to last for one week at the most but often lasted longer. To ease the aching hours, especially at night or after

---

[10] As a result many later sanatoria were deliberately sited to be as inaccessible as possible by public transport.

[11] Quoted in Smith, F. B., *The Retreat of Tuberculosis, 1850–1950* (London, 1988), p. 116.

[12] Ibid., p. 120.

"useful but painful" intramuscular injections of calcium chloride and galvanic cautery to the larynx, morphia and heroin were freely prescribed.

The early results Paterson claimed for Frimley looked impressive on paper, though they were always difficult to verify and are today almost impossible to understand. Of the 297 patients admitted from the Brompton Hospital before the end of 1908 197 had been discharged in "working capacity", forty-three were "improved or stationary", two had died and fifty-five "left early", often because of insubordination. Three years later only 246 of the 297 patients were "well and able to work", nineteen were "at home" and thirty-one were dead. A count of patients discharged through a later five-year period, 1912–17, showed that 37 per cent were "well and at work", 14 per cent were "alive" and the remaining 46 per cent were dead. It was never officially admitted that all cases referred from the Brompton Hospital had been carefully vetted beforehand for their promise of recovery and their likelihood of adjusting to Frimley.[13] They were "of the better working-class type of the London area, respectful and orderly in character" and had "clean and careful homes to support them after their return". None were in an advanced state of the illness. How the Frimley authorities determined "well" and "better" and "at work" is uncertain: it would probably be factually correct to say that about half the patients survived after their discharge and were able to find work for five years or more; and that, by and large, their chances in life would not have been significantly worse had they never set foot in the Brompton Hospital or in Frimley.

If the advantages that accrued from Paterson's regime to patients remained problematic, the sanatorium benefited hugely. "The patients, even those previously engaged in clerical and sedentary occupations, have carried out much useful work", Powell and Hartley's authoritative textbook stated.[14] "A reservoir capable of holding 500,000 gallons has been excavated and concreted. Trees have been cut into firewood. The main building has been painted, a kitchen garden has been trenched and cultivated and the grounds have been kept in order." To put it more crudely, it was estimated that patients did among other things the work of four gardeners, two window-cleaners, two general repairs men, a firewood supplier and a poultry keeper: or, as the governors of the Brompton Hospital reported in 1920 with some satisfaction, they saved the hospital (which was supported entirely by voluntary contributions) about £3000 per year in wages and some £1000 in capital outlay, both large sums at the time.[15] It must also be added that

[13] Keers, R. Y, *Pulmonary Tuberculosis* (London, 1978), p. 104.
[14] Powell, D., Hartley, P. H. S., *Diseases of the Lungs and Pleurae* (London, 1921), p. 624.
[15] Trelaine, J. ed., *Brompton Hospital Report, 1920* (London, 1920).

Paterson was a charismatic leader as well as a delightful luncheon guest at the Athenaeum; and when he reported in one of his papers that "there was little grumbling: most of the patients were justifiably proud of their achievement" he was probably not far removed from the truth.[16]

Frimley with its distinctive ethos and well-orchestrated publicity was unusual. The rapid spread of other less well-known sanatoria in England ended decades of muddled thinking, paralysis and despair about how to cope with tuberculosis. In 1900 those who could not afford private treatment either at home or abroad could seek admission to one of the specialised hospitals: they had grown from the London four to about ten, including ones in Liverpool, Manchester and Newcastle-upon-Tyne. In contrast, there was no provision of any kind in Birmingham, Leeds or Bradford, and none in Wales. By 1910 sixty-one public and twenty-nine private or semiprivate sanatoria in England and Wales offered a nominal 4000 beds, of which around 2800 were classified by independent inspectors as efficient.[17] In fact they varied from basic or worse to elaborate and even comfortable, mirroring the country's class structure.

The barest and most numerous establishments were offshoots of the Poor Law infirmaries.[18] They were funded by local authorities on medical prompting as a way of concentrating tuberculous patients – at least tuberculous men – and reducing the chances of infection and nursing difficulties in the workhouse. Small trade unions and trade associations often erected special isolation huts in the grounds of infirmaries, much as they used to do during the typhoid and smallpox outbreaks of the past. Larger and more affluent unions founded self-contained and self-sufficient clusters of pavilions outside the towns. These tried to implement something of the Nordrach ideal.

Heswall in Liverpool set a kind of pattern.[19] The men were admitted through the workhouse and slept in dormitories. Food, heating and bedding was provided: strict economy was claimed to advance the curative process. Like all English sanatoria, the institution was conceived as preventative rather than curative: it was to admit only early cases, heal them, make them fit for employment and keep them off the rates. Since early cases were by definition ambulant – that is capable of dressing and feeding themselves – nursing requirements were deemed to be minimal. The policy never worked: most consumptives entered the workhouses only because their ambulant stage had passed. On the other hand, even exercising extreme economy,

[16] Paterson, *Lancet*, no. 1, 216.

[17] *Tuberculosis Year Book* (London, 1912–13), 89.

[18] Manby, E. P., Seymour, F. R., *Report on the Poor Law Infirmaries and Tuberculosis* (London, 1923); Ministry of Health. PRO, MH 55/145, 23.

[19] Marriott, C. L., *Heswall* (Liverpool, 1956).

Heswall was too expensive to have beds kept empty waiting for "suitable young men ... likely to derive some permanent benefit from early treatment", and increasingly the beds were filled with the more advanced and terminal cases. Inexorably, like most Poor Law sanatoria, the establishment became a staging post of the dying. By the end of 1904 of the thirty-eight cases transferred from the workhouse during the previous year eight had been "lost", twenty-six were "dead", "dying" or had been been discharged, or had discharged themselves (inevitably to end up in the workhouse again where the company was better and supervision less strict), one had died of alcoholism, one had died at home and one survivor had been arrested. Sanatorium statistics never quite added up and the above leaves one admission silently unaccounted for.

Heswall and institutions like it provided food, a roof and a bed for the starving, the friendless and the homeless. They may have helped to contain the infection in the community; but they made no pretence at providing treatment, let alone the prospect of cure. By 1909 44 per cent of all London male and 32 per cent of all female tuberculous deaths occurred in such Poor Law sanatoria: the average survival after the patient's last admission was 133 days. (In Dublin the corresponding figure was seventy days.) [20] Later these establishments benefited from Lloyd George's 1911 National Insurance Act which required local government boards to contribute to their upkeep; but this provision ended in 1921, just when the influx of 35,000 tuberculous ex-servicemen, about half of whom were in public sanatoria, was crushing the system. The treatment costs, but not capital works, were then underwritten by the new Ministry of Pensions; but that support too was discontinued in 1924.

Easby sanatorium near Skipton, built by the Bradford Guardians, aimed at patients slightly higher in the social scale than the clientele of Heswall. Inspired by Nordrach, it housed its inmates in largely unheated temporary wooden pavilions divided into wards. Since it had no sewage system patients were required daily to excavate and cover earth closets. Medically, the Guardians reported, the main difficulties were the endemic sore throats and stomach upsets.[21]

The Hull and East Riding sanatorium was partly maintained by subscribers, mostly by enlightened employers who could nominate patients on payment of a £13 admission fee. Once admitted, inmates could stay for three months, generally recognised as too short, but as long a stretch as even enlightened employers could be expected to keep jobs open for recovered invalids. They

[20] *Report of the Medical Officer of Health for the London County Council* (London, 1909), 60.
[21] *Tuberculosis Year-Book* (London, 1913–14), 234.

were not in fact numerous. Of the 183 discharged between 1902 and 1905 only twenty-three maintained some improvement or did not not actually deteriorate by 1907: the rest were "worse", "dead" or "unaccounted for".[22]

Some institutions made an effort to make use of what were conceived as scientific and medical advances. At Maiden Lane Sanatorium in Manchester, previously a smallpox hospital, tuberculin was administered and inhalations of antiseptics were prescribed in suitable cases. Maiden Lane was also unusual in having two of its five pavilions reserved for women and children. The children received lessons and "musical societies kindly assisted at giving concerts". Even here sewage was emptied into local streams which were soon blocked. They were still blocked in 1926.[23]

Keiling in Norfolk and Barrasford near Newcastle-upon-Tyne were typical of sanatoria created by private, mostly London-based, charities. Their proclaimed aim was to "intercept" tuberculosis "in medically suitable [that is early] patients on their way to pauperdom". Patients had their fare, dressing gown, slippers and toiletries paid for by the society; they shared two-bedded cubicles clustered in pavilions built of unheatable, uninsulated concrete slabs. Between the walls and the ceiling there was a three-inch wide unblockable gap. The mainstay of the active treatment was exposure to the sun (when available) in board and canvas shelters. "Visiting members of the Society also provided much cheer." The average length of stay was three months set by the £18–20 maximum allocated to each referral. Keiling pioneered the system of putting patients to work which came to full bloom in the later village settlements. Skilled workers were encouraged to stay.[24]

The Devon and Cornwall sanatorium at Didworthy was created by subscribers in 1903 for "necessitous patients" but, prompted by the Reverend John Clark, the board was exceptional in declaring that it would also admit "hopeless cases". The latter were never welcome and many were discharged when their death was imminent. "These unfortunates died twice", Dr Arthur Latham observed, "their true death being preceded by the moment when they were arbitrarily sent home." [25]

In England only one self-help project, as distinct from charitable or private enterprises, achieved institutional form. Benenden was inspired by the German insured workers' sanatoria and funded by the Post Office Workers Union. They hoped that other unions – the Teachers and Railway Servants and the Hearts of Oak Friendly Society in particular – might join them. They

[22] Bullstrode, H. T., *Report on Sanatoria for Consumption* (London, 1908).
[23] Manchester Health Corporation Reports, January 1926, PRO, MH 52/343.
[24] Lister, T. D., *Lancet* (1911), no. 1, 738.
[25] Latham, A., Garland, C. H., *The Conquest of Tuberculosis* (London, 1910), 59.

never did. Benenden's declared purpose was as much to educate as to cure.[26] By 1910 40,000 Post Office employees had sought cover at 2s. a year, deducted at headquarters from their wages. This entitled them to a six-month stay if the need arose, on full pay and with travel and establishment expenses. Benenden did well, mainly perhaps because Post Office workers were hand-picked with a relatively low tuberculosis rate of about 1.8 per 1000. There were only 153 admissions during the six-year period leading up to 1910 and no waiting list. Surplus beds were taken up by local authorities and funding was available to employ a full-time medical officer. The food was ample. Patients did graduated work around the grounds and attended lectures on hygiene and other improving topics. Benenden maintained an approximately 80 per cent discharge rate "fit for duty", a credible figure even though no information is available about subsequent relapses. Its achievement was quoted (with slight cosmetic distortion) by Lloyd George in his parliamentary oration in support of his National Health Insurance scheme.[27]

Some sanatoria for white-collar workers, such as teachers, insurance clerks and low-grade civil servants, a notch at least above the employees who entered Benenden, were show-cases of private or corporate philanthropy. Pinewood Sanatorium in Wokingham in Berkshire was opened in 1904, its Edwardian baroque facade a visible expression of the public-spirited munificence of the diamond cartel of Wernher, Beit and Co. By 1913 it contained sixty-four rooms heated by radiators, a bold innovation; it housed two resident physicians and boasted an X-ray appliance before the First World War. (It was used to select desirable early cases rather than to monitor patients' progress.) Walking in the grounds rather than manual work was the basis of the physical exercise prescribed as part of the therapeutic regime: the institution could exist without the extra income generated by the cheap labour of patients. Even so, in 1932 50 per cent of discharged patients were dead within five years and another 25 per cent were unfit for employment.[28]

Crossley at Frodsham in Cheshire, endowed by the engineering magnate Sir William Crossley, was a less wealthy cousin of Pinewood. It too had an imposing three-storey main block with a colonnade, on which a substantial proportion of the original endowment had been spent, and well-maintained grounds with an artificial lake. Ten out of the hundred beds were for poorer patients subsidised by Manchester Corporation. Every self-respecting sanatorium, even those for the very poor, had a kind of house speciality: in Crossley it was hydrotherapy. This meant frequent showers, baths, wet

[26] Ibid., p. 76; *Transactions of NAPT* (1909), 36.
[27] *Parliamentary Debates*, July 12 1911, vol. 28, col. 421.
[28] *Tuberculosis Year Book* (London, 1913–14), 201.

blankets and the actual drinking of the local spring water: according to Dr James Cross, the medical superintendant, all this "promoted the healthy action of the skin in eliminating effete material". Visitors – not more than two at a time and no children – were allowed for two hours on the last Saturday of each month, the usual allowance for sanatoria. Breaking sanatorium rules (such as the unauthorised perusal of reading matter) entailed the prompt withdrawal of visiting privileges. Private patients could receive visitors more frequently.[29]

In addition to pioneering hydrotherapy Crossley also advertised that the floors were covered with linoleum, "a new, polishable impervious material which makes it possible to guard against the fluff and dust in the joints of floorboards notorious for enfolding dried sputum and preserving the bacilli". It was a foretaste of the great lino boom of the 1920s and 1930s and indeed of the effect of sanatorium design on everyday life. More than a decade before Bauhaus produced its sophisticated simplicities sanatorium doctors and architects were working on eliminating hiding places for dust, producing shapes and textures that were to become part of the modern movement and still dominate styles in the 1990s. Ceilings were stripped of mouldings; picture rails, pelmets, window ledges, carved head-pieces of wardrobes were jettisoned. The much-prized textured wall-papers, which collected organisms and dirt, were replaced with renewable or washable paint usually of a pale neutral colour. Plush curtains gave way to wipeable Venetian blinds which could also be adjusted to admit more sunlight. The Victorian profusion of objets d'art, commemorative china, mementoes of the Raj, ornamental ferns and elaborately framed pictures on walls, side-tables, piano-tops and mantelpieces, and the jumble of dust-collecting, hard-to-shift furniture with their velvet drapes and lace covers, began their stately migration into the storerooms of the burgeoning antique trade.

Sanatoria also changed personal habits and fashions. Sanatorium doctors instructed male patients to shave off their beards and trim their moustaches to a thin line in order to avoid catching phlegm from their cough This seemed the more radical since one reason for growing bushy beards in Victorian times was partly to guard the chest and to make it easier to draw breath. Consumptive women were told to bob their hair, wear lighter dress material and raise their hems above ankle level to avoid gathering dust. It was a welcome change.

What induced the Wernhers, the Crossleys, the Beits and the Cassels (but not the Cecils, the Percies, the Grosvenors or the Seymour-Conveys)[30] to

---

[29] Ibid., p. 203.
[30] Who presumably disapproved of such ostentatious charity outside the family.

invest in sanatoria was a new development: for the first time around the turn of the century tuberculosis became a fashionable target for philanthropy. In 1898 the Prince of Wales had been induced to take an interest in consumption: "if preventable why not prevented" became a widely quoted pithy royal wisdom. (The phrase was cribbed from William Withering, the discoverer of digitalis; but original pithy royal wisdoms were always in short supply.) Later the King's banker and financial adviser, Sir Ernest Cassel, donated £250,000 towards the initial cost of a sanatorium in Midhurst in Sussex to be named after the portly monarch; and the famous-to-be establishment was opened by the King Emperor with all pomp and circumstance in 1906. It was intended for officers of the army and navy, clergymen, civil servants and teachers, "ladies and gentlemen in the early stages of the disease whose means do not permit of their becoming inmates of one of the private sanatoria" but "who cannot conveniently make use of public institutions". Applicants who had been in domestic service or were obviously working class were excluded, although an exception was made for the under-housekeeper of the Duke of Devonshire. The usual fee was two guineas a week. (Some of the 104 beds were originally reserved for those who might be able to pay four guineas and upwards, but patients who could afford that kind of money usually went to Davos or Mentone.)

Midhurst was a cross between Nordrach and a minor public school. The sound of a gong at approximately half-hourly intervals, starting at 7.30 a.m. ("Patients rise; take temperatures per rectum; proceed to hydrotherapy bath"), signalled every meal-time and treatment or leisure period. The gong at 9 a.m. announced the opening of the library for half an hour: it was well stocked – but exciting and taxing books and books on tuberculosis were excluded. The gong at noon instructed patients to proceed directly to their bedrooms or balconies for an hour's rest: "talking strictly forbidden". The gong at 2 o'clock signalled the beginning of the period devoted to the weaving of raffia bags and coverlets, tray making, basket weaving, crochet work for coat hangers, doilies and men's ties, hand-painting of shoe-trees and other useful and diverting craftwork as prescribed for individual patients. (Painting by numbers did not come in until after the Second World War.) A last gong at 9.30 p.m. commanded patients to repair to their rooms: all lights were extinguished at 10 p.m.[31]

By the 1920s the originally targeted class of patients had largely ceased to apply and "with some reluctance" the managers began to admit "clerks, shop assistants, commercial travellers and low-grade civil servants of good character". The period of stay was shortened from over six to four or five months.

[31] Smith, E. B., *The Retreat of Tuberculosis* (London, 1988), p. 132.

The medical superintendent, Dr Noel Bardswell, was slightly less sanguine about the results than most of his colleagues: he calculated that those discharged in the first stage of the disease had one-sixth of the life expectancy of a healthy person of the same age and those discharged in the second stage one-twentieth.[32]

The only sanatorium in England designed for the rich who did not want to travel or were advised against it was Mundesley on the coast of Norfolk. Begun in 1899 as a private venture by a consortium of doctors, it prospered almost from the start. By 1903 the minimum weekly rate for the thirty-seven guests (rather than patients) was five guineas a week; and, although the prospectus insisted on a strict medical regime, the "comforts of life and the curative effect of cheerfulness were not forgotten". Mundesley early acquired an X-ray machine and was quickly into chest surgery; but the main source of recuperation was arguably the food: it was excellent and varied, "the table forming the subject of the medical director's constant personal attention". A golf course was available for health-giving exercise, the only sanatorium in England to be so equipped. Mundesley never published medical statistics but by the early 1930s it was netting its proprietors over £8000 a year.[33]

[32] Bardswell, N. D., *Tubercle,* 34 (1920), 16; Watt, J., *Lancet* (1932), no. 1, 428.
[33] *Tuberculosis Year Book* (London, 1912–13), p. 365.

16

Saranac Lake and Riverside

More than anywhere in Europe, the question of how to confront tuberculosis in the light of Koch's great discovery provoked controversy in the United States.[1] America was not yet weighed down by social hierarchies and deference to professional wisdom; but it was dedicated to two often conflicting ideals. On the one hand, it was, as the grand old lady (not so old then) in New York Harbour proclaimed, the citadel of individual freedom:

> There's freedom at thy gates and rest
> For Earth's downtrodden and oppressed.[2]

On the other hand, it was intensely proud of its youthful vigour and determined to safeguard it. Though the identification of the tubercle bacillus had no immediate practical implications, American physicians understood its potentially alarming as well as hopeful import. In contrast therefore to Europe, where doctors were, by and large, too busy congratulating themselves on yet another momentous medical scientific advance, the first response in the United States was to try to reassure ordinary citizens.

The Story of the Bacteria and their Relation to Health and Disease was not a homely health manual in the Mrs Beeton tradition but a serious attempt by a leading academic bacteriologist, T. Mitchell Prudden, to explain tuberculosis to the public and discuss the precautionary measures which all health-conscious citizens should adopt.[3] It described how tubercle bacilli can "gain access to the various organs if conditions are favourable to them ... how they tend to multiply and form about them little masses of new tissue called 'tubercles' and how these can gradually erode and replace normal tissues". It made clear that the major source of the organism was sputum coughed up from the lungs of the tuberculous person and it emphasised that the bacillus could survive for weeks or months in dust particles. But – and this was the book's real message – "the healthy body is not good soil for the

---

[1] Landis, H. R. M., "The Reception of Koch's Discovery in the United States", *Annals of Medical History*, 4 (1932), 531.

[2] Lazarus, Emma, *Give Me Your Tired* (New York, 1885). The statue was dedicated in 1886.

[3] Prudden was professor of bacteriology at Columbia University, New York, and one of Trudeau's teachers. His book was published in 1899.

tubercle bacillus: even those living with consumptives can avoid contracting the disease". The best defence was not medicine but a strong natural resistance: "eat plain properly cooked food and plenty of it ... Get all the fresh air you can ... Keep clean". Though the organism could survive in dust, "sunlight will kill it in a few hours". The most important public-health precaution was that those infected should restrain from promiscuous spitting. This, as Sir John Smith-Cuckle of the London Chest Hospital observed, was "perhaps talking a little too freely to the uninformed public".[4] The book's optimistic tone was reinforced by the popular physician and writer S. Adolphus Knopf of Philadelphia, who suggested that "the threat of contagion can be reduced if people strive to be as much as possible in the open air, drink plenty of pure clean water, keep early hours, live a regular life and avoid the saloon ... Just from coming into contact with clean conscientious tuberculous invalids nothing whatsoever is to be feared". His pamphlet, *Tuberculosis as a Disease of the Masses and How to Combat It*, grabbed attention: it was quickly translated into twenty-seven languages, including Chinese and Thai, and for some years enjoyed a circulation in the United States second only to the Bible. Knopf spoke to doctors, politicians and the lay public equally in a way inconceivable at the time in Europe: "to combat consumption successfully requires the combined action of a wise government, well-trained physicians and an intelligent people".[5] Carrying the gospel as far as it would go (and perhaps further) Edward von Adelung, a health officer in Oakland, California, called tuberculosis "a ministering angel in disguise for it tends to force better drainage, better dwellings, better modes of living, more fresh air, sunshine, cleanliness, rest and recreation".[6]

Education and a positive attitude were not quite enough, however. As wave after wave of fresh and usually poor immigrants added their quota of tuberculosis to what was already endemic, the task of isolating invalids and carriers as well as of defeating the disease had to be faced.[7] The American version of the sanatorium idea was one possible strategy.

[4] Smith-Cuckle, J., *Lancet* (1900), no. 2, 543.

[5] Knopf, A., *Tuberculosis as a Disease of the Masses* (4th edn, New York, 1907), 86.

[6] Adeling, E. von, *California State Journal of Medicine*, 1 (1903), 292.

[7] The term "carrier" was beginning to come into use in medical jargon – not yet among the public – in the early 1900s. The first United States Immigration Act of 1882 was followed by the more stringent Undesirable Persons Act of 1891, which provided for "every person arriving from abroad ... to be examined and prohibited from landing if found to be a convict, a lunatic, an idiot, a cretin, an epileptic, contagiously diseased, a pauper, a polygamist, a prostitute or an anarchist". Subsequent legislation stiffened the conditions and in 1921 the first Quota Law specified a long list of illnesses which were supposed to bar entrants. But, however comprehensive the conditions of entry, it was, in Senator J. D. Burns's phrase in 1904, easier to spot an anarchist or a prostitute on physical examination than an early tuberculous. Chest

Dr Paul Kretzschmar had been a patient and later a disciple of Peter Dettweiler in Germany and spent much of his working life looking after poor German immigrant families in Brooklyn. As a recovered consumptive himself he had a particular interest in tuberculosis and he was dedicated to his flock; but for the American Do-It-Yourself ethos he had no use. Of course he agreed with prevailing opinion about the importance of building up resistance and the value of cleanliness and good food; but, like his master Dettweiler, he saw the doctor as a pivotal figure in the antituberculous regime.

> The smallest details of the patient's life [should be] controlled by the supervising physician and nothing of any importance should be left to the patient's unsupported judgement. The daily exercises in the open air, the use of lung gymnastics, the administration of stimulants, even the changing of garments are matters for close scrutiny by the physician, not matters to be decided by patients ... It is essential that the physician should have the widest possible control over everything that might influence the condition of the patient either favourably or unfavourably ... and such supervision cannot be maintained outside well-regulated sanatoria.[8]

Kretzschmar suggested that in such sanatoria a physician who had achieved complete authority (based of course not on coercion but on the patients' trust) could produce many cures. "If the disease has not made too much progress and if the treatment is continued for a sufficient length of time more than one-half of all bacillary phthises will be cured and will remain so if the patient will live according to prescription."[9] Kretzschmar himself never had the chance of putting his vision to the test; but his ideal was to become the inspiration of the American sanatorium movement. It was in the sanatoria that the American sick (like their European cousins) first ceased to be invalids and became patients in the original sense of the word, passive recipients and executors of decisions made by their doctors. Every hour, indeed every minute was regulated and supervised, if not by a doctor or nurse personally then by the spirit and provisions of the sanatorium rule book. "We are going to make you well and the shortest distance between two points is a straight line. This book is that line. Either follow it or get out." These were the characteristic opening sentences at The Pines, Betty MacDonald's sanatorium. Others were terse and biblical – "Ego sum Via, Veritas et Vita" – but with a dash of prison standing orders added to the mix. "Patients must not read. Patients must not write. Patients must not talk. Patients must not laugh. Patients must not sing. Patients must relax. Patients ..." Prohibitions on keeping non-washable,

X-ray screening did not become part of the medical routine till 1926 and was then widely criticised for picking up old and inactive lesions and missing small but active ones.

[8] Kretzschmar, P. J., *New York Medical Journal*, 47 (1888), 175.

[9] Kretzschmar, P. J., *Transactions of the American Clinical Association*, 5 (1988), 69.

non-sterilisable, non-essential personal belongings were especially strict and rigorously enforced: the teddy-bear of a newly-admitted young patient going up in flames to the sound of uncontrollable sobbing was the image that imprinted itself on the mind of one inmate. Compared to such institutions many prisons were liberal, humane and permissive.

The sanatorium doctrine did not go unchallenged; and Kretzschmar's opponents too had spokesmen with excellent credentials. Samuel Fisk, President of the Colorado State Medical Society and a physician who had found a cure for his own tuberculosis in the west, cited both his personal and his patients' case histories with great eloquence. Of course diagnosis, including laboratory investigations, and medical treatment were important and only a fool would not want to benefit from the experience of a wise physician relating to exercise, diet, clothing, ventilation, hours of sleep and indeed all physical aspects of life.[10] But he bridled at the idea that this required "a system running with clock-like regularity". Anyone afflicted with a disease was surely entitled to remain "his own master, to live without constant surveillance and interference in a boarding house of his own choice or in his own home". Fisk's attitude was thoroughly American and western and his platitudes did not seem platitudinous at the time. Nor were they. "I think we should never forget that a phthisical invalid is a human being ... who values his independence as we all do ... who chafes under discipline of any sort and who detests being treated as a school-child or herded together with other invalids like a flock of sheep." Fisk could draw on his own experience and did so with passion. "I have been a consumptive invalid myself ... And I appeal to you that I would rather live as a man under the plan pursued in Colorado than be caged in with a crowd of hollow coughing consumptives in a so-called sanatorium however beautifully designed and salubriously situated."[11]

Fisk and his followers were fighting a losing battle. In 1900 the United States had thirty-four sanatoria with 4485 beds. Twenty-five years later the numbers had risen to 536 sanatoria with 73,338 beds. The man who, more than anybody else, was responsible for this development was, like Laënnec, a victim of the disease himself.

The ancestors of Edward Livingston Trudeau had came to Louisiana from French Canada at the end of the eighteenth century and prospered: they were physicians, governors, congressmen, soldiers, artists.[12] His father, a

---

[10] All agreed on the importance of laboratory tests in striking contrast to medical opinion in England.

[11] Fisk, S. A., *Transactions of the Colorado State Medical Society*, 14 (1889), 830.

[12] Meade, G. M., "Trudeau", *Tubercle*, 52 (1972), 229.

physician, artist and linguist, was acclaimed as "the most learned and accomplished man in the State". Edward's childhood was unsettled though not unhappy. He was born in 1848 and his parents separated when he was three. He spent most of his boyhood in France with his mother. Back in the United States at seventeen he was on the point of entering the United States Naval Academy when his much-loved elder brother, Francis, fell ill with rapidly advancing tuberculosis. In more senses than one it was a turning-point in Edward's life. "I took entire care of him from the time he was taken ill in September [1865] until he died on December 23rd, occupying the same room and often the same bed. I bathed him and brought up his meals and when he felt well enough to go downstairs I carried him down on my back ... This was my first introduction to tuberculosis and death." 13 Did he know about Keats and his brother? Probably not at the time: his interests were rowing, sailing, shooting, and exploring the wilderness, not poetry.14 But he changed his mind about his future career and enrolled to study medicine at the College of Physicians and Surgeons of Columbia University, New York. He also married Lotte Beare, a doctor's daughter.

His career as a medical student was undistinguished but, as an intelligent and personable young man with the right background, he had no difficulty in obtaining a junior partnership in a fashionable New York practice. His marriage was fulfilled: a daughter, Charlotte, was born in 1872. Life seemed full of joy at present and promise for the future: a cold abscess on his neck which he had developed on his honeymoon in Liverpool was dismissed as a nuisance. One night, after walking from Central Park to the Battery in forty-seven minutes as a bet, he started another vague illness; and within a few days more cold abscesses appeared on his neck. The relationship between cold abscesses and tuberculosis was still not understood: "it had been explained to me as a medical student that tuberculosis was a non-contagious generally incurable disease due to constitutional peculiarities, perverted humours and various types of inflammation: and there was nothing to connect scrofula with pulmonary phthisis".15

Two years after the first signs of ill-health he began to suffer from attacks of debilitating fever which did not respond to quinine and his friends insisted that he should have himself examined.16 In February 1873 he at last agreed

---

13 Trudeau, E. L., *Autobiography* (New York, 1912).

14 Later in life he became an avid reader and impressed Robert Louis Stevenson with the catholicity of his taste and the breadth of his reading.

15 Trudeau, *Autobiography*, p. 32.

16 Intermittent fever was automatically attributed to malaria at that time and treated with quinine.

to consult Dr Sam Janeway, a colleague noted for his skill in physical diagnosis.

> The examination concluded Janeway said nothing. "Well, Janeway, you can find nothing the matter?" I said buttoning my shirt. Gravely came the reply, "Yes, the upper two-thirds of the left lung is involved in a tuberculous process and the right lung is touched". I think I then knew something of the feelings of the man at the bar who is told that he is to be hanged on a given date, for in those days pulmonary consumption was considered an absolutely fatal disease. I pulled myself together and escaped from the office thanking Janeway for his examination. When I got outside I felt stunned. It seemed to me the world had suddenly grown dark. The sun was shining and the street was filled with the rush and noise of traffic but to me the scene had lost every vestige of brightness ... Had I not seen all the horrors of consumption in my brother's case? It meant death and I had never thought of my death before. Was I ready to die? How could I tell my wife whom I had just left in unconscious happiness with the baby in our new house? And my rose-coloured dreams of achievement and professional success in New York, all lay shattered now; and in their place only exile and the inevitable end remained.[17]

Further on in his *Autobiography* he added: "How little could I have realised then how many times it would fall to my lot to tell other human beings the same dreadful truth. I think my own experience that day was never forgotten and helped, every time I made a positive diagnosis of tuberculosis, to make me as merciful as was compatible with truthfulness and the welfare of the patient." [18]

At first he followed what was the generally accepted as the proper course in such a situation, seeking improvement in the south and in prolonged exercises on horseback; but as this brought no improvement he returned to New York where his general condition continued to deteriorate. Then, believing that his end was near, he retired to the Adirondack Mountains in upper New York State, an almost pristine wilderness of forests and lakes where he had spent some of the happiest days of his youth. The choice was not prompted by the climate: the region was not only rough and inaccessible but also windy and cold for much of the year. But it was a paradise for hunters and fisherman: and "if, as I was sure, I had only a short time to live, I yearned for the wilderness which I loved". Burning with fever, weighing no more that a "dead lamb's skin" after an arduous six-day journey by train, boat and stage-wagon, he arrived at Paul Smith's Inn on Saranac Lake on a sunny June day. There he spent the summer, resting, floating over the lake, fishing and and even hunting from the boat. Within a few months he had gained fifteen pounds, recovered his usual vigour and was ready to return

[17] Trudeau, *Autobiography*, p. 83.
[18] Ibid., p. 122.

to New York. Or so he thought. After a few weeks back in town the fever returned; and early next spring, once again tired and wasted, he returned to the Adirondacks with his wife, daughter and a baby son, Ned. The miracle repeated itself: "little by little, lying out under the green trees and looking out onto water and the hills in tranquillity, my fever subsided and my health – and with it my desire to live – began to return".[19]

The year 1882 was a critical one. Now permanently settled in a small rented house on the lake, he had not given up medicine: as the only doctor in the region he looked after the fishermen, guides, trappers and their families, travelling by horse, buggy, sleigh and boat in all seasons, as well as after a trickle of tuberculous who had followed him from New York. He had also in a desultory way kept up with medical literature; and it was in an old issue of the *English Practitioner* that he came across an article describing the Brehmer-Dettweiler regime in Germany. The emphasis of the German doctors on pure air, rest, graduated exercise and a rich diet almost exactly mirrored his own experience and he fancied (mistakenly as it happened) that the atmospheric conditions of Göbersdorf and Falkenstein closely resembled those of Saranac Lake. A few weeks later he read about Koch's discovery and intuitively grasped its significance. "Every step", he wrote of Koch's research, "was proved over and over again; and the ingenuity of the new methods of staining, separating and growing the germs read like a fairy-tale to me." He himself owned a microscope from his medical student days – an exceedingly primitive one but no more primitive than Koch's had been in Wollstein – but he had completely forgotten how to use it.

Neither his illness nor his ignorance would deter him. He travelled to New York to ask his former teacher, Mitchell Prudden, to give him a crash course in Koch's methods. Prudden was courteous but sceptical, gave Trudeau a specimen culture of the bacilli and instructed one of his laboratory assistants to show the visitor where the stains were kept. "For days the pinks and the blues ended up on my fingers, my clothes and my shoes while the germs remained determinedly invisible";[20] but eventually Trudeau mastered the technique of staining and was ready to study some of his doubtful cases by looking for organisms in the sputa. On his return to the Adirondacks he also set up a research laboratory of sorts to "determine how far extremes of environment might favour or arrest the progress of the germ infection".[21]

In 1887 he reported his findings to a meeting of the American Climatological Association.[22] He had divided fifteen rabbits into three groups. Group

---

[19] Ibid., p. 184.
[20] Ibid., p. 198.
[21] Ibid., p. 203.

One he had inoculated with the bacillus and kept "confined in a small box ... in a dark cellar ... deprived of light, fresh air and exercise, and fed limited rations". Four of the animals died within three months. Group Two had not been inoculated but were confined to a freshly dug hole in the middle of a field and fed small amounts of food through a trap-door. Three months later they were emaciated and their coats were rough but none had developed the disease. Group Three had been inoculated but had at once been turned loose on a small island near the Trudeau camp. For the next three months they lived "in the midst of conditions well adapted to stimulate their vital powers to the highest point attainable". One rabbit died a month after the inoculation but the other four were in apparently perfect health after three months: their point of inoculation could not be located. This fairly rudimentary experiment was hailed by Dr Alfred Loomis, originally a leading sceptic, "as one of the most valuable and carefully prepared papers we have had before this Society":[23] it was in fact – oddly perhaps – the first and last attempt to provide experimental evidence to support the idea of sanatorium treatment on either side of the Atlantic. The proverbial garden shed where Trudeau carried out his experiments eventually grew into one of North America's most prestigious medical research institutes.

It was not plain sailing. In accepting the Brehmer-Dettweiler model Trudeau encountered a problem which did not trouble the German pioneers: how to attract patients. In Germany spa-going was an entrenched habit of the well-to-do; and the well-to-do were the people Brehmer and Dettweiler wished to attract. But who would come to Saranac Lake? Loomis now encouraged his wealthier and more sporting patients to go to the Adirondacks but in 1882 a modest hotel with twenty guest-rooms was adequate to accommodate them all. In any case Trudeau had other ideas; and putting them into practice he was to discover in himself a previously unsuspected gift. What he wanted was a sanatorium not for the rich but for the poor, constructing a few simple cottages, providing medical care free, and subsidising rather than charging patients; and what he discovered in himself was a talent for fund-raising.

He first approached men and women who, like himself, had had personal experience of tuberculosis. When he met Anson Phelps Stokes, a wealthy banker sailing on Saranac Lake, Trudeau immediately outlined his plan "to let some poor invalids shut up in cities have the opportunity for recovery in the setting which has done Mrs Stokes and me so much good". Stokes at once pledged $500 and some weeks later Mrs Stokes held an open-air

[22] Trudeau. E. L., *Transactions of the American Clinical Association*, 4 (1887), 131.
[23] Loomis, A., ibid., 142.

fund-raising fair which was to become an annual event. Through the Stokeses, Trudeau also gained an entrée to the salons of the benevolent rich of New York and became a star attraction at charity tea-parties and musical soirees. His task was not always easy. "Many people argued that it was well known that tuberculosis could not be cured ... that an aggregation of dying invalids would be so depressing that nobody would want to stay ... that the region was inaccessible (forty-two miles from the nearest railroad at the time) ... that the climate was rough ... in short, that the plan was completely visionary".[24] Yet they could not deny the fact that here was a seemingly frail physician, once given no more than a few months to live, back in town after spending years in the Adirondacks, bursting with life and energy.

Like all successful fund-raisers, Trudeau tailored his appeal to his potential donors. To some he emphasised the need for testing Dettweiler's method scientifically. To others he underlined the humanitarian aim of helping the deserving poor. To some he offered the chance to endow and have named after them a self-contained cottage where patients might retain a measure of independence. Others were invited to contribute to the erection of a larger building and perhaps to the cost of a library and laboratory. "I had in fact no knowledge whatever of what sort of buildings to plan: nor was such information available in books." Yet by 1900 the Adirondacks Cottage Sanatorium consisted of twelve substantial buildings, including a large administration block, a library and a well-equipped laboratory. It was to to grow to ten times that size over the next few decades.

Trudeau's professed aim (as that of all sanatorium doctors in all countries) was to cure tuberculosis by catching the disease early. This was universally accepted as reasonable: indeed, however beset with arguments were the methods of attainment, the objective itself was never questioned. (There is hardly a learned paper on sanatoria before the 1920s where the concept of diagnosing "early tuberculosis" does not crop up prominently and frequently.) In truth, though early was never clearly defined, in any meaningful pathological sense the expectation was misplaced. Not until the advent of skin testing and X-ray screening a quarter of a century later did early detection become a practical possibility. Until then the term "early" could mean no more than that the patient was still generally fit, not visibly losing weight and showing no sign of anaemia. Even repeated haemoptyses and daily peaks of moderate fever were often referred to as "premonitory" signs; and the most experienced clinical diagnosticians of the day could detect abnormal sounds in the chest only when there was advanced tuberculous infiltration and the beginning at least of cavitation. In other words, even under ideal

[24] Trudeau, *Autobiography*, p. 205.

conditions and for those who could afford the best available treatment, the philosophy underlying sanatorium care was flawed. Trudeau himself probably came to suspect this and so probably did others; but nobody would openly admit it or even speculate about the implications. This remained true for some time even after X-ray examination of the chest became relatively common in the 1920s and proved that early signs on physical examination usually meant already extensive tissue destruction. Like Trudeau himself, most patients did not seek medical advice until at least a third of one of their lungs had been destroyed and the prospect of eradicating the disease was virtually non-existent. Lack of evidence alone cannot be blamed. Even before X-rays and tuberculin screening, experienced pathologists had demonstrated the frequency of relatively advanced tuberculous lesions in subjects unsuspected during life of harbouring the infection and dying from some other cause. The evidence was ignored.

Such self-delusion was not unprecedented in the history of medicine but none had lasted for so long or was so defiant of the facts. For this, in retrospect, it is tempting to blame the vanity and self-interest of doctors. Many, of course, were guilty of both. Trudeau himself was neither vain nor self-seeking. Far more compelling in his case and in that of many others was the wish to cure the incurable. The need to be deluded was shared by the overwhelming majority of patients.

However bitter and frequent the disappointments, Trudeau's faith in the Brehmer-Dettweiler method held firm. He instructed his patients "to very gradually accustom themselves to an outdoor life ... increasing short walks in the open air little by little until the entire day could be spent out of doors in almost any weather". Second only to graduated exercise in importance was the need for a rich diet – three full meals every day supplemented by a glass of milk every four hours. Most importantly perhaps, he insisted on a physician monitoring every patient's progress every day. "Patients", the Saranac Sanatorium rule book stated, "will be informed by the physician how much exercise their case requires each day."

Trudeau was all the more prepared to empower physicians because many of his first patients were poor immigrants unfamiliar with American ways. Charity was a cornerstone of his sanatorium policy; but charity imposed a rigid code of behaviour. "Patients are reminded that the sanatorium is not run for profit but only for their own benefit and they should therefore do all in their power to keep the place looking neat and protect the furniture and other property from injury." Anyone whose behaviour was "obnoxious to others [or] who violates the rules of the establishment" would be discharged. Even in Saranac Lake disobedience trumped cure.

After the early 1900s Trudeau's professed faith that most victims of tuberculosis could be cured, once they were safely ensconced in a well-run
sanatorium, became the basic tenet of America's battle against the disease;
and sanatoria mushroomed. Many were lavishly or at least generously funded
by churches, professional bodies, trade associations and charitable organisations. All looked to the Adirondacks for inspiration: no physician could hope
to be placed in charge of a new establishment until he had made at least a
token pilgrimage to Saranac. Although numerous and flourishing, these
philanthropic institutions could never hope to stem the tide of tuberculosis
among the poor of the big cities. This was a task which devolved on the
tax-funded city, county and state sanatoria. Their responses varied.

Some tax-funded institutions tried to emulate the charitable foundations
and charged a small weekly fee, not so much to balance the books as to keep
out the riff-raff. As always and everywhere, the result of such a strategy was
two-edged. It raised the standard of the fee-paying establishments. It also
left the non-fee-paying ones to look after the most chronic, hopeless and
generally undesirable patients. It was not an assignment they relished.

To European visitors Hermann M. Biggs, New York City's long-serving Public Health Officer, was in his way as American a phenomenon as Trudeau.
He was energetic, ambitious and invincibly optimistic.[25] "Public health", he
firmly believed and repeatedly proclaimed, "is purchasable. Within a few
natural and unimportant limitations any community can determine its own
death rate from tuberculosis." [26] He was also and unashamedly as much
concerned with safeguarding the health of the hardworking and fit majority
as he was with the relief of the infirm few. The trouble was that the infirm
few were never few enough. First – in 1893 – he tried to reserve a ward in
every municipal hospital for tuberculosis; but the number of tuberculous
who now demanded admission (as an alternative to starving or freezing in
the streets) soon exceeded the number of reserved beds; and the "lungers"
quickly became scattered throughout the non-tuberculous wards. Next, he
took over a recently vacated lunatic asylum on Blackwell's Island in New
York's East River. Renamed the Tuberculosis Infirmary of the Metropolitan
Hospital, it admitted anyone with the disease; but there too the beds were
soon blocking the corridors, even though at least one-third of new admissions
died within a month.

Biggs was no fund-raiser in the Trudeau mould, but he finally persuaded
the city fathers to fund the opening of Otisville in the Catskills, a modified
version of a real sanatorium dedicated to the city's poor. Inevitably the

[25] Wimslow, C. E. A., *The Life of Hermann M. Biggs* (Philadelphia, 1929).
[26] Biggs, H. M., New York City Dept of Health Reprints, series 7 (New York, 1914).

emphasis was on the modification. Convinced that a "rest cure" had no place in a facility for the "incorrigibly poor", Biggs substituted for it what he called a "work cure". "In my judgement", he wrote, "the treatment by long-continued rest has been carried too far. It often returns patients with the disease arrested but physically unprepared for any useful manual occupation ... The working invalid is often transformed into a healthy loafer." [27] Instead of the customary six months' treatment period, he set a three months' limit of stay, except for the "most diligent workers who provided exceptional service". Biggs's problem, however, was never the numbers who wished to stay but the speed with which most of the inmates left. Many were gone within days of their admission, almost always against medical advice.

Supplementing the Tuberculous Infirmary and Otisville was Biggs's Riverside Hospital. It was established to confine, voluntarily or not, tuberculous individuals whose "dissipated and vicious habits" endangered the health of the community. Biggs and his advisers (like so many of their professional brethren in other city halls) never quite decided how this was to be achieved. Riverside was short even of such basic medical supplies as sputum cups; and even elementary hygiene could never be enforced. Discipline was supposed to be strict but patient-inmates spent their days "playing cards and wandering around the corridors and in and out of the hospital grounds. Fights were common and dying was no bar to drinking and partying." Serious infractions of the rules were supposed to be punished with solitary confinement; but, as Superintendent Robert J. Wilson noted in 1913, "we have neither the police officers nor the cells needed to put such a policy into effect. All we can do is to try and persuade".[28] It worked – sometimes. Riverside was too much of a prison to be a hospital and too much of a hospital to be a prison.

In the meantime Saranac flourished, if such a term can be applied to an establishment which in fact though never in name was devoted to the care of the dying.[29] It was also changing. Just as Trudeau felt that the poor should not be deprived of the benefits of Saranac because of their poverty, so the wealthy could not be excluded because of their wealth. As the fame of Trudeau's sanatorium spread, the rich and then the super-rich started to come. Of course they kept themselves to themselves, congregating in separate neighbourhoods with strict zoning laws and regulations about waste disposal and other communal matters, most especially about keeping undesirable elements out. In these enclaves the niceties of polite behaviour were strictly observed: new arrivals paid established residents courtesy calls; guests were

---

[27] Quoted in Wimslow, *The Life of Hermann M. Biggs*, 189.
[28] Wilson, R. J., *Journal of the Outdoor Life*, 11 (1914), 102.
[29] Taylor, R., *Saranac: America's Magic Mountain* (Boston, 1985).

expected to dress for dinner; butlers buttled. Invitations to high tea, a Saranac ritual, with prominent residents were in demand; and all who were strong enough and many who were not attended.

Both the rich and the merely well-to-do cultivated "serious gossip": "it enabled strangers to share experience by sharing stories". Knowing who else in or on the fringes of the Social Register was in Saranac made the disease more tolerable or at least more respectable. Among the rich, even more than among the poor, outdoor living became a fetish. "We all like zero better than thirty or forty above", a Du Pont sprig reported home. "I have not foregone my walk a single morning on account of the cold." Proficiency in winter sports was highly esteemed: the toboggan runs were carefully main-tained and the weekly ice-skating exhibitions were well attended. High living and the cult of the outdoor culminated in the spectacular winter carnival in February. The cost (which was considerable) was borne by a few rich patients. Their families and friends came from New York, Boston, Philadelphia, the Midwest and even the West Coast for the occasion; and the non-tuberculous townspeople – the "pioneers" – for once mingled with the inhabitants of the cure cottages and even with patients from the sanatorium.

It was a strictly one-day break. For most of the year what struck visitors most was the eerie quiet of the place. "We arrived after midday during the rest period. We thought that the President had died and put the town in mourning. Our room faced the main street but even with the window open not a sound came to us. Nothing. From two to four in the afternoon dogs were kept indoors: somehow or other children, even babies, were kept quiet. There was no talking, not even whispering. No reading. No writing. Only silence." [30]

In Saranac, as in many other sanatoria, the less wealthy made increasing use of the "cottage system". These were small boarding houses, or enlarged family homes, where patients were looked after by their own doctors who had access to hospital laboratory and later X-ray facilities and specialist consultation. By 1920 there were about 1500. Every social and ethnic group was catered for: there were Jewish (of all degrees of orthodoxy), Greek, Cuban and German cottages; there were cottages for lawyers, writers, frater-nal orders, actors and circus performers; there were cottages for ambulant patients ("up cottages") and for those confined to bed ("nursing cottages"). Representatives of the local Anti-Tuberculosis Society met arriving trains and directed those who had made no advance booking to a suitable estab-lishment. Homogeneity helped alleviate the feeling of separation – or was supposed to.

[30] Quoted in Sandstone, D. A., *Saranac Diary* (New York, 1914), 289.

What linked the social strata was the regard in which Trudeau was held. When his daughter Charlotte died of tuberculosis, in March 1893, the town mourned with him. "I have just come from Miss Trudeau's funeral", Philip Washburn wrote to his mother. "There was no school this morning, all shops were closed. The church was filled with flowers: where they all came from I do not know. She was mourned by the whole community." Yet by then death of the young was commonplace in Saranac.[31]

Trudeau himself never attended a carnival or a party, not even in a good cause. Ascetic by temperament and limited by his own illness, he spent what strength he had on his patients. Hundreds of surviving letters testify to his ability to make each invalid feel special, not least those about to die. "This is my last letter", one of them wrote. "You have been a rock in this dreary land to my wife and me. Good bye and God bless you." Robert Louis Stevenson, who disliked sanatoria, stayed on for several months for his sake alone and inscribed copies of all his own books that he had with him to the "best of doctors".

If his nobility and compassion brought comfort to many, Trudeau's therapeutic victories remained few. He himself was rarely free from symptoms and he felt distressed about his long periods of sick-leave. "I am sorry to say that I am in the grip of the enemy again", he wrote to a friend in 1908. "Once again life is ... made up of my bed, my room, my invalid chair, my little porch and last but not least that dreadful spit cup I know so well. But however well one knows it, I don't think that one can ever get used to this illness." Most of his patients fared no better. Yet they kept arriving and all wished to be seen by him personally. "One woman", he wrote shortly before his own death in 1916, "had come all the way from New Orleans ... to be seen by me. I told her that I was sick and could not examine her. 'Well, what is the matter with you?' I said: 'If you really want to know, pulmonary tuberculosis.' Then she threw her hands in the air and exclaimed in despair: 'And you have such a reputation! Why don't you cure yourself?'"[32] She had a point.

[31] Ibid., 378.
[32] Meade, G. M., "Trudeau", *Tubercle*, 52 (1972), 229.

17

Doctor, Patient, Writer

Tuberculous Grand-Dukes went in search of their lost health to mock-rococo villas on the Riviera. Ordinary Russians, including modestly successful writers and doctors, went to Yalta. The climate and the setting there – a narrow, cypress-strewn strip between the Black Sea and the majestic Crimean mountains – was not unlike that of Nice: both were natural havens for refugees from the north. When Anton Chekhov built his *belaya dacha* (white cottage) there, it was still barely more than a village, entirely without the glitz and glamour of its Mediterranean counterpart.[1] He had been told by his doctors, shortly after the disastrous first night of *The Seagull* in St Petersburg in October 1896, what he had suspected already: that he was gravely ill and unlikely to survive another winter in Moscow or Melikhovo,[2] anywhere in fact outside a benign and warm climate. He was thirty-seven and reluctant to move; but "this terrible, godforsaken place known as Yalta of the Damned" gave him another six years of life and the chance to write his greatest plays.

He was born not very far away (by Russian standards), in the declining port of Taganrog on the Sea of Azov, the third of six surviving children of a struggling and eventually bankrupt grocer and his gentle, long-suffering wife. Pavel, the father, was a pious martinet, master of the cathedral choir, who beat and bullied his offspring but who made sure that they obtained the best education available locally.[3] Whatever else was crammed into Anton's head, it was at the Taganrog *gimnaziya*, writing and producing school plays and charades, that he developed his love for the theatre. At eighteen he followed his impoverished family to Moscow, partly to help to support them,

---

[1] Ever since Alexander II had made nearby Livadia his summer residence the coast was dotted with exclusive aristocratic villas and estates; and a fast and luxurious train service connected Yalta to Moscow and St Peterburg. The town itself had also become a favoured holiday resort for artists and writers: Tolstoy, Gorkij, Chaliapine and Rachmaninov were all occasional visitors at Chekhov's *dacha*. In Chekhov's day this was situated well outside the centre of the town; now it is a museum dedicated to the writer, engulfed by hotels, sanatoria and workers' convalescent homes.

[2] Melikhovo was a small-holding about fifty miles south of Moscow which he purchased in 1892 when he was becoming well known as a writer. He still practised medicine there, especially during the cholera epidemic of 1895.

[3] Pavel himself was the son of a serf.

partly to enrol as a medical student. The next five years were arduous: moonlighting from his medical studies, he was churning out hundreds of short humorous pieces for popular magazines to make ends meet.[4]

As soon as he was qualified he established himself in practice: a brass plate still announces Dr A. Chekhov on the house where he had his surgery in Moscow. But, though he practised on and off till his departure for Yalta, his heart was never in it. Perhaps he had enough of medicine looking after the sick in his own family. His feckless but gifted and charming elder brother, Nikolay, died of tuberculosis in 1889. By then Anton knew that he too was "touched".

For ten years short stories, some of them only a page or two long, others short novels, were Chekhov's main literary output. He was to be known outside Russia as a master of the genre before he achieved fame as a dramatist. Some of his tales were autobiographical and in several he explored the experiences of the physically ill. In "The Schoolmaster" poor Sinoviev feels a trifle weary but on no account will he miss the banquet given in his honour, the realisation of a life-time's dreams. Putting on his spotlessly polished boots exhausts him so much that he has to rest for a while; and in front of the director's apartment he is seized by a bad bout of coughing. So bad that he flings his stick to the floor and his cap drops off his head. When, alerted by the noise, his host and fellow teachers and even the school inspector hurry out of the flat, he is sitting gasping at the top of the stairs covered in sweat. "An unfortunate and undignified contretemps", he muses when eventually he gets home. He gazes at his drawn, shadowed face in the mirror. "Ah, but I'm making a fuss. My colour is better than it's been for months. If only the gastric catarrh wouldn't bring on this wretched cough." He decides to spend the summer in the south – if only he can scrape up the necessary funds.

The stories established Chekhov's reputation, but he was always drawn to the theatre. He jumped at a commission offered by a Moscow impresario, F. A. Korsch, for a four-act play, "a kind of a farce". The result, Ivanov, was more than Korsch had bargained for: at its first night the cheering and the whistling were more or less evenly matched.[5] A year later, between the debacle

---

[4] The facts of Chekhov's life are well described in the recent biography by D. Rayfield, Anton Chekhov (London, 1997), but Chekhov remains an elusive character.

[5] Today Ivanov seems the most conventional and conventionally moralising of Chekhov's plays; but it did not seem so to the first-night audience in Moscow. The play's main character, a landowner in his thirties, Nicholas Ivanov, has a Jewish wife, Sarah, who is dying of tuberculosis. Instead of taking her to a warm climate, her only chance of recovery, he is busy seducing the daughter of a neighbouring landowner. Sarah dies and Ivanov commits suicide; but, far from pillorying him as a spineless scoundrel, the writer seemed to be more in sympathy with him than with the virtuous but priggish Dr Lvov.

of the *The Seagull* in St Petersburg and the play's triumphant Moscow opening, Chekhov was confronted with the truth.

Most critics, those at least with no ideological axe to grind, have found it easier to analyse the seemingly timeless appeal of Chekhov's last plays in negative terms, to emphasise what they are not.[6] They are clearly not conventionally exciting, tempestuous, larger than life, desperately tragic, uproariously funny, emblematic of anything outside themselves, purposeful, instructive, politically relevant, morally crusading or socially prophetic. Some commentators have come to the conclusion that they are studies in moods or states of mind.[7] They are in fact not in the least negative: they are unique insider studies of the tuberculous destiny without once mentioning the illness. Of course tuberculosis could be any other ailment – if such existed – which struck down the young and crippled and shortened their physical but often enriched their spiritual life, which excluded them from many of the most intensely pleasurable pursuits yet made them abnormally responsive to some of the mundane beauties and sadnesses of the world around them. Most surprisingly perhaps, it undermined the bedrock of most young people's daily existence, the planning for a future, and could yet sustain unquenchable hope.

Why, if Chekhov's last great plays are about tuberculosis, does he never mention it? That of course would not only have robbed his plots of their inner tension – there was no dramatic mileage for Chekhov in acts of God – but would also have been a denial of the essential character of the disease. The tuberculous in real life – Chekhov himself among them – rarely referred to their illness to outsiders (that is to the healthy), hardly ever by name. Even in his daily correspondence with Olga Knipper, symptoms and signs of the disease were mentioned only in the most desultory way, like the weather but as less interesting.[8] The only one of his mature plays in which

---

[6] There have been many attempts at transforming plays like *The Cherry Orchard* into sociological and political tracts. The results have generally been unconvincing. Chekhov himself was often reproached by his friends for not being politically more committed, though he did in fact break his friendship with his patron, the newspaper proprietor Suvorin, over Suvorin's anti-Dreyfus stance.

[7] Chekhov, A., *Five Plays*, introduced by Ronald Hingley (Oxford, 1977).

[8] Olga Leonardovna Knipper was born in Glasov, a small provincial town in Central Russia: her parents were of German extraction, the father a respected chemical engineer, the mother an accomplished musician. She received a conventional middle-class upbringing except for her determination to become an actress. This was not easy: they were not rich and she had no influential "protector". After her father's death the family moved to Moscow and her mother's artistic friends secured her a place in the Philharmonic Society Actors' School. Three years later Konstantin Stanislavski, one of the founders of the Moscow Arts Theatre, auditioned her

tuberculosis is a feature of the plot and is actually named, *Ivanov*, was written before he was himself engulfed by the illness and began to experience life in exile. *The Seagull* spans the divide. The first play written after his realisation of the truth is his most profoundly tuberculous.

Good productions of *The Three Sisters* can hold an audience spellbound without either the audience or the actors being aware of the pervasive presence of a physical illness: indeed, as physical illnesses are usually per-ceived – encrusted with symptoms, signs, diets, injections, drugs, operations – any hint at it would destroy the impact of the play. Yet the lives of the children of the late General Prozorov only make sense on the assumption of some insuperable underlying though unstated physical impediment. Andrew Prozorov would have liked to be a professor in Moscow but he works in a a humdrum job for the municipal council of which his wife's lover is chairman. His three sisters are all disappointed in love: Olga regrets being an old maid, Masha has married the wrong man, Irina's fiancé – unloved – is killed in a duel in Act Four. Olga dislikes being a schoolmistress, Masha dislikes being a schoolmaster's wife, Irina dislikes working in a post office. All their problems would, they fervently believe, magically disappear if only ... if only, if only ... they could return to their childhood home in Moscow. Why can they not? Because they are, like their creator, banished to their provincial Yalta by something irremovable, something which does not stop them from speaking, feeling, thinking and dreaming (seemingly like the unspeakably healthy people outside their private universe) but which stops them from trying to enact any of their thoughts, feelings and dreams.

All four of the great Chekhov plays abound in suicidal moods, despairing utterances, unhappy love affairs and careers in ruins, exactly as did the lives of the exiled tuberculous in Yalta – and in the hundreds of Yaltas around the world. There is – as there was in Chekhov's reality – always a touch of playfulness about the tragedies, a wrapping up of the heartbreak in gentle teasing and badinage: if the grand love affairs are always doomed, humdrum affections and friendships bloom. Even in small externals the plays recreate

and promptly gave her the role of Arkadina in *The Seagull.* She must have been much too young for the role but she triumphed and soon became a firm favourite with Moscow audiences and later with audiences in other Russian cities.

The Chekhov-Knipper correspondence was published in Moscow between 1934 and 1936 by the Soviet State Academy of Sciences, an edition widely hailed at the time as a monument of scholarship. In fact, comparing it to the complete Chekhov edition of thirteen volumes published in 1914, both George Forgach, the Hungarian Chekhov scholar, and Jean Benedetti, a more recent editor, have shown up many instances of Soviet censorship, especially deletions of any critical reference by Chekhov to Stanislavski and of any praise for Meyerhold. The present extracts are from Jean Benedetti's excellent volume *Dear Writer ... Dear Actress: The Love Letters of Olga Knipper and Anton Chekhov* (London, 1996).

the tuberculous existence of Chekhov's days more truly than any other work of art or literature. There is the constant preoccupation with time, the more absurd since nothing on the face of it depends on it. "It's exactly a year ago today since father died." "In twenty-five years' time everyone will work." "What time is it? – Nearly two o'clock." There are the opening sentences of *The Cherry Orchard*: "It's already light." "How late was the train then?" "A couple of hours at least." (What makes them so memorable?) There is the low-key self-obsession, the ruminations about missed opportunities, the desultory monitoring of the patient-characters' seemingly long drawn out and yet purposeless existence. Purposeless? Well, that of course needs to be re-examined once again. And again. There is also the hope that something will change for the better after all – a hope that never becomes an expectation. There is also the patient-characters' dislike for the fit and the successful, the only people for whom Chekhov himself could never summon up any sympathy. If only Natasha in *The Three Sisters*, Serebryakov in *Uncle Vanya* or Irina Arkadin in *The Seagull* were ever so lightly touched by the disease they would be less insufferable.

Chekhov's correspondence with Olga Knipper reads today like jottings for an unwritten Chekhov play, perhaps his best.[9] They met at a rehearsal of *The Seagull* at the Arts Theatre in Moscow in 1898: she was twenty-one, he thirty-eight, already in the grip of tuberculosis. "I never forget how overcome with fright I was when I read Nemirovich-Danchenko's notice telling us that the author would be at the rehearsal the next day. But at once we were captivated by his subtle charm, his inability to teach but also by the wonderful way in which his remarks, half-joking and half-serious, gradually sank in." [10] The fascination was mutual; and when Chekhov left a few days later to return to Yalta they promised to write to each other from time to time. In fact they were to exchange more than a thousand letters over the next five years inconsequential, jocular, loving, ardent, sometimes a little petulant, only rarely about great events and hardly ever about details of his illness.

> Greetings, dear Actress ... It suddenly turned freezing cold in Yalta ... how I would like to be in Moscow! I didn't send you my photograph because I haven't received yours yet, oh snake! I certainly didn't say that you were "biting as a snake" as you write. You are a great, big but wonderful snake. Isn't that flattering?

[9] There was something of the writer in many of the characters of the plays, especially the doctors like Dr Astrov. In *The Seagull*, Trigorin's invincible untidiness too, like his passion for fishing and his obsessive note-taking, are clearly fragments of a self-portrait.

[10] Olga Knipper's memoirs were published in Moscow as volume one in the Chekhov-Knipper correspondence in 1934 and are quoted by Jean Benedetti in *Dear Writer ... Dear Actress.* See also Pincher, H., *Chekhov's Leading Lady* (London, 1979).

So, be healthy, dear actress, wonderful woman. God keep you. I kiss both your hands and bow. Don't forget me.[11]

And from her a few days later:

Greetings, dear Writer. Yesterday we performed our beloved *Seagull*. We played it with delight. The theatre was packed ... The acting was good, light, as you like it. Stanislavski says my performance has never been better. Even the scene with Trigorin has improved. But I am not quite happy with Act I – I get tense, I play a little jerkily. But you can calm down, dear writer, yesterday Roksanova was much better: she cut down on the "pregnant pauses", didn't snivel so much, and Meyerhold told me that the audience listened in quite a different way. The third act, as usual, broke the audience's heart ... On Monday we shall really set to work on *Uncle Vanya* ... Why don't you write to me more often? ... Be healthy, go for walks, enjoy yourself, breathe the fine southern air. I press your hand in mine.[12]

And much more in the same chatty vein: the correspondence became for Chekhov – as similar correspondences were for thousands of tuberculous marooned in their Yaltas – a life-line, a tenuous link with the real world. He had hoped to attend a performance or two of *Uncle Vanya* and then the first night; but he developed "my usual accursed October cold" and could not. It was almost a flop, which Olga, Nemirovich-Danchenko and other friends tried to conceal from him. His antennae were too sensitive and his intelligence too acute to be taken in.

Dearest Actress, telegrams started arriving this evening when I was already in bed and kept arriving all night. They were read out to me over the telephone: the first time my own fame kept me awake. All the telegrams talked about curtain calls and dazzling success but there was a nuance, a hint of something from which I concluded that the mood was not entirely positive. The papers today confirmed my suspicion. But that does not matter ... You actors and actresses in the Art Theatre have become a little spoilt by success ... That happens very easily and is not good for you.[13]

In fact, after the disappointment of the first night, the play became a resounding success: many Muscovites went to see it three or four times and its author was elected to the Academy of Language and Literature.

In March 1900, the Arts Theatre troupe went on a tour of the Crimea, performing *The Seagull*, *Uncle Vanya* and Ibsen's *Hedda Gabler*. Olga was enchanted with the writer's *dacha* and especially with the garden: he was, like his character Dr Astrov, a passionate gardener with a natural feel for plants and soils. She was back for a month during the theatrical summer break in

---

[11] Benedetti in *Dear Writer ... Dear Actress*.
[12] Ibid., p. 130.
[13] Ibid., p. 148.

July, this time on her own. During that stay they became lovers.[14] Then she returned to Moscow and their separate lives and the daily correspondence started up again. He was also, in short sharp spells, writing *The Three Sisters*, hoping but not certain that he would be able to finish it. His doctor, the dependable and commonsensical but slightly melancholic Azov, urged him to try to recoup his strength in Nice or Italy. Eventually he decided to go. From the Riviera and then from Florence he dispatched sections of the new play as he completed them, with copious explanatory notes. She too wrote at length. Their love and longing for each other was as ardent as ever but there was also growing tension. What would the future bring? What future?

After three months in the west he was back in Yalta, feeling slightly stronger. She was on tour in St Petersburg with the company, the first of what was to become a regular annual event. She wrote to him about every performance, every reception, every newspaper article, every fascinating tit-bit of theatrical gossip. He urged her to come to Yalta over Easter – if only for a few days. "But how can I, my dearest? There is no Easter in the theatre. Stanislavski would howl if I left." But ... but ... long letters, explaining, expressing sorrow. Eventually a telegram: "Coming to Yalta tomorrow, Olga." She stayed for two weeks and they decided to get married.

Inevitably the correspondence reads like a long drawn out dialogue between two leading characters in one of the post-tuberculosis Chekhov plays. The plays themselves are never dialogues: there is always a cast of four or five of equal importance (or, in worldly terms, equal unimportance). It was so in life as well. Above all – though barely mentioned in the letters to and from Olga – there was the writer's sister, Masha, who looked after him day in and day out. Very little is known about her: almost nothing after her brother's death. During his last years he needed almost full-time nursing, apart from the cooking and other household chores; and Masha continued to provide those even after his marriage to Olga in June 1901. After the couple's honeymoon, travelling down the Volga and ending in a sanatorium in Aksynovo in the Caucasus, he returned to Yalta, Olga to Moscow. She busied herself with looking for a flat, buying furniture, having old pieces reupholstered, getting new curtains, even acquiring a cat; but there was never any question of her giving up her career. Of course she went on writing every day, asking for his advice about armchairs and bathroom fittings. "You see what a good wife I am, my darling husband, writing to my lord and master every day ... asking for his opinion, his commands." She eventually found a flat: "of course there is a room in it for

---

[14] Neither the Chekhovs nor the Knippers were Bohemian and the liaison was never openly referred to.

Masha too".[15] None of Masha's letters survive: at least none are included in the six volume edition of the Chekhov-Knipper correspondence published under the aegis of the Soviet State Academy of Sciences. Perhaps she did not write any. Who would she have written to? Yet the Mashas – thousands of them – were essential adjuncts of the tuberculous universe; and in a variety of guises they live on on the stage in Chekhov's last plays.

In November 1901 he spent three days in Moscow, attending rehearsals of *The Three Sisters*. It was too much for him. After a small party with theatrical friends he had another severe pulmonary haemorrhage; it took him two weeks in bed to recover sufficiently to brave the journey back to Yalta. Then the correspondence resumed. Olga was pining for him:

> I can see my beloved Anton everywhere in the flat. But everything is so spick and span, none of your beloved disorder. I didn't tidy your bed. I couldn't. I pretended that you're still here beside me, perhaps trying to go to sleep while I bustle about noisily. But ...[16]

And a few days later from him:

> Good day my darling wife ... I am healthy though since my arrival back I haven't been quite my usual bubbling self. So I took litres of cod-liver oil yesterday. Ough! what revolting stuff. Gorkij says that even the thought of it gives him nightmares. Yes, I would terribly like you to have a little half-German. He or she would surely amuse you. More than your wretched husband can.[17]

Reports about clothes, shoes, haircut, guests, trying to work; declarations of love, a million kisses. She was soon pregnant but had a miscarriage during another tour in St Petersburg and then spent three months in Yalta and Perm recovering.[18] She was also beginning to be tormented by guilt. "Oh, what sort of a wife I am? Pursuing my own selfish career instead of looking after my dear, dear Anton." But there was no question of her moving to Yalta. He would have to come to Moscow.

In all the Chekhov plays there is an "event" in Act 4, usually offstage, eliciting revealing responses from the characters, leading to a kind of muted climax. This was true of many tuberculous lives as well. It usually took the

[15] The flat she found was in fact wholly unsuitable for the invalid writer. When he eventually got to Moscow Dr Schuller, a friend and one-time colleague, was horrified to see him struggling with the stairs. "He was a physical wreck: it took him half an hour to get from the street to their front door."

[16] Benedetti, *Dear Writer ... Dear Actress*, p. 189.

[17] Ibid., p. 192.

[18] Their roles were temporarily reversed, he looking after her. They eventually accepted an invitation from Sava Morozov (the collector of Picassos and Matisses) to spend time on his estate in Perm. It was there that he began writing *The Cherry Orchard*.

form of a last determined and almost always doomed effort to ignore the illness and try to make a come-back into the real world. Stanislavski had been nagging Olga to press Chekhov to get on with the next play. It was slow in coming: his strength was ebbing away. There was a first reference to a title – "not very good, only temporary" – in a letter dated 24 December 1902: *The Cherry Orchard*. A few weeks later the author expressed the wish to attend the rehearsals and the first performance in person – even if it meant spending the winter in Moscow against medical advice.

Both Chekhov and Stanislavski were to be promoted as Marxist-Leninist ikons in Stalin's philistine empire; but their relationship was far from the creative idyll portrayed by Soviet literary sycophants. It is true that the director, a great survivor, recognised and admired Chekhov's genius and was determined to make use of it; but it was to be used as much as a vehicle for his own directorial ideas as to demonstrate the greatness of the writer. Soon it became a real-life enactment of the dislike Chekhov's tuberculous heroes (and probably he himself) felt for the ostentatiously fit, self-centred and successful.[19] *The Cherry Orchard*'s prospects seemed increasingly dim as rehearsals proceeded. Chekhov insisted that the play was a comedy, almost a farce, both in fact inappropriate terms for a work which cannot be squeezed into any traditional category. What he was appealing for was a lightness of touch, a casual manner, the abandonment of the traditional ponderous style of Russian (and not only Russian) theatre. Here was Stanislavski serving up "not a soufflé but a suet pudding", an orgy of tiny but meaningful details, gloomy pauses, smouldering looks of frustration and regret, secret – but not so secret – displays of suppressed emotions. The latent antagonism – Chekhov was too weak physically to thrash out his objections in the open – had to reach a suitably dramatic and tuberculous climax; and it did.

The play's first night was to be "the great writer's finest hour", the moment when he was to receive ecstatic recognition for a lifetime's achievement. That was not all. What better occasion could there be (according to Stanislavski) than one of those jubilee celebrations so beloved of both theatrical folk and first-night audiences? Though Chekhov's literary debut was in 1880, making any celebration at least one year premature, such little discrepancies were to be no bar to a spot of publicity. His twenty-fifth anniversary in the theatre would be celebrated on the first night, 17 January 1904; and, undeclared, the occasion was to be made more poignant by the fact that (as everybody knew) he was dying.

Even when in robust health Chekhov detested schmalz; and what was in store for him was therefore kept a secret. He was not well enough to be

---

[19] Stanislavski died in 1938, aged seventy-six.

present during the first and second acts; but when the ovation in the second interval signalled the play's success, Nemirovich-Danchenko sent him a note begging him to come. A little alarmed Chekhov complied – he suspected a flop: the cast obviously needed a bit of morale-boosting – only to be dragged onto the stage in the last interval. There was tumultuous applause though it was obvious to many that he was near fainting and several members of the audience called out that at least a chair should be provided for Anton Pavlovich. Though convulsed with coughing and unable to say a word, he endured the lengthy speeches and the presentation of bouquets, swaying but standing. Only in Olga's dressing room did he collapse.

Shortly after the event and back in Yalta he developed painful cramps in the limbs to add to his chest pain, cough and sore throat He was also losing weight and his hair was falling out.[20] He continued writing playful letters to Olga who was urging him to come back to Moscow (after her own return from the Arts Theatre tour in St Petersburg): she had found a lovely *dacha*, all on the ground floor. In April he did return but at once became feverish. His Moscow doctor, Dr Taube, recommended that they go to Badenweiler, a sanatorium in the Black Forest which "specialised in just this kind of complaint". In Berlin on the way they consulted the famous Professor Ewald. "He came to our hotel", Olga wrote later, "examined him, but could do no more than shake his head and shrug his shoulders and depart. I'll never forget Anton's gentle bewildered smile." In Badenweiler he seemed at first to improve and liked the doctor in charge, Dr Schwörer, a recovered patient himself. (He usually hated seeing doctors: Dr Altschuler in Yalta had always to find some non-medical pretext – however transparent – for his visits.) "We stayed at the Hotel Sommer", she later recorded,

> a pleasant, homely place. We even went to Freiburg to buy a white flannel suit. The journey took a whole day and next day Anton felt very breathless. But he was eating a little and all the time when he had the strength he was making up wonderful funny stories to make me laugh. On the last night night he woke up with severe stabbing pain in his chest. We sent for Dr Schwörer who came at once. Anton sat up and said in Russian "I'm dying". Then he turned to Dr Schwörer and translated "Ich sterbe". The doctor gave him an injection of camphor and ordered champagne.[21] Anton smiled and whispered: "It's a long time since

---

[20] This was not infrequent, probably the result of high concentrations of heavy metals in many preparations used for treatment.
[21] The tranquilliser of the age.

I drank champagne". He drained the glass and lay back quietly and I had just time to run to him, lean across the bed and embrace him. Then he stopped breathing and was sleeping peacefully as a child.[22]

[22] Benedetti, *Dear Writer ... Dear Actress*, p. 260. Like others who have lost loved ones, Olga went on writing letters to him for a long time after he died. She survived him by fifty-seven years, never remarrying. In old age she lived in Moscow, honoured as an historic personage but declining all official roles. In fact, most people were unaware that she was still alive until she attended a gala evening at the Moscow Arts Theatre in 1960. The programme included the scene of parting between Masha and Vershinin in *The Three Sisters*. At the climactic moment a strong deep voice rang out from one of the boxes, Olga speaking "her" great line, "Good bye, dear", before the young actress on the stage could get it out. After a moment's dumbfounded silence the young actress started to clap and the audience, realising who the interrupter was, burst into thunderous applause which lasted many minutes.

18

Advances

Modern microbiology was born in the laboratory; but the achievements of its dazzling first decades were quickly translated into clinical practice.[1] Pasteur and his team had hardly announced their discovery of the transmission of rabies by a submicroscopic virus and the successful attenuation of the killer in the laboratory when an Alsatian farmer's son, Joseph Meister, was mauled by a mad dog and his mother begged the scientists in Paris to try to save him. With some hesitation Pasteur agreed – medical colleagues assured him that otherwise the boy had no chance of surviving – and Joseph became the first to receive the anti-rabies vaccine and to be saved. (It earned him a statue in front of the Institut Pasteur in Paris, one of the lamentably few public monuments erected to pioneer patients.) A few months later nineteen illiterate moujiks from Smolensk in Russia who had been savaged by a rabid wolf eighteen days earlier – too long a time-lapse in Pasteur's own estimation for the vaccine to be effective – were sent by their Little Father, the Tsar, to Paris to be treated by Pasteur's team; and the newspaper-reading world waited with trepidation and France with pride and bated breath to see whether any of them would survive. Sixteen did. No sooner had Walter Reed and his human guinea-pigs revealed the mode of transmission of yellow fever and made the eradication or at least the control of the disease possible than work on the Panama Canal was resumed and this time carried to a triumphant conclusion.[2] Von Behring's isolation of the diphtheria bacillus quickly

---

[1] Over the thirty-year period 1873–1903 the causative organisms of almost every common disease was identified, starting with the spirochete causing relapsing fever (identified by Obermeyer in 1873) and ending with the spirochete of syphilis (identified by Schaudinn in 1903). Additional advances were the discoveries of Pasteur, Roux, Behring and others in the field of immunisation, Metchnikoff's work on phagocytosis and dozens of methodological advances any of which would be hailed as a break-through today. There has been nothing comparable in the biological sciences before or since.

[2] The first attempt by a French consortium presided over by Ferdinand de Lesseps of Suez fame collapsed in financial ruin and political scandal in 1889. The culprit (other than greed and mismanagement) was yellow fever, which was endemic in Central America and which virtually wiped out the imported work force. Once Reed and his colleagues had established the mosquito, *Culex fasciatus*, as the carrier of the causative agent (later identified as a virus), the knowledge enabled Captain William C. Gorgas of the US Army to organise prophylactic

led to the production of an antitoxin, the first preparation so named, and was widely (though not universally) acclaimed as a life-saver.[3] In general, all the prodigious feats of the early microbe-hunters were fuelled by the expectation of saving thousands or millions of lives within their own lifetime, and events by and large vindicated their hopes.[4] There was one exception. No practical cure emerged in the wake of what was acknowledged as the most important microbiological discovery of all, Koch's identification and isolation of the tuberculosis bacillus.

The rush of tuberculous patients to Berlin ended in shattered hopes and tearful recriminations. The tragic farce of tuberculin tainted the reputation of the most admired medical scientist of the age. Nor did the next few decades fulfil the high hopes raised by his discovery. Statisticians and public-health experts continued to assure the public that mortality from the disease was slowly but surely declining (except in such hopelessly backward countries as Ireland); but a diagnosis of clinically advanced pulmonary tuberculosis still spelled death in much the same way as it had to John Keats in 1818; and other forms of the infection were not much more merciful. Yet these decades were not without significant advances.

The initial excitement aroused by Röntgen's discovery, to many as near to science fiction as was compatible with the image of a bearded and be-spectacled German professor, was inevitably followed by a reaction. Röntgen had hardly resumed his seat after delivering his memorable lecture to the Würzburg Scientific Society when the eminent Professor Peter Schönborn from Munich rose to warn doctors in the audience – not many – that the method, though interesting in itself, "scarcely promised to be of much value in the diagnosis of internal diseases since the X-ray appearances of abnormal organs probably did not markedly differ from those of normal ones". With a slightly more open mind, if not with an excess of prophetic afflatus, the *Boston Medical and Surgical Journal* opined that "the discovery, whatever future it may have, will inevitably fall short of the oversanguine hopes that have been expressed by some".[5]

---

measures and eventually to make the region mosquito free. The digging was restarted in 1905 under US aegis and the canal was declared open by President Wilson in 1920.

[3] Von Behring's other success in the field was the tetanus antiotoxin; but his many attempts over several decades to find an antitoxin against tuberculosis failed. He died in 1917, aged sixty-three.

[4] *Microbe Hunters* was the title given to a best-selling book of potted biographies by the American doctor-writer Paul de Kruif. His matey and relentlessly upbeat style, anticipating the editorial manner of *Readers Digest*, makes his book almost unreadable today, but in its day (1927) it was a landmark establishing medical researchers as popular heroes.

[5] Brown, L., *The Story of Clinical Pulmonary Tuberculosis* (Baltimore, Maryland, 1941), 214.

The technique, however, was too explosively exciting to be smothered by professorial caution and editorial wet blankets. Less than a year after Röntgen's initial announcement, at a meeting held on the premises of the premier British medical insurance company, the Medical Defence Union,[6] a group of surgeons, physicians and scientists resolved to form an X-ray society, the first in the world. A month later Silvanus Thompson, a Fellow of the Royal Society and professor of physics at the City and Guilds of London Technical College, opened its inaugural meeting with the resounding if somewhat vacuous announcement that "November 8th, 1896, will forever be memorable in the history of science: a light was then seen which had never before been seen by man on land or sea".[7] Significantly the speaker referred to science, not medicine: it was scientists, engineers and the lay public who first appreciated the potential of Röntgen's rays. (Röntgen himself had coined the term "X-rays" to express – with characteristic modesty – his own mystification about the origin of the phenomenon.) Newspapers and magazines catering for photographic enthusiasts were bombarded with enquiries as to where one of the new "cameras" could be obtained and how much they would cost. Engineers speculated about their use in detecting hidden faults and fractures in metal castings and weldings. The prospect that the technique might be capable of spotting imperfections in golf-balls was enthusiastically discussed in the pages of the *Illustrated London News*. No such unseemly squeals of excitement emanated from the tenebrous plush and mahogany consulting rooms of Harley Street.

Despite a Bill introduced to the Legislative Assembly of the State of New Jersey prohibiting the use of X-rays in opera glasses and all similar contrivances, the American scene was more lively. In 1897 Francis H. Williams of Boston conducted chest X-ray examinations on several hundred patients and reported his findings in a well-argued and well-illustrated article. He pointed to the close correspondence between the physical signs elicited by orthodox methods, like percussion and auscultation, and X-ray appearances. More controversially, he suggested that X-rays could reveal more extensive disease than could be diagnosed on physical examination. Most alarmingly, in some patients in whom only one lung had been suspected of being touched, X-rays showed that the companion lung was also affected. His conclusion, that X-rays would prove to be a more powerful tool in detecting early stages of the illness than fingers and ears,[8] was the first salvo in what was to escalate

---

[6] Perhaps the venue was prophetic. By the 1920s X-rays would provide the most crucial evidence in most cases of disputed medical negligence (as they still do).

[7] Thompson, S., *Archives of Roentgenology*, 2 (1897), 23.

[8] Williams, F. H., *American Journal of Medical Science*, 114 (1897), 665.

into a battle royal between "listeners" and "viewers". It would rage for the best part of half a century.

Even among those who quickly grasped the potential of the new technique, much argument – and hot air – was expanded on the relative merits of fluoroscopic screening versus radiographic pictures. Fluoroscopy was less time-consuming, less expensive and better able to demonstrate the effect of chest movements; but its true though undeclared attraction was that it was less sensitive. In particular, the fluoroscopic screen barely showed up normal lung markings, notoriously confusing to beginners (who were inevitably the majority of actual and potential early users), and generally did not reveal "unnecessary details which ... make the detection of abnormal features difficult and sometimes wellnigh impossible".[9] To the more adventurous this argument was unconvincing. Eventually Lewis G. Cole, initially a partisan of fluoroscopy, pronounced the verdict that "to discard radiography in favour of a slightly easier but less informative technique would be like discarding high-powered modern microscopes because they showed up too many confusing details".[10] Cole later became consulting radiologist to the New York Board of Health and went on to teach that radiology not only made it possible to diagnose early tuberculosis but could also determine with reasonable certainty whether the lesion was active or inactive, advancing, static or resolving. First attempts were also made to use X-rays in the diagnosis of tuberculosis of bones and joints, though the need for diagnostic aids was generally perceived to be less pressing in the extrapulmonary forms of the illness. (It took some years for it to be realised that X-ray changes in bones could lag behind clinical signs.) Among sanatorium doctors Edward Trudeau was a pioneer in embracing the new technology: Saranac Lake became the first institution to have all new admissions X-rayed routinely.

France was not far behind. In 1902 Albert Beclère, a leading tuberculosis specialist in Laënnec's old hospital, La Charité, declared that "examination by radioscopy and radiography will soon totally supersede percussion, auscultation and all other methods in the diagnosis of early tuberculosis of the lungs";[11] and, so far as his own country and much of German-speaking Europe and Scandinavia were concerned, his slightly exaggerated, probably deliberately provocative, forecast soon proved accurate. By 1902 at least four university hospitals in Vienna, and two in the Dual Monarchy's second capital, Budapest, had up-to-date chest X-ray facilities; and, significantly for

[9] Minor, C. M., *Tennessee Medical Journal*, 5 (1908), 56.
[10] Cole, L. G., *American Journal of Medical Science*, 140 (1910), 29.
[11] Beclère, A., *Transactions of the British Society of Tuberculosis*, 3 (1902), 278.

the future, a training scheme for special X-ray nurses and X-ray engineers was inaugurated in Berlin. By 1908 Germany had twenty-five X-ray departments in hospitals and in sanatoria, Davos in Switzerland alone had three and the Scandinavian countries had at least five. Added to their clinical use there was soon another incentive: both France and Germany began to manufacture X-ray machines on a commercial scale and by the 1930s they had become big business.

By contrast, medical opinion in England, after the initial burst of enthusiasm of the X-Ray Society, remained for long unconvinced. When in 1901 John McIntyre, a Glasgow laryngologist, used an X-ray apparatus rigged up for the occasion by the physics department of his university to locate a small coin wedged in the gullet of a patient, the *Lancet* hailed his report as "at last a useful application of the new rays we have heard so much about but whose value has so far eluded most of us".[12] A correspondent added whimsy to idiocy by describing the recovery of the coin as "at any rate profitable". At the International Congress on Tuberculosis in London in the same year a short discussion on the "possible uses of roentgenograms" was squeezed into the programme in the last minute in deference to the venerable Professor J. -L. Bouchardon of Bordeaux who had made radiology his hobby in retirement and who threatened the organisers with a tantrum if he was prevented from showing his "exceedingly pretty pictures". ("Let us hope they're not improper", the secretary of the meeting, Dr John Augustus Prowie, scribbled on a note passed to the chairman.) In fact the occasion was used by Beclère to reaffirm his view that radiology was the diagnostic method of the future, a claim which provoked an acid comment from Dr Hugh Walsham of the Brompton Hospital about "the often short-lived enthusiasms of our French colleagues".[13]

The reasons for the scepticism were mixed. Although tuberculosis and chest diseases in general were gradually becoming a respectable as well as a profitable branch of the profession, they never in Britain attracted the intellectual elite as they traditionally had in France. What little the British top echelon had to offer was their expertise in making elaborate topographical diagnoses based on traditional methods of tapping and listening. Sir William Osler, a generally benign figure but not without a sarcastic streak, treasured a referral letter, sent to him by an eminent London chest physician, describing a tuberculous cavity in the apex of the patient's lung diagnosed entirely by auscultation as being the size of a walnut without the shell. Not many were

---

[12] *Lancet* (1901), no. 2, 465.
[13] Johnson, M., *Dispensary Doctor* (Edinburgh, 1938), p. 87.

prepared to admit that such egregious skills were becoming redundant and might in time prove to be illusory if not fraudulent.

There was a little more to the resistance than a Luddite fear of obsolescence. With clinical pathology not yet perceived as a menace, radiology was the first diagnostic technique which foreshadowed – foreboded was the correct word in the opinion of many – the rise of middleman specialists. Of course the reading of a chest X-ray plate would eventually become part of a chest physician's bedside skill: once a few not very complicated if rather shadowy appearances were mastered none would need another specialist (who often knew nothing about skodaic resonances and sybillant breath sounds) to pontificate about translucencies and striations. Nor would orthopaedic surgeons need radiologists to point out to them bone erosions and hairline fractures. The taking of high-quality X-ray pictures and, even more, the development of new techniques, on the other hand, would inevitably become the domain of a new breed of experts, not an additional clinical skill like auscultation or, more recently, laryngoscopy.[14] This became even more apparent as the potential risks of exposure to X–irradiation became known. Understanding basic radiation physics was not an accomplishment to which leaders of the medical profession aspired; but nor, it seemed, could the matter be left to a few medically unqualified mechanics. It was rather vexing.

In the 1900s the division of labour between several specialities in establishing any but the most complex diagnoses was still far from being the norm. Physicians or surgeons would gather in solemn *consilia* to pool their wisdom around the bedside of important patients; but none saw the need to consult backroom – that is laboratory – technicians, let alone the lead-clad creatures from outer space who had taken charge of the dangerous new X-ray machines. In 1903 Shaw's royal physician, Sir Ralph Bloomfield Bonnington in *The Doctor's Dilemma* would still nonchalantly drop in on his colleague's "lab boys", to borrow a few drops of opsonin with which to pep up his patient's sluggish phagocytes, without feeling the need to ask the advice of somebody who might know something about either opsonins or phagocytosis. Many sensed that the new speciality of radiology heralded the end of these happy days.[15]

[14] A Spanish singing master practising in London, Manuel Garcia, invented this clever instrument in 1854. Laryngoscopy soon became a routine part of the examination of patients with pulmonary tuberculosis. Often it revealed secondary tuberculosis of the larynx.

[15] In fairness to the Sir Ralph Bloomfield Bonnington and the Sir Percival Horton-Smith Harveys (the latter the real name of a real person whom Shaw might have blushed to invent), the multiplicity of specialists now deemed necessary to make a single diagnosis may not be an unmixed blessing.

Scottish doctors were, by and large, more adventurous than their English colleagues. One who foresaw the diagnostic potential of the method was the pioneer of sanatorium regime in Scotland, David Lawson. Having opened Nordrach-on-Dee in Aberdeenshire (in the face of vigorous but unavailing protests from Dr Walther of the original Nordrach in the Black Forest), he acquired in Germany the equipment necessary to take X-ray pictures and even appointed an electrotherapist, R. Hill Crombie, to the staff of his establishment. In a paper published by them jointly in the *Lancet* in 1903, they described what were to become classic X-ray appearances – the roof-tiling of the ribs associated with unresolved pneumonia, cardiac enlargement in emphysema, cavity formation and the opaque bands of scarring in tuberculosis – leaving no room, it might have been thought, for argument about the value of the method.[16] But there is always room for resisting the new.

By the turn of the century putting a needle into the chest under local anaesthesia to aspirate an effusion or pus from the pleural cavity had become well established as a useful and sometimes even life-saving procedure; but the intervention was not without risk. The main difficulty lay in distinguishing the dull sound on percussion and the absent breath sounds on auscultation due to fluid in the pleural space from the not dissimilar aural effects of inflammatory consolidation of the underlying lung. It was nevertheless essential to do so: in an already sick patient the attempted aspiration of the latter could prove fatal. This was a conundrum for which X-rays might have been invented: "a diagnostic greenhorn", as Lawson a little tactlessly put it, "could better distinguish the X-ray shadow cast by fluid in the pleural space from that of lung consolidation than a physician, however eminent, equipped with nothing but his fingers and ears".[17] He made little impression; or rather, he put backs up. Perhaps the very simplicity of the method militated against it: perhaps, on the contrary, it was too complicated for elderly doctors with knighthoods. Whatever the reason, Harley Street consultants continued to thrust trocars into their patients' chests guided by nothing but their well-attested clinical acumen; and the other ranks duly followed. Despite important advances in X-ray technology before the First World War, most notably the introduction of the Coolidge bulb in 1913, capable of generating far more penetrating rays than Röntgen's original tube, the *Tuberculosis Year Book and Sanatorium Annual* of 1920 reported that out of twenty-two local authorities who operated tuberculosis dispensaries only five had access to X-ray facilities; and of the ninety-six sanatoria listed only

[16] Lawson, D., Hill Crombie, R., *Lancet* (1903), no. 2, 65.
[17] Lawson, D., *Practitioner*, 32 (1906), 17.

seven had an X-ray machine. In 1916 Lawson retired from medicine, a disappointed man, to devote his energies to his family business. The value of X-ray diagnosis in tuberculosis was not generally accepted in England until the introduction of collapse therapy in the 1920s.[18]

The revelations by radiology of tuberculous lesions far earlier than could be diagnosed clinically, and X-ray evidence that such lesions might be more common than had been suspected, were reinforced by the advent of skin testing. That a tuberculin-like preparation might be useful in diagnosis even if it proved ineffective in treatment was foreseen by intelligent observers of the tuberculin debacle: indeed, the original material was quickly and success-fully introduced into veterinary medicine for the detection of bovine tuberculosis.[19] The unlikely trail-blazer who adapted the method to routine human use and in the process shed new light on the nature of tuberculosis was a quietly-spoken children's specialist, the scion of an aristocratic Walloon family which had settled in Austria at the time when Habsburg domains were scattered all over Europe. Clemens von Pirquet (1874–1929) was brought up by the Jesuits in Graz and proceeded to study theology in Louvain with the idea of becoming a Jesuit Father himself. Then, though he remained a deeply religious man, he fell in love with his future wife and turned to medicine. He graduated from Graz in 1900 and became an assistant to Professor Escherich, the director of the Vienna Children's Hospital, the first institution of its kind in Europe. After several years of quiet experimentation in his spare time he announced on 8 May 1907, to a meeting of the Berlin Medical Society, the discovery of a safe cutaneous tuberculin test.[20] He made no extravagant claims, merely suggesting that the procedure might help to recognise the initial stages of tuberculosis without putting healthy individuals at risk or even to serious inconvenience and that, hopefully, it might lead to other similar and indeed more sensitive tests. He was right on both counts.[21]

[18] The sixth edition of Sir Douglas Powell's and Sir Percival Horton-Smith Harveys' standard and authoritative textbook, *On Diseases of the Lungs and Pleura*, published in 1921, still states that "in our experience the diagnosis of early phthisis can be made on physical signs long before the appearance of characteristic X-ray changes". This contradicted hundreds of well-documented papers published over the previous twenty years establishing the opposite.

[19] It was often positive in affected cattle even when both sputum and milk were negative for tubercle bacilli.

[20] Pirquet, C. von, *Wiener klinische Wochenschrift*, 20 (1907), 1223.

[21] A year after von Pirquet, Charles Mantoux of Lyon introduced an intracutaneous test (as distinct from von Pirquet's subcutaneous one): though slightly more elaborate, it was capable of better standardisation and became the more widely favoured procedure in most European countries by the late 1920s. It received the blessing of the Medical Research Council in England in 1933. A further refinement, the so-called "percutaneous test", described by E. Moro in 1909, never gained wide popularity. There were many other similar tests, all short-lived.

The Pirquet test was based on the subcutaneous injection of minute doses of a preparation based on Koch's original tuberculin. The original material – insofar as the material was capable of being standardised – had been tried but quickly abandoned. Not only was the injection unpredictably painful, or at least unpleasant, but it could also whip up a fierce local reaction and was not above suspicion as a cause of activating previously quiescent lesions. Various other more or less bizarre routes of administration – including by enema or as eye-drops – were then tried with results equally dismal. Von Pirquet's important realisation was that live or even dead bacilli were not essential for a positive reaction: what mattered was the altered sensitivity of individuals exposed in the past to chemical substances originally elaborated by the organism. As befitted a Jesuit-trained classical scholar he coined for this state the term "allergy".[22]

The Pirquet test was simple, safe and positive (as he had predicted) not only in individuals who were suffering from clinical tuberculosis but also in those who had been exposed to tuberculous infection in the past but in whom the invasion had been ostensibly overcome. In 1912, in the first population survey carried out with the test, 60 per cent of children between the ages of twelve and fifteen resident in one of the inner-city districts of Vienna were found to be positive responders.[23] Even before the outbreak of the First World War put a temporary stop to such studies, several similar surveys on both sides of the Atlantic carried the same message.

The significance of this was not immediately appreciated. "Our awakening began so gently", the American physician, A. K. Krause, wrote in 1919,

> that most of us refused to be stirred up. We may date the dawn of this new day to the Pirquet test. This simple manoeuvre innocently put forward to aid us in diagnosing consumptives even before they are aware of the impending trouble did not fulfil its original purpose. It did not point out who were tuberculous enough to need to be treated and who were not: indeed from this point of view it was a failure. But rarely did failure lead to more significant results. After several years ... the Pirquet test taught us as much about the nature and natural history of tuberculosis as did the discoveries of Laënnec, Villemin or even Koch.[24]

What in a nutshell it did teach doctors was that tuberculosis, the invasion of the body by the tubercle bacillus, and tuberculosis, the clinical disease,

---

[22] From the Greek ἄλλος (other), plus ἐργόν (work).

[23] After a short spell as professor of paediatrics at Johns Hopkins University, Baltimore (appointed at the recommendation of Sir William Osler) and a few years at Breslau (Wroclaw), Von Pirquet had succeeded Escherich as professor of paediatrics in Vienna.

[24] Krause, A. K., *American Review of Tuberculosis*, 2 (1919), 637.

were causally related but not synonymous; and that to understand their relationship the basic pathology of the disease would have to be rethought.[25]

---

[25] His own life ended in tragedy. His wife became a severe manic-depressive a few years after their marriage and a source of constant anxiety to him. He was himself a much-loved figure in Vienna and it came as a shock to his colleagues and pupils when, on 28 February 1929, he and his wife were found dead in their flat from cyanide poisoning.

19

The New Pathology

Some of the rethinking had in fact begun even before Koch's discovery. The primary complex of childhood tuberculosis was described by a French pathologist, Joseph Marie-Jules Parrot, in 1876, and in fine detail by another Frenchman, George Küss, around the turn of the century; but it was Anton Ghon, a Prague doctor, who devoted a whole book to the subject and earned with it eponymous fame.[1] "Ghon's focus" consisted of a tuberculous lesion, rarely more than a centimetre in diameter, too small to be detected in life by percussion or auscultation but demonstrable on post-mortem examination and easily seen on a good-quality X-ray plate. The last was especially striking when, after a lapse of years, the focus calcified and became, like bone, radio-opaque. It was always at the periphery of the lung, just under the pleura, but it was characteristically associated with a conspicuous enlargement of the regional lymph-nodes around the hilum, the site of entry of the main bronchus and blood vessels into the lung. This too could be seen on X-ray plates. But the most striking fact about the complex was its good prognosis in most cases, at least in the short run. Though it signalled the exposure of the child to the bacillus, and it sometimes coincided with a transient minor illness, only rarely did it progress and threaten life.

In some cases, however, months or years later a different kind of lesion developed, apparently caused by the same organism but entirely unlike the primary focus. It occupied the interior of the lung, for some reason never explained almost always the upper lobe.[2] There was no further enlargement of the regional lymph nodes but this time the illness was associated with fever, loss of weight and anaemia, recognisably the Captain of the Men of Death of old.

Inevitably, a learned and sometimes acrimonious debate developed as to whether the second coming was a recrudescence of the primary complex or a reinfection: in 1917 a German pathologist, K. E. Ranke, even proposed a

---

[1] Ghon, A., *The Primary Lung Focus of Tuberculosis in Children*, translated by D. B. King (London, 1916). In his introduction Ghon paid tribute both to Parrot and to Küss.

[2] Why the preferred location is near the apex is still a mystery: posture can have little to do with it since the favoured localisation also applies to quadrupeds.

complicated three-stage progression, comparable to what was by then well established as the primary, secondary and tertiary stages of syphilis.[3] It was more important – and far more difficult – to define the role of Koch's bacillus in two such seemingly different pathologies.

That it was the underlying cause was by the late 1900s no longer in doubt. Its microscopic appearance had become familiar to most doctors and even to laymen. It was a slender, elegantly curved rod, so small that a dozen or more could be accommodated inside a medium-sized tissue cell. It was not easy to stain but Koch had worked out a method, using an alkaline solution of methylene blue, which showed up against a pale background of Bismarck brown.[4] His pupil, Paul Ehrlich, a virtuoso of dyes and stains, improved on his master's method by substituting hot fuchsin as the primary stain and decolourising everything except the bacillus with 30 per cent nitric acid. Characteristically, once stained the colour could not be removed from the organism by flushing the slide with strong acid or alcohol: hence the code by which doctors came to refer to it when speaking in hushed whispers – acid-alcohol-fast. Although acknowledged as the cause of tuberculosis, its mode of action, and even more its frequent mode of inaction, remained a puzzle.

Of course instances of lethal pathogens causing no illness had long been known; and they were not always saintly miracles. Amid screams of horror from his audience the eccentric Professor Max Pettenkofer of Munich, determined to disprove the existence of the cholera bacillus – "the figment of a fevered and uneducated mind" – swallowed a culture teeming with live organisms (sent to him by Koch himself), a gesture which should have killed him in agony within forty-eight hours. He did not turn a hair. Yet by and large the sequence of a bacterial invasion and the corresponding illnesses

[3] Ranke, K. E., *Berliner klinische Wochenschrift*, 54 (1917), 397. The three stages of syphilis (primary chancre, secondary rash with systemic illness, and tertiary gummata and cardiovascular and neurosyphilis) were well established; but tuberculosis never really fitted into such a pattern. Nevertheless, Stages One to Three were widely used as rather imprecise indications of how advanced the disease was thought to be. A cure was thought to be possible in Stage One and problematic in Stage Two. Patients in Stage Three were reckoned to have less than a year to live.

The controversy of recrudescence versus reinfection continued well into the late 1940s when (unsurprisingly) consensus came down in favour of both mechanisms being possible. The answer was by then of no practical importance.

[4] The staining method used for demonstrating the tubercle bacillus today is associated with the names of Ziehl and Neelsen, who introduced minor modifications to Ehrlich's technique, the first the use of carbolic acid and the second the use of sulphuric instead of nitric acid. Eponyms in medicine often bear no relationship to the importance of the workers or the work commemorated.

could be predicted with reasonable certainty with most organisms. But tuberculosis was different.

Some of the differences were obvious. For a creature that was still, at the turn of century, the chief killer of young people in the western world, the organism lacked most of the traits which pioneer microbiologists had already recognised as characteristically lethal or at least aggressive. Though it was hardy in the sense of surviving in dark dusty corners and cracks in the floor-boards for months or even years, in the laboratory, under conditions carefully designed to provide it with all a bacillus might reasonably be expected to desire, it grew and multiplied many times more slowly than most other organisms. Indeed, Koch's heroic persistence in looking at his original cultures for signs of growth for weeks, after other pathogens would have shown up as luxuriant colonies and other researchers would have given up in despair, had become part of the mythology of microbiology.[5] Even more remarkably, the bacillus neither elaborated nor contained within its substance obviously noxious agents. It did not, for example, produce haemolysins which caused the destruction of red blood cells in infections with the haemolytic streptococcus (the causative agent of scarlet fever and of other grave illnesses) or with *Clostridium welchii* (the causative agent of gas gangrene); nor did it produce toxins which in minute amounts could paralyse the brain or the heart, as did the organisms responsible for diphtheria or tetanus.[6]

Yet if Koch's bacillus did not behave as a killer, neither was it easily killed. One explanation put forward by an otherwise obscure Austrian pathologist, Johannes Lange, and still accepted today, was that the organism possessed a fatty envelope or capsule which was uniquely impermeable to antibacterial enzymes.[7] This could partly at least account for its unusual natural history. Carried by inspired air inside liquid droplets or particles of dust to the microscopic air-sacs of the lung, or penetrating through minute cracks in the gastrointestinal mucosa, the organism could lie for a few days or weeks inactive but unharmed in the tissue spaces. It would then be picked up by a wandering cell vaguely referred to as a mobile histiocyte and later renamed

[5] If Koch had never discovered any new organisms he would – or should – still be remembered as a technical innovator. In 1882 he introduced the first of the now standard culture media, gelatin enriched with a sterilised meat broth, followed by agar enriched with egg yolk, serum and eventually whole blood. One of his assistants, R. J. Petri, introduced what he described as a "slight modification", the still standard "Petri dish".

[6] Exotoxin was the technical term coined for the group of poisons which are synthesised by organisms and are active outside them. Toxic substances which are part of the chemical structure of organisms and are released only when the organisms disintegrate are known as endotoxins.

[7] For decades the presence of the capsules also inspired a sense of nihilism among research workers since it was widely held that no chemotherapeutic agent or antibiotic would pass through it.

a macrophage. The reference was vague because the origin of these cells was (as it still is) uncertain: though seemingly ubiquitous, they were, like the wind when it is not blowing, difficult to detect when not homing in on microbes or other foreign material. Wherever they came from, they could engulf and often destroy intruders: in other words they belonged to a class of cells recognised – even celebrated – by the turn the century under the name of phagocytes.[8]

The process of phagocytosis had been expounded and actually demon-strated under the microscope by the brilliant (if according to many more than slightly mad) Russian scientist Elie Metchnikoff in the late 1890s.[9] Almost inevitably, it became the flagship of the medical avant-garde. Here at last was the key to the body's defences against the ubiquitous microbes. What Metchnikoff had shown (more or less) was that the invasion of a living body by harmful organisms triggered off a complex but purposeful reaction. Activated by a chemical signal (not clearly identified then or since), the bone marrow stepped up its rate of production of a certain kind of white cell at least a million-fold. Metchnikoff called these cells polymorphnuclear leuko-cytes. Within minutes billions of them, some obviously hastily assembled and only half-finished, were carried by the bloodstream to the site of the invasion. There they would squeeze through the lining of the capillaries and actively propel themselves – again nobody knew how – to confront, engulf, consume and destroy the invading microbes. There was a sequel to this. Although the polymorphnuclear leukocytes destroyed the bacilli, the leuko-cytes too were destroyed. The debris of the battle would constitute the bulk of what for centuries had been known as pus and had often been referred to as laudable pus.

Compared to this heroic scenario (not far from reality in the case of such common pathogens as the *staphylococci* and *streptococci*), the sequence of events in tuberculosis lacked drama. The progress of the mysterious tissue

[8] Literally "cells which eat up".

[9] He was born in Ivanovka in Moldavia in 1845, the son of a Jewish businessman (whom he later in life tended to describe as a major general of noble Moldavian descent), and became professor of zoology in Odessa in 1874. After travelling widely and teaching at several European universities, a laboratory was set up for him by Pasteur at the Ecole Normale (later hived off to become the nucleus of the Institut Pasteur) in Paris in 1888. There he continued to work for the rest of his life. He wrote in three languages on an extraordinary range of subjects, among them intracellular digestion (in which he described phagocytosis), the comparative pathology of inflammation, immunity, the nature of man and the prolongation of human life. In the last he ranged rhapsodically over every aspect of the decrepit state known as old age, maintaining – probably rightly – that it should be regarded and treated as an abnormal process in its own right rather than as the sum total of a host of separate degenerative diseases. Many of his extraordinary insights are still not widely enough recognised. He died in 1916.

phagocytes wherever they came from was stately and their number remained small. What distinguished them most clearly from Metchnikoff's polymorph-nuclear leukocytes was their relationship to their target organism. Though the tubercle bacilli were engulfed – that is phagocytosed – neither the cells nor the organisms showed much inclination to destroy the other. Indeed, the organisms continued to multiply inside the macrophages,[10] their fatty capsules soon imparting to their host cell a slightly bloated, ground glass appearance. Because this appearance reminded pathologists of the wholly unrelated cells of the skin known as epithelial, the altered macrophages were called epitheloid. For reasons unknown – a monotonous refrain in the pathology of tuberculosis – these epitheloid cells had a tendency to fuse, forming the second characteristic microscopic structure, a blob of cytoplasm with a dozen or so nuclei lined up horseshoe fashion along the periphery. Though not in fact particularly big, these became known, after the German pathologist who described them, as Langhans giant cells.

Though in many respects atypical, the events so far could be understood and interpreted in terms of cellular pathology, the majestic and all-inclusive system elaborated by the great Rudolph Virchow, and his disciples.[11] (By the 1880s they occupied all the important university chairs in pathology in Germany.) The system was based on the idea that individual cells were the units to which both the normal and the abnormal functions of the body could be traced: without a cellular explanation, in other words, there could be no disease (or, for that matter, no health). Since cells could be seen and studied under the microscope, this made microscopic pathology the touch-stone of truth both in diagnosis and in research. The concept delivered the coup de grâce to such ancient and discredited but still lingering notions as the four humours and even to Bichat's more recent idea of tissues. Within a few decades it shed new light on a host of fundamental processes, including inflammation, cancer, hypertrophy, atrophy and hyperplasia, and clarified the origin of a wide range of diseases in almost every organ of the body.[12] The revolutionary findings of microbiology required adjustments but could be accommodated within the overall design: microbes were, after all, cells themselves. Even phagocytosis was an essentially cellular if somewhat out-landish phenomenon. Yet the more majestic and comprehensive a biological

[10] The term "macrophage" was to distinguish these cells from Metchnikoff's smaller poly-morphnuclear leukocytes (occasionally referred to in the early literature as "microphages").

[11] See above, chapter 12, note 11.

[12] Inflammation: tissue response to injury. Cancer: inadequately controlled (autonomous) proliferation of cells. Hypertrophy: enlargement of an organ due to enlargement of individual cells. Atrophy: the reverse. Hyperplasia: enlargement of an organ due to increased number of cells. Aplasia: the reverse.

system, the more likely it is to be full of holes; and at the very moment when the humours seemed to join the ranks of historical curiosities, humoral mechanisms began to crop up in a new guise.

In 1889 Richard Pfeiffer, a thirty-year-old assistant of Robert Koch, devised a method of distinguishing two morphologically similar organisms. One was *Vibrio cholerae*, the causative agent of cholera, the other the harmless *Vibrio metchnikovi*. The test was based on injecting the organisms into the peritoneal cavity of guinea-pigs and watching the organism multiply. During the 1892 cholera epidemic in Hamburg, Pfeiffer noted that when vibrio were injected into animals previously exposed to the infection the organisms did not multiply: instead they swelled and burst. He was more puzzled to note that this did not seem to involve any cellular activity, almost a contradiction in terms. Before reporting his findings, and more for the sake of completeness than expecting a positive result, he added to a suspension of vibrio in a test-tube a few drops of cell-free serum from a previously infected animal. The serum produced the same swelling and lysis within a few minutes as occurred in the living animals. The observation was commended as interesting but pronounced an anomaly.

A year later a young English graduate, H. E. Durham, was awarded the Gull studentship at Guy's Hospital in London and joined the bacteriology department of Professor Max Gruber of Vienna. Gruber was an authoritarian figure who harboured the soul of a rebel. To the surprise of his own staff, he suggested that his visitor might like to study the mechanism of what was known as "Pfeiffer's phenomenon" – known but not approved of. Indeed, Gruber made it clear that it was probably a freak and would therefore leave enough time for the young Englishman to sample the pleasures of the Prater, the Wienerwald, Hietzing and, since he was a music-lover and an admirer of Richard Wagner, the Opera. In the event, the project left Durham little time for anything else but proved to be as full of surprises as the score of *Tristan*. The paper embodying his findings,[13] not published until after his return to London, was short; but, coupled with Pfeiffer's original observation, it paved the way for the new science of immunology.[14]

---

[13] Durham, H. E., *Proceedings of the Royal Society*, 54 (1896), 224. Durham later became professor in Cambridge. He died in 1945, aged seventy-nine.

[14] Durham's aims were and remained essentially practical, to show how the specific sera could be used in the diagnosis of obscure fevers, in tracing carriers and in epidemics; alternatively how the interaction of patients' sera with known bacteria could help in making individual diagnoses. Other important papers, among them reports by Ferdinand Widal of Paris (on the diagnosis of typhoid), R. C. Cabot of Boston, A. E. Wright at the time of the Army Medical School at Netley (on the diagnosis of Malta fever) followed within the next few years. The complement fixation test, an ingenious elaboration of Pfeiffer's phenomenon devised by

Immunity – or, more precisely, the effects of immunity – had been recognised for centuries. The teachers of Salerno stated that individuals who had by the grace of God survived a fatal pestilence were less likely than others to succumb to that pestilence when it struck again. During the great plague of Venice in 1576 the Doge and his Council searched for elderly doctors who had themselves survived the illness to look after the sick: however frail, they had the best chance of surviving for a second time. The experience led to several deliberate prophylactic schemes, most notably to Edward Jenner's breathtakingly audacious programme of inoculating against smallpox with the relatively harmless cowpox.[15] It was the microbiological revolution, however, which made it necessary to put that experience on a general and experimental basis.

Even before Durham's paper gave support and general validity to Pfeiffer's phenomenon and provided the opening to a new methodology, diagnostic serology, Koch, Pasteur and many of their immediate collaborators began to discern a new biological mechanism. It was to prove as important in the long run as their discovery of disease-causing germs. It seemed that most vertebrates possessed a microscopically invisible but extraordinarily efficient system of protection against outside invaders. By the turn of the century the system – beginning to be known as immunity – took on recognisable outlines. It could do three things. First, it could recognise material that was foreign (non-self in the ugly jargon of the 1950s) when such material was introduced into the body. Secondly, it could mount a purposeful and often astonishingly quick and effective response to such an intrusion. Thirdly, it remembered the event long after every visible trace of both the invasion and the response had disappeared. This last capacity was shown by a second response markedly different from the first when the same material was introduced again.

In the paper in which he described tuberculin and hinted at its potentially healing properties (which inevitably stole the show), Koch also referred to a less immediately newsworthy observation. It presaged many subsequent developments. He had found that when tubercle bacilli were injected under the skin of a guinea-pig for the first time there was no reaction for ten to fourteen days. Then a nodule developed at the injection site which, when excised,

---

J. Bordet, prompted A. P. Wassermann and G. Sachs to try serological diagnosis in tuberculosis. The results were too unpredictable; but in 1905 the work led to the famous Wassermann reaction, the standard diagnostic test for syphilis for sixty years.

[15] Jenner, a country practitioner, published his epoch-making article on vaccination in 1798. It is not perhaps widely known that so certain was he in his own mind that *vaccinia* (cowpox) would protect against *variola* (smallpox) that he followed up his first vaccination of a farmer's son with scratching the subject a month later with fluid from a smallpox vesicle. At the time the experiment does not seem to have raised an ethical eye-brow. Jenner became highly acclaimed in his lifetime and died in 1823, aged seventy-four.

showed under the microscope an aggregation of tubercles. If it was not excised, it usually ulcerated and became secondarily infected. Meanwhile the bacilli were carried to the regional lymph nodes where they produced necrotic lesions. If the injected dose was big enough, the animal soon died of disseminated tuberculosis. If the dose was small, however, and if the animal survived for a few months at least, a second inoculation at a site distant from the first elicited an entirely different response. At the site of the second injection a nodule began to form within a matter of hours; it went on to ulcerate within a day or two; and, most surprisingly, it then healed.

Instead of a simple explanation the next decades brought further confusing evidence. There existed, it seemed, not only immunity but also abnormal immunity. Indeed, by the turn of the century Koch and others began to suspect that what killed many tuberculous individuals was not the bacillus itself but the body's protective response to the bacillus, which had somehow gone wrong. This was a disturbing concept. Not surprisingly, it gave rise to much heated argument.

First, there was the question of terminology. It seemed reasonable to describe the body's protective – that is beneficial – reaction to microbial invasion (or reinvasion) as the immune response. The term became blatantly inappropriate, however, when, under different circumstances, the reaction led not to healing but to more tissue destruction and even, on occasion, to death. Under these circumstances, it was felt, the response should be described not as immune but as hypersensitivity. Semantic distinctions in themselves did not overcome the basic difficulty. Nobody could predict when, why and in what way the different circumstances were different. Neither hypersensitivity nor immunity came with a label attached to it. The only thing that made it possible to make the distinction was the outcome. If the response helped the individual to overcome the disease, it was immune. If it made the disease worse and even killed the patient, it was hypersensitivity. This fell well short of a practical breakthrough.

In the meantime the actual mechanism of the response – whether immune or hypersensitivity – was further investigated. Both responses were shown to depend on a special property of the invading foreign material. This property was beginning to be labelled antigenicity.[16] A wide variety of substances could be antigenic. Others, often quite similar, were not. Nor was the property fixed. It could vary depending on the individual exposed to them. It could change even in the same individual with the passage of time.

---

[16] This nonsensical coinage (whose exact authorship is difficult to ascertain) followed the already widespread use of terms like "antitoxin" and "antibodies" in the 1890s to describe property X which would provoke anti-X.

Even more confusingly, both immunity and hypersensitivity manifested themselves by two different mechanisms. By the 1920s these became known as the non-cellular and cellular responses. "Non-cellular" later became "humoral" and "cellular" became "cell-mediated".

The non-cellular or humoral response involved the elaboration of antibodies. These were large molecules belonging to the globulin class of proteins. The cells responsible were identified in the 1920s and early 1930s. They were not particularly distinguished looking but had special staining properties. They could best be demonstrated in the bone marrow but were distributed in several other organs as well. Originally called plasma cells, they became known in the 1960s as B lymphocytes.[17] Changes in medical nomenclature sometimes have a hypnotic effect. They suggest a better understanding of observed but mysterious phenomena. After a lapse of time the benefits become less obvious. Whether called plasma cells or B lymphocytes, most of the key questions remained unanswered or incompletely answered. What was the signal which switched on the antibody synthesising activity of the plasma cells or B lymphocytes? How was the signal conveyed? And how were the antibodies tailor-made to interact with distant antigens?

The non-cellular or humoral response was demonstrable within minutes or even seconds. The antibodies were carried to the antigen by the bloodstream. Ehrlich's idea that their interaction was analogous to acids and bases forming salts was soon shown to be simplistic; but nobody could suggest convincing alternative. Whatever the mechanism, it was generally assumed to be protective in character, neutralising or destroying harmful antigens. Yet this too could go wrong. Individuals exposed to an antigen sometimes collapsed and died. Was this anaphylactic shock caused by the antigen? Or by the antibody? Or both? Nobody knew.[18]

---

[17] The inelegant terms B lymphocytes and T lymphocytes first came into use following the discovery of two distinct types of lymphocytes which could not be differentiated by conventional morphological examination. The thymus, a vestigial organ in adults but active in foetal life, was shown to provide the precursor cells of lymphocytes active in cell-mediated immunity: hence the term "T" lymphocytes. From this it seemed (to some) reasonable to argue that a similar precursor organ must exist for the lymphocytes responsible for the production of antibodies, that is for humoral immunity. Unfortunately, the only species in which such an organ appears to exist is the chicken. The bird is said to possess a localised mass of lymphoid tissue in close proximity to an anatomical outpouching in the region of the cloaca long known (to veterinary anatomists) as the Bursa of Fabricius. The word bursa begins with b: hence "B" lymphocytes. As various methods developed, none of them foolproof, to distinguish T from B lymphocytes, it became apparent that some lymphocytes belonged to neither category. It has been suggested these should be described as "null lymphocytes".

[18] Individuals dying of true anaphylactic shock (fortunately extremely rare) show no specific abnormality on post-mortem examination.

Since antibodies were too small to be visible under an ordinary microscope, humoral immunity spelt the end of the total dominance of microscopic pathology. The study of the newly discovered phenomena demanded – and got – a range of new indirect techniques, many based on the work of Pfeiffer and Durham. Red blood cells or inert cell-sized particles, for example, could be coated with a known antigen. They would be added to serum suspected of harbouring the corresponding specific antibodies. A positive antigen-antibody interaction could be observed by watching the clumping of the antigen-coated cells or particles. The tests grew in complexity and created a new laboratory speciality – diagnostic serology. There was no branch of medicine that was not affected.[19]

Cellular – later cell-mediated – immunity differed from non-cellular – later humoral – immunity in several respects. Humoral immunity could be initiated by a wide variety of different organic and even inorganic antigens. It was an immediate response. Cell-mediated immunity required the antigen to be a protein. It also required the antigen to remain fixed in the tissues for some time. In tuberculosis the response did not begin to show itself for twenty-four to seventy-two hours. The trigger was supposed to be the engulfing of the tubercle bacilli by macrophages; but nobody knew for certain. Whatever the signal, cells (known later as T lymphocytes) began to migrate toward the lesion from nearby and distant parts of the body.[20] The migration was obviously purposeful but what directed it and what its exact purpose was remained uncertain. The migrant cells were not overtly phagocytic. They resembled lymphocytes: perhaps they *were* lymphocytes – but perhaps not. Their congregation in and around the tuberculous lesion would be described in countless pathology reports as small round-cell infiltration. Soon the small round cells and their cousins, cells not so small and not so round but of equally uncertain provenance, came to make up a significant portion of the tuberculous lesion. Some attached themselves to free-lying tubercle bacilli. Many more clustered around the macrophages inside which tubercle bacilli multiplied. Their attachment often resulted in the cells and bacilli being killed. This was to be applauded, but it was not the only effect. In a way, and for reasons mysterious when first described and almost as mysterious today, the round cells were also instrumental in the break-down of apparently normal or at least still living tissue.

Usually this first became apparent near the centre of the tuberculous lesion.

---

[19] Apart from its value in bacterial illnesses, diagnostic serology opened the way to safe blood transfusion, allowing the identification of the major blood groups. This in turn led to tissue grouping and organ transplantation and much of modern surgery.
[20] See note 17 above.

What at one moment was an area packed with a variety of more or less clearly defined cells – macrophages lymphocytes, giant cells and structures still recognisably belonging to the parent organ – suddenly coalesced into an amorphous mass. Because the consistence of this mass reminded Matthew Baillie in the eighteenth century of cheese, in the seemingly unalterable tradition of describing deadly tissue changes in culinary terms, he called the event caseation.[21] As the tuberculous nodule grew, so often did the caseating area. In some situations – in lymph nodes, for example, or in bone – it was sometimes referred to as a cold abscess.

One other element in the tuberculous process had long attracted attention. Inflammation is a biological phenomenon even more ancient and universal and basically even less well understood than the immune response. It is the reaction of all living things – plants as well as animals and humans – to any kind of injury. Its main clinical manifestations in man were summarised by a Roman physician, Aurelius Cornelius Celsus, in the first century AD: *rubor, calor, tumor, turgor* and *dolor* (redness, heat, swelling, turgidity and pain). The list soon became one of the hallowed litanies of medicine.[22] Celsus also described how the inflammatory response merged with another complicated process – the process of healing. This was later shown to be largely the function of another kind of ubiquitous cell which seemed to emerge from nowhere around an injury. In deference to their main function, the elaboration of collagen fibres, Virchow named them fibroblasts.[23] In acute lesions (like a staphylococcal abscess), fibroblastic activity tended to follow tissue destruction and the inflammatory response. In contrast, in chronic infections tissue destruction, inflammation and fibroblastic activity often proceeded side by side and at the same time. Once again, tuberculosis was special. As Sylvius had noted in the seventeenth century, healing by scar formation in

---

[21] Baillie was the son of a professor of divinity in Glasgow and the nephew of John and William Hunter. He was appointed to the staff of St George's Hospital, London, in 1787 at the age of twenty-seven. He described caseation in his famous textbook, *The Morbid Anatomy of Some of the Most Important Parts of the Human* Body (London, 1793). He died in 1823. The fatty capsules of tubercle bacilli may be partly responsible for the "cheesiness" of what is in effect tuberculous pus.

[22] It has been suggested (perhaps because he wrote so well) that he was not a practising doctor but a popular writer on medical topics. His great work, *De medicina* (of about AD 30) seems to have been lost sight of in the middle ages but became the first medical book to be printed (in 1478 under the title *De re medicina*). Thereafter it enjoyed immense popularity, being reprinted at least fifty times by the mid eighteenth century. Celsus's sonorous list omits one important cardinal sign of inflammation (added in the eighteenth century): *functio laesa* or impaired function.

[23] Generically "blasts" mean young cells. Fibrocytes, theoretically adult or old fibre-producing cells, are not readily identifiable.

consumption could become so vigorous that its consequences, some of them undesirable, overshadowed those of the active disease.[24]

One of the cardinal properties of collagen is that after a time the fibres interlink and contract. This is usually beneficial, indeed essential. It pulls together the edges of a wound and obliterates gaps and cavities. But in tuberculosis thick bands of scar tissue surrounding a lesion were capable of causing terrible deformities. These were most conspicuous in the skin and around joints; but the consequences were even graver inside the body. In tuberculous peritonitis they accounted for the matting together of coils of intestine and the nightmare sequence of acute obstruction, operation, more scarring and further episodes of obstruction. In the pleura they would assume critical significance with the introduction of collapse therapy.[25]

The fact that tubercle bacilli could not be shown to produce toxins deepened the mystery of the systemic effects of the disease. Why did patients with tuberculosis in almost any organ begin to develop spikes of temperature in the evening, sometimes months before any localising symptom or sign? Why did they lose weight? Why did they feel at times overwhelmingly tired? Why at other times did they feel irrationally and exuberantly gay? Why did they become anaemic – that is white? For want of a better explanation all these were now ascribed to cell-mediated immunity. This was pure guesswork. Medical oracles of the past were no more inclined to dwell on what they could not explain than are recognised authorities today; and by the 1930s cell-mediated immunity had become the dumping grounds of conceptual rubbish.

At the clinical level one fact began to crystallise. In the natural history of slowly progressive tuberculosis there was usually an event which reduced or even extinguished the chances of spontaneous recovery. It was not caseation as such: small caseating lesions could heal and even calcify. The point of no return – or very unlikely return – varied from organ to organ but was best documented in the lung. Inevitably, as a pulmonary tuberculous focus expanded, it would begin to encroach on a branch of the bronchial tree. For a time the bronchus might offer resistance; but sooner or later its wall would crumble. It was then only a question of time before the caseous material from the centre of the lesion would burst into the air passages. Some of it would be coughed up; but the event would leave behind a space lined with ragged tuberculous tissue. It was known as a cavity.

Although cavitation had been recognised as a calamity by Bayle, Laënnec

---

[24] Nobody knows the reason why tuberculous scarring is so gross: only some burns leave comparable scars.

[25] See below, Chapter 22.

and especially by Skoda during the first half of the nineteenth century, only after Koch's discovery did the reasons for this become clear. Apart from indicating a diseased area of considerable size, it meant that henceforth the lesion would be well-aerated. Koch had shown that the tubercle bacillus was a strict aerobe: it could survive but not grow and multiply without a generous supply of oxygen. Since cavities communicated directly with the outside world, organisms in the lining of cavities could flourish. Even more alarmingly, the bronchial tree provided a ready-made conduit for the infected material to spread. From now on caseous necrotic tissue, often teeming with bacilli, would be coughed up: in clinical parlance the patient became an "open" case. That would transform his or her relationship to the outside world. In hospitals it often meant a separate ward, masked nurses and doctors, restricted visiting. The patients would be conveyed to other parts of the hospital – the lecture theatre perhaps or the X-ray department – on special trolleys enclosed in large tent-like structures. At home they would be isolated as far as possible. Isolated or not, they would be shunned by all but their closest family. To them they would be a menace. On the way up the bronchial tree caseous material would often lodge in the throat, setting up tuberculous laryngitis. Coughing then became not only dangerous to contacts but also intensely painful. In the late stages the power of speech could be reduced to a hoarse, agonising whisper.

This was not all. However conscientiously patients used sputum cups, some of the coughed up material would be swallowed. In the stomach it would act as an irritant and sooner or later set up a superficial gastritis. This could cause overwhelming nausea, almost impossible to alleviate. The patient's breath often became foul smelling. Superficial gastritis could progress to tuberculous ulceration. Abdominal pain, vomiting and diarrhoea would then add their share of suffering to the illness.

Spread of the infected material in the opposite direction could set up new, more peripheral lesions in the lung. Any of these could impinge on the pleura and start a tuberculous pleurisy. This was one of the most feared complications. Not only coughing but the taking of every breath became painful, "side-stitches that shall pen your breath up".[26] Disturbed nights turned into nightmares: no pain-killer, not even laudanum or later morphine, could entirely cope with them. In generally enfeebled patients an empyaema, the accumulation of tuberculous pus in the pleural cavity, and disseminated tuberculosis, including tuberculous meningitis, was now an ever-present danger.

Before cavity formation, slowly-growing tuberculous lesions surrounded

---

[26] Shakespeare, *The Tempest*, Act I, Scene 2, line 326.

by scar tissue tended to cause thrombosis in the blood vessels with which
they came into contact. This meant that massive haemorrhage (as distinct
from streaks of blood in the sputum) was comparatively rare. Once a cavity
had formed, growth often outstripped such protective thromboses. From
then on relatively large blood vessels could be suddenly eroded. This could
precipitate massive, dramatic bleeds. One of these was often a terminal event.
Perhaps, after months or years of suffering, the end was not always wholly
unwelcome. The thought sometimes comforted grieving relatives.

20

Blip

Throughout the nineteenth century industrious pathologists filled tomes or more often multitomes with erudite speculations about the causes of tuberculosis, an ever-lengthening list. After Koch there should have been no need for this. The cause was known. The *Mycobacterium tuberculosis* fulfilled Koch's own rigorous postulates. For those determined to search for a cure it provided a target to shoot at. In practice the change was more semantic than real. One key question replaced another. Nobody asked what caused tuberculosis any more. Everybody wanted to know what determined the outcome of the infection. Why, to put it differently, did the disease progress in some patients and cause death; while in others the organism remained a seemingly harmless fellow-traveller.

The possibilities fell into two categories. First, it was reasonable to blame variations in the inherent nature of the bacillus. Even in the early years of bacteriology such variations were well recognised. The ancient term virulence was used to describe them. Nobody understood its mechanisms; but there was no doubt that in the case of many, apparently identical organisms, including some of the commonest, it could determine whether an infection would kill, cause a minor illness or never even be noticed. Yet nobody was able to demonstrate such variations in the bacillus causing tuberculosis. This did not mean that the bacillus could not be attenuated in the laboratory. Attenuation, that is loss of virulence, was not only possible: it was soon to acquire great practical importance. Yet it was not part of the natural history of the illness. It could certainly not explain the differences in the clinical picture in different individuals, different families, different races and different historical periods.

The second category involved variations not in the bacillus but in the hosts. Although this could be described as varying susceptibility or resistance, it was clearly not a single characteristic. At least no single characteristic could be shown to account for it. It implied the operation of a large number of variables – the term aetiological factor was gaining currency around the turn of the century – whose interplay was subtle and complex. Yet, if such variables did exist – and if virulence did not change they *had* to exist – what were they?

One unwelcome answer soon emerged. All statistics agreed that by 1914 mortality from tuberculosis in western countries was declining and had been declining at least since the 1870s. (It was said – but nobody at the time tried to compile statistics – that the incidence of the disease rose sharply in Paris during and immediately after the siege of 1871.) The reasons for this were obvious to some, less so to others. Philanthropists, public-health workers and politicians pointed with satisfaction to the steady improvement in the material and moral welfare of the masses – the blessings of wise government and generous private benevolence. It was undoubtedly true that fewer people in Europe starved in 1914 than had half a century earlier and that new-born infants in the slums of London and Paris (though not of Dublin) had a better chance of surviving their first year of life. Doctors claimed to have made great strides in their understanding of the disease (which was true) and in the treatment of patients (which was questionable); and hospitals were less lethal than when Dickens was a young man. In short, those in positions of authority and influence could – and did – claim that ordinary folk had never had it so good. It is true that, much to the irritation of those in positions of authority and influence, cynics maintained that wise government and private benevolence had nothing to do with the improvements, but even they had to admit that, if the prevailing trends continued, by the 1940s death from tuberculosis in the civilised west would be a thing of the past.

But the prevailing trends did not continue. Among the historically least often considered but starkest consequences of the shots fired in Sarajevo in the summer of 1914 was the end of the steady downward trend in the mortality from tuberculosis. The curve did not, as had occasionally happened in the past after a bad harvest, just flatten out for a year. Between 1914 and 1918, for the first time since more or less reliable statistics had begun, mortality from the disease actually rose. The figures varied. In England the rise was by about 17 per cent, in Italy by about 34 per cent, in Austria by about 44 per cent, in Germany by about 62 per cent, in Hungary by about 58 per cent and in Denmark by about 30 per cent. Of these the last was perhaps the most surprising.

Denmark was not in the war and escaped many of the material deprivations of countries which were. Its economy rested largely on the export of meat and dairy products; and demand for these by the belligerent powers rocketed. The consequences at home were mixed. The high prices paid for farm produce abroad benefited farmers, an important minority but still only a minority of the population. Since wages in general did not keep pace with prices, the rest of the Danes starved. (Despite the war, this was still the golden age of liberal economics and the idea of restricting exports or regulating prices by government action was unthinkable.) By 1917 the British blockade of Germany and Germany's unrestricted submarine warfare combined to curtail and eventually to stop Danish exports. The country was forced to live off its own produce; and shortage of fodder led to the wholesale slaughter of pigs and cattle. On paper this was a disaster and was universally lamented by economists. There was a precipitous fall in the income per head of the population. But almost unnoticed amidst the wailing and wringing of hands the consumption of milk, milk products and meat, now once again affordable, rose to acceptable levels. This was immediately reflected in the mortality figures from tuberculosis: toward the end of 1918, while abroad the war was still raging and tuberculosis mortality rising, in Denmark it fell from its 1917 level of 176 per 100,000 to the 1914 level of 128 per 100,000. (Denmark had one of the best statistical services in Europe; and these wartime fluctuations were among the first to show how quick and sensitive properly collected and analysed data could be in reflecting social and economic changes.)

It is still not known what were the critical components in the shortages and hardships of the war which drove up the death rate from tuberculosis elsewhere in Europe.[1] Just as urban squalor during the Industrial Revolution was a combination of many evils – malnutrition, overcrowding and alcoholism perhaps the most deadly – the causes were obviously multiple. Nor did the question attract much attention at the time. What mattered was winning the war. Tuberculosis was – or was perceived to be – a civilian and therefore an irrelevant problem. Even well-advanced antituberculous legislation and campaigns started before 1914 were put on hold.[2] In Austria-Hungary to raise

---

[1] Despite a cataract of words, inconclusive research and statistical juggling, the undoubted correlation between tuberculosis and general nutrition has never been convincingly traced to any particular food. Even "general nutrition" should perhaps to be between quotation marks since its decline never occurs in isolation.

The experiences of the First World War were patchily repeated during the Second. In Britain, Germany, France and in most of German-occupied Europe the rise in civilian mortality from tuberculosis (to the very limited extent that these were reported in official statistics) was not nearly so dramatic as it had been during the First World War but was nevertheless real. The most striking and by and large the most reliable statistical evidence relates to Japan, where in 1945–46 mortality from tuberculosis was more than twice as high as the official figures recorded for 1938.

[2] An Inter-Departmental Committee on Tuberculosis had been set up in Britain in 1912 under the chairmanship of Waldorf Astor, MP (later Viscount Astor) "to report at an early date upon considerations of general policy in respect to the problems of tuberculosis in the United Kingdon in its preventive, curative and other aspects which should guide the Government and local bodies ... in making provisions", etc. The committee reported in 1913 and its recommendations were broadly accepted by the government and Parliament as the basis of official antituberculosis policy; but all projected schemes were halted in July 1914 "for the duration of the Conflict". While the rise in mortality from tuberculosis in Britain during the war years was slightly less than in most continental countries, it was still, by 1918, alarming enough to call for action. Special concern was felt (or so the government professed) for tuberculous ex-servicemen who by 1919 numbered over 35,000. Goaded by public opinion,

the subject was considered unpatriotic. The editor of the German-language Budapest newspaper, *Pester Lloyd*, went to prison in 1917 for protesting against the evacuation of the tuberculosis sanatoria and lunatic asylums to make room for the wounded (but not the shell-shocked). The lack of public interest was not perhaps surprising. Compared to the carnage of young men in Flanders and Russia, compared even to the depredations of the Spanish Flu which began to sweep over Europe in the wake of the war, the rise in tuberculosis mortality was a blip. But unlike the shooting and the influenza virus, the effects outlasted the end of hostilities by several years. Two artists, one from each side of the trenches, can provide illustrative case histories.

Amedeo Modigliani, Dodo to his family and Modi to the many friends who did little to help him in life but wrote best-selling first-hand accounts of his struggles after he died,[3] was born in the prosperous Medici port of Livorno in Italy in 1880. Because of a wonderfully civilised law dating back to the Emperor Trajan which forbade bailiffs to seize material possessions from the bed of a woman in labour, he first glimpsed the world from under a mound of his mother's heirlooms, furs, silver and jewellery piled onto the bed. Both the Modiglianis and his mother's family, the Garsins, were Sephardic Jews who had settled in Italy in the early nineteenth century and had waxed in popularity and esteem but not in wealth. They were artistic, generous and eccentric; but, though they called themselves bankers, financial prudence was not among their virtues. All these qualities, together with their predisposition to develop tuberculosis and to die young, Flaminio and Eugenia Modigliani passed on to to their fourth and youngest child, Amedeo Clemente.

At fourteen Amedeo developed his first attack of pleurisy for which he was dispatched to relatives in Naples and Capri. He returned after a year apparently cured but determined to become an artist. His student works, mostly carved African heads, he later destroyed.[4] In 1906 he arrived in Paris, "gare centrale debarcadère des volontés, carrefour des inquiétudes" as his friend,

the government reconvened the 1912 committee, again under the chairmanship of Waldorf Astor (who owing to the pressure of parliamentary business delegated the role to his deputy, Sir Montague Barlow). The investigation revealed that of the 35,000 ex-servicemen needing residential treatment only 22,000 had received or were receiving it and that in most cases it was for "far too short a period".

[3] Few artists have been claimed to have been the "intimate friends" of so many after so short a life. Unlike many such reminiscences, the biography by C. Mann, *Modigliani* (London, 1980), is both sympathetic and well-informed.

[4] The news item in 1928 that many of them were recovered from the sea turned out to be a student hoax which the artist might have appreciated. The curator of the Municipal Museum of Livorno, who had just published a long article extolling the master's inimitable touch, did not.

Blaise Cendrars, was to describe it, and became part of the artistic and literary landscape of Montmartre. Everywhere in Europe, but nowhere more than on the windy slopes of the hill, this was the heroic decade of modern art,[5] the most dazzling efflorescence of talent since fifteenth-century Florence. Unlike fifteenth-century Florence, however, it effloresced in conflict with the world around it. It was indeed the contrast which later generated the legends. On one side was the brilliance, the poverty, the excesses, the drink, the drugs, the debaucheries and the fun of creative Bohemia; on the other respectable middle-class society was nearing the zenith of its material power and spiritual constipation. Perhaps because Modigliani never lived to enjoy the wealth and acclaim which came in middle or old age to many of his friends – Matisse, Derain, Picasso, Chagall, Braque, Brancusi, Bonnard, even Soutine – he became in countless personal memoirs the incarnation of the former. In fact he was much too individual to incarnate anything but himself: he was witty, cultivated, fastidious, crudely contemptuous of anything he considered phoney or meretricious, irresponsible in matters financial and sexual, kind to friends, the best of companions, the worst of debtors. For most of the prewar years a small allowance from home, and the odd ten-francs sale of portraits executed on the pavement terraces of cafes,[6] kept him in drink, drugs, cigarettes, models and even food; there is no record that his cough bothered him. It was the war years which broke his health.

Even from their low peacetime level the price of new paintings plummeted in 1914. Many artists and small-time dealers were called up. Their families, legitimate or not, trying to keep body and soul together, were selling works of art for a pittance or, more often, bartering them for bread and fuel. Even so, with German shells exploding around the Madeleine, buying works of art seemed neither prudent nor patriotic. Even more depressing was the later arrival of the vultures, entrepreneurs cashing in on what they recognised as the art bonanza of the century. Corrupt policemen were in the vanguard: many of the artists still working in Paris – Chagall, Foujita, Lipchitz, Soutine and others beside Modigliani – were foreigners who could always be black-mailed with threats of internment or deportation.[7]

[5] As it was of modern music, science, medicine, political thought, literature, economics and philosophy: in retrospect the concentration in time of seminal works and events is stunning.

[6] Between 1908 and 1912 the artistic and literary community, Modigliani among them, migrated from Montmartre to Montparnasse. La Rotonde became the hub of international Bohemia during the war years. See Douglas, C., *Artists' Quarters: Reminiscences of Montmartre and Montparnasse* (London, 1941).

[7] Legendary pillars of extortion like Police Inspector Caveau and Superintendent Zamaron amassed thousands of masterpieces. After the war their enterprise made them not only multimillionaires but also acclaimed patrons of avant-garde art. The spectacle was repeated almost exactly twenty years and one world war later.

In contrast to paintings, the price of food began to soar even before the German army reached the Marne. To a far greater extent than London (which was still a great port), Paris had always depended on the provinces for its basic necessities; and those without rural brothers, uncles or cousins (which meant most of the flotsam of Montparnasse) were at the mercy of Les Halles. By the autumn of 1915, when at Poincaré's insistence the first feeble attempts were made to control food prices, the price of milk, sugar and salt had risen to five times their peacetime level. Alcohol and drugs, now more essential than ever to keep hunger and despair at bay, were also getting expensive.[8] Restaurant meals were unaffordable.[9] The price of soap went through the ceiling. Children of the ghettoes, like Soutine, brought up on starvation and pogroms, took the deprivations more or less in their stride; those used to changing their shirt like Modigliani found them more difficult. It was in 1916 that he began to show to his friends the blood stains on his handkerchiefs, with a laugh. He had always been a bit of a show-off.[10]

If his finances were in ruins and his health was obviously threatened, artistically he soared. The double portrait of the Lipchitzes, the wonderful first portrait of Soutine and some of the greatest nudes date from 1915; the portraits of Beatrice Hastings belong to 1916; the book on African art, written jointly with Derain, Matisse, Picasso and de Chirico, was published in 1917; the *Blonde Nude* was painted in 1918. To the fabulous nudes and the adult portraits were now added the children, serene in their wide-eyed innocence, working-class and peasant youths, gazing into the world tranquil and trusting. This was genius coming into full bloom, the beginning of a career of immense promise. Only it was not the beginning but the beginning of the end. In the corner of one of his preliminary drawings for his portrait of Lunia Czechnowska he scribbled: "La vita è un dono dei pochi ai molti de coloro che sanno e hanno a coloro che non sanno e che non hanno". ("Life is a gift from the few to the many, from those who have and who know to those who have not and who do not know".) He was and would remain to the end a giver.[11]

---

[8] The drug laws were lax and opium derivatives were much cheaper and more easily accessible than they are today. Absinthe was still legal and wine was cheap.

[9] The arrival of American troops early in 1918 gave the upward spiral its final twist.

[10] By then tuberculosis was rampant (more than it had been in living memory) among the avant-garde. One who died from it, at about the same time as Modigliani started to cough up blood, was Picasso's beautiful mistress, Eva Gouet. Her lover drew her on her death-bed and mourned her in one of his blue-period Harlequinades. (In his magisterial book Picasso's biographer, John Richardson, expresses the view that she probably died from some form of cancer. This may be so; but she almost certainly suffered from tuberculosis as well.)

[11] The lines, based on d'Annunzio's *Convito*, were not entirely his invention.

Tuberculosis killed more young artists than any other illness and it might be expected that the shadow of death would sometimes be detectable in their last creations. So it is – but the effect is different in every case, incapable of being encapsulated in a single trait. Yet there are minor and superficial changes which do crop up with some regularity.

To Modigliani, as to several others who knew or sensed that this was their last creative period, finishing a work to their own satisfaction assumed overriding importance. Before the war, taking his cue from Cézanne, he used to warn sitters that a portrait might take anything up to a hundred sittings. It never did; but he disliked working in a stretch for more than an hour and was trying to make sure that he would not be hurried. This was no longer so during the war years.[12] "He was so excited that at first I was terrified", Lunia Czechnowska, one of his sitters, later described an occasion.

> But as the hours passed I was no longer afraid. In his shirt-sleeves, his face drenched in sweat, his breathing often laboured, he seemed obsessed but no longer frightening. From time to time his left hand would extend towards a bottle of what smelt like cheap brandy and he took a swig without taking his eyes off the canvas. Every ten minutes or so he would cast a glance at me. Now and then he was convulsed with a fit of coughing. I noticed the blood on his handkerchief. At times his brushwork became so violent that the canvas kept falling on his head. But when I exclaimed a little frightened, he became all gentleness and started to sing an Italian song. He had a beautiful whispering voice: it was like hearing somebody from a great distance. We had started about nine o'clock. At two in the afternoon he suddenly stopped. "Finito", he said. He collapsed into an armchair and went to sleep.[13]

In July 1917 he met Jeanne Hébuterne, an art student at the Académie Colorassi, the daughter of devout Catholic petit-bourgeois parents. She was nineteen and a virgin but within a month they were living together, first in cheap hotels, then in their first and last home, a studio apartment Zborowski, Amedeo's Polish friend, dealer and admirer found for them. She loved him deeply but made no attempt to curb his drug or drink habits. He often seemed brutal – "like a madman" as a friend described him after an all-night drinking session at La Rotonde – but after countless casual affairs he was now deeply in love; and his portraits of her are among his most beautiful. His one and only one-man show at Berthe Weill's gallery in 1917 was,

---

[12] Knowing that he charged for portraits per session and anxious to help him financially the Lipchitzs (passing through a relatively affluent phase) tried to persuade him that the double portrait he painted of them in 1915 in one sitting needed a "second look". Tired of arguing with his friends and perhaps sensing their good intentions, Modigliani spent another hour gazing at the canvas a week later: at the end of the session he added the inscription "Lipchitz" to the canvas.

[13] Mann, *Modigliani*, p. 166.

however, closed by the police after a few hours for "blatant immorality":[14] when the news was brought to him he was too drunk to care.

After the Armistice Zborowski and other dealers arranged an exodus of underfed artists from Paris to the south of France. Modigliani avoided Nice, where most of them congregated, and with Soutine rented an annex to a farmhouse near Cagnes. His health seemed to improve – he gave up spirits for a few weeks – and he painted his only known landscapes. Or rather his known-about landscapes. They were in arrears with the rent when they left – he was homesick for Paris, Jeanne and their baby daughter, Giovanna, who had been born in the last month of the war – and the farmer confiscated their canvases and used them to cover his chicken coops and rabbit hutches.

Back in Paris his material circumstances began to change. He became an almost charismatic figure. Perhaps it was the perception that he was dying, always a boon in the commercial art world. Perhaps it was part of the hectic postwar enthusiasm for modern art which started in Revolutionary Russia and swept over Europe like a benign epidemic. Articles appeared about him in glossy magazines. At a group exhibition at the Hill Gallery in London, organised by Zborowski, three of his paintings sold for prices beyond his dreams. Patrons like Roger Dutilleul began to assemble collections of his work. More surprisingly perhaps, an air of near-domesticity descended upon his private life. Jeanne was expecting their second child. They were planning to get married. Even a tiresome future mother-in-law was hovering in the wings. There were clearly moments when he himself had hopes of surviving or made himself believe that he had them. In a letter to his mother he promised to spend his and Jeanne's next holiday at home in Italy and bring the *bambina*. Ah, she was stupendous, a real Garsin. He enclosed clippings of recent favourable reviews, and wrote about future plans, but he was still totally reckless, drinking away the night with Utrillo at La Rotonde, wandering about in the bitter winter of 1919 in shirt-sleeves, rounding on friends in a rage if they suggested that he should wear a coat. They probably did not insist too strenuously: in Montparnasse doomed geniuses were two a penny and past experience suggested that while their spirit was unquenchable, their bodies were wretched and beyond help.

The end was not unexpected but more sordid than was perhaps necessary. In the first days of January 1920 Modigliani was stricken with violent pains in his back. Uncharacteristically, he took to bed. Zborowski was ill himself and could not visit him. When Modigliani failed to turn up at La Rotonde

---

[14] The criterion (more or less the equivalent of an erect penis today) was visible pubic hair. Dedicated boot-lickers like Kees van Dongen (in both world wars), patronised by fashionable society and later by the Nazis, got away with it; but not Modigliani.

for two days running Ortiz de Zarate, another *copain*, and Moise Kisling decided to investigate. The door to the flat was open. He was lying delirious in bed, alternately screaming with pain and lapsing into unconsciousness. The stench was terrible. On the easel was the beginning of a portrait of Jeanne, his only unfinished work. The bed was littered with empty and half-empty bottles of wine and spirits, overflowing ashtrays and dripping tins of sardines. Jeanne was sitting in the middle of this desolation in a state of catatonic paralysis. When asked whether she had sent for a doctor, she silently shook her head. When the doctor arrived he declared that the patient was dying of tuberculous meningitis.[15] He administered morphine. Ortiz de Zarate carried the sick man downstairs. By the time they arrived at the hospital he was in deep coma. Two days later, on 9 January 1920, a Saturday, he died in the evening.

Next day Jeanne, now nine months pregnant, came to see the body and gazed at it for a long time. Then her brother, André, took her home to their parents who banished her to the maid's room on the top floor. André sat up with her most of the night but dozed off at dawn. She then threw herself from the window and died instantly.

If the quality of the exhibits and the number of paying visitors are the two criteria by which the success of an art exhibition can be judged (and it is difficult to think of better ones), then Hitler, Goebbels and Hitler's favourite painter, the unspeakable Adolf Ziegler,[16] can be credited with staging the most successful art exhibition ever. Two million people are said to have visited the show of *Entartete Kunst* – Degenerate Art – in Munich in the summer of 1937 to mock, giggle and shout abuse at the artists whose works only a few months earlier had been the prized possessions of the country's leading museums and private collections. Prominent among the unwilling exhibitors – along with Nolde, Grosz, Dix, Kokoschka, Chagall, Barlach, Klee, Munch, Picasso, Gaugain and other degenerates – was Ernst Ludwig Kirchner, his *Peasants at Midday* bearing the label "Germans workers as seen by the Yids".[17]

Kirchner was born in Aschaffenburg in Bavaria in 1880 into a cultivated middle-class family: his father was an authority on the chemistry of paper manufacture. There was no record of tuberculosis in the family. As a twenty-one-year-old student of architecture at the University of Dresden he and three fellow students, Erich Heckel, Karl Schmidt-Rottluff and Fritz Bleyl, founded the group *Die Brücke* (The Bridge) which, together with Kandinski's

[15] The post-mortem examination confirmed the diagnosis. It also showed extensive tuberculosis of the urinary system.

[16] He was known among his pupils as the Master of the Pubic Hair. His *Judgement of Paris* hung over the Führer's desk.

[17] The occasion is well described in Ian Dunlop's *The Shock of the New* (London, 1972).

and Marc's *Blaue Reiter* (Blue Horseman) in Munich, launched Expressionism in Germany. Nolde, Pechstein and others joined a few years later. In 1908 the group moved to Berlin.

The movement met with the same kind of ridicule – or at least pained disapproval – as had the Fauves and the Cubists in France, and like them it drew strength, inspiration and a good deal of enjoyment from scandalising the bourgeois. Though professedly internationalist, it was also intensely and self-consciously German, acknowledging Cranach and Grünewald as artistic ancestors.[18] It was probably this which struck a chord with a few rich bankers, industrialists and academics. While the group was venomously attacked in print and the Kaiser was unsparing in his disapproval, they never lacked patrons or actually starved.

The outbreak of the First World War came as a shock. Kirchner in particular hated uniforms and the thought of soldiering filled him with existential dread. A self-portrait painted at the time shows him as an artilleryman with his right forearm and hand replaced by a bleeding stump. His training period as a gunner justified in his own mind his worst fears: within a few weeks he was a mental and physical wreck. (By his own later account he was unable to summon up enough energy to end his life.) He was saved by the providential intervention of one of his officers, a professor of Greek literature in civilian life who happened to be an admirer of *Die Brücke*. When the artist was marched – or rather dragged – in front of him on a charge of insubordination, the prisoner was referred for a medical report. The army doctor was also an academic in civilian life and a friend of Nolde's and had no difficulty in diagnosing pulmonary tuberculosis with the involvement of the right kidney and bladder. Tuberculosis was the one illness which meant prompt sick-leave (usually followed by discharge) from the army; so Kirchner spent some months in a recuperation centre. This was followed by a year in a requisitioned civilian sanatorium in East Prussia to which his war service entitled him. Every time he seemed to improve and was sent for a check-up, with a distant view to returning to military duty, he had a nervous breakdown. Again friends and former patrons pulled strings and he ended the war in a sanatorium in Davos in neutral Switzerland.

Physically he was still in a pitiful state, as shown in several self-portraits of the period. A little fancifully perhaps they have been described as artistic documents of tuberculosis. Tuberculosis was in fact only one of his ailments.

---

[18] Germanness was an artistic attribute which had no equivalent in other countries at the time. Many people hated Matisse's daubs in France but nobody accused him of being un-French; and while Augustus John was popular in Britain nobody praised the Welshness of his draughtsmanship.

By the time he arrived in Switzerland he was – like most sufferers from tuberculosis of the urinary tract – heavily addicted to morphine. It was a habit he never shed completely. He was also subject to fits of depression which would mentally paralyse him for days or weeks. He had nevertheless survived the war. As Davos became too noisy and too expensive, he and his companion, Erna Schilling, moved to the small village of Frauenkirch on the other side of the valley. There he remained for the rest of his life and there his tuberculosis remained comparatively well controlled. Only on his forays to the "terrible lowlands" – to Zurich, Basel and, on three occasions, to Germany – did his breathing become difficult.[19] He never got rid of his urinary symptoms either; and at times he found his nocturnal frequency almost unbearable. Insomnia drove him to increase his dose of morphine and the drug made him painfully constipated.

Ironically, in the meantime, German Expressionism underwent one of its startling changes of fortune. Before the war Kirchner and his friends claimed to give shrill voice to the hidden anguish of the supremely self-satisfied Wilhelmine establishment – and perhaps they did – but officially they were a mentally deranged minority not worthy even of formal persecution. All this now changed. Amid the degradations of the postwar years their fevered imaginings suddenly became the rancid reality, truly the *Neue Sachlichkeit*.[20] Official recognition was a side-effect of the new perception. Professorships, presidencies of academies and directorships of museums went to former figures of fun and execration, including Kokoschka, Hofer, Schmidt-Rottluff, Dix and Nolde; and Kirchner's name became revered as one of the founding fathers of modern German art.

Being famous and with his work being sought by museums and private collectors, the invalid of Frauenkirch was now financially secure, even affluent; and financially secure and affluent artists were always welcome in Switzerland. It added to his popularity that his subjects were now mostly the mountainous landscapes of the Engadine and its peasant inhabitants, some recognisable enough to be put on posters advertising the health-giving charms of the region. Some commentators regarded these creations as a natural progression, comparable to Picasso's classical phase; and to historians of tuberculosis views of Davos by a good artist at his second best will always have a certain documentary interest. In truth – in his own estimation as well – his postwar work never recaptured the punch and zest of the prewar years.

---

[19] This was a common experience of those living in mountain resorts (described among others by Thomas Mann in *The Magic Mountain*). It is difficult to think of a simple and convincing medical explanation.

[20] New objective reality is an approximate translation.

Perhaps it was the result of his illness: perhaps he needed a challenge. In fact, few of his now celebrated Expressionist colleagues found material success an inspiration. Between bouts of depression he tried to recapture the elan of his revolutionary youth by experimenting with Cubism and trying to emulate Matisse and Picasso. The results were dismal.

The penultimate turn in the Expressionists' wheel of fortune came with the advent of Hitler.[21] Uniquely among twentieth-century monsters he regarded the visual arts as important: unfortunately his taste oscillated between academic bombast and pornokitsch. By 1936 he felt secure enough to order the wholesale purge of Expressionist and other degenerate works from Germany's museums and private collections. Over 600 paintings and drawings by Kirchner alone were removed from view and either destroyed or auctioned abroad; he was expelled from the Prussian Academy of Fine Arts; and his name was expunged from books on contemporary art. His friends and colleagues fled or went into internal exile.

As often happens with highly-strung individuals, Kirchner's physical health reflected outside events. After being more or less stable for some years, he began to suffer from attacks of severe abdominal pain, nausea and bowel disturbance: he was convinced, perhaps rightly, that it was the beginning of gastrointestinal tuberculosis. He also had several episodes of chest pain, perhaps angina, perhaps pleurisy. (He regularly consulted doctors but refused to go to hospital for investigations or even to have a chest X-ray or a blood test.) His pictures were no longer selling: corrupt Nazi officials were offering many of his confiscated prewar paintings on the open market in Switzerland, which depressed the price of his current work. Swiss tourist agencies too felt it unwise to offend Aryan patrons in the Third Reich by displaying the posters of a degenerate Jew. Acting as a fine barometer of his new status, officials in Berne began to express concern about the validity of his residence permit.[22]

He forced himself to go on working but it was an effort. In March 1938 Hitler's troops marched into Austria. Swiss Nazis, whose headquarters happened to be in Davos (only some thirty miles from the frontier), confidently expected the Führer in Switzerland within a year. Judging by the posters plastered on the walls and the flags fluttering from every picturesque wooden chalet in Frauenkirch, his reception would have been as delirious as it had been in Vienna. It was too much. Kirchner had always kept his army revolver. On 15 June 1938 he shot himself through the heart.

---

[21] The ultimate one (so far) has been the revival of interest in the period and style which began in the 1960s and is still going strong.

[22] Hounding the exiled and mortally ill Klee to his death had whetted bureaucratic appetites.

21

Peacetime Aetiologies

War was not the only aetiological factor which replaced cause in discussions about clinical tuberculosis. Indeed, the First World War was not yet over when the Spanish Flu epidemic rammed home another. It had long been recognised that tuberculosis often behaved as an opportunistic infection: in other words it tended to flare up in the wake of some other illness. Measles and whooping cough in particular were feared as much for predisposing to consumption as for themselves. Nobody counted, but it was estimated that a quarter of survivors of the Spanish Flu were later discovered to be suffering from tuberculosis.[1] By the mid 1920s several non-infectious ailments were added to the list. Most famously, no sooner did diabetes mellitus become manageable if not curable – insulin became widely used after 1923 – than it also emerged as the most important predisposing factor among chronic diseases.[2] In hospitals for many years every newly diagnosed diabetic was immediately and routinely X-rayed, and a significant number proved to be tuberculous. The only question was whether this was a reflection of the poor nutritional state of diabetics or the relish of Koch's bacilli for the high sugar content of diabetic tissues.[3]

Later opportunistic associations depended on lowered immunity induced by drugs. In the 1950s tuberculosis became a dangerous complication of steroid and other forms of immunosuppressive therapy in rheumatoid arthritis, other collagen diseases and acute leukemia. It was a distant – or not so distant – rumble of what was to come in the 1970s.[4]

Nor was the debate over the importance of heredity laid permanently to

---

[1] Conversely, the influenza struck the tuberculous with particular ferocity. At least one tuberculosis sanatorium near Vienna was virtually depopulated.

[2] F. G. Banting and C. H. Best performed their first animal experiments demonstrating the effect of insulin in 1921 and injected their preparation into their first human subject, a fourteen-year-old schoolboy, on 23 January 1922; but insulin did not become commercially available for another two years.

[3] Several organisms, including the *Staphylococus aureus*, the commonest cause of boils and carbuncles, grow more quickly in media enriched with glucose. Boils are also abnormally common and sometimes the presenting feature in diabetes. Egg yolk is the standard enrichment of media used for culturing the tubercle bacillus.

[4] See below, Chapter 33.

rest by Koch's discovery. For some years after the emergence of the bacillus there was, it is true, a reaction against aetiologies crudely based on the inherited diathesis. In 1870 Sir William Jenner, physician to the Queen, had stated that "tuberculous parents invariably transmit the disease to their offspring, the participation of both heightening the tendency to a degree exceeding the sum of the tendencies of each parents, just as occurred with insanity".[5] Such pontifications, repeated with minor modifications in text-books, official memoranda and the lay press, were for a time out of fashion. "No child is born tuberculous", Dr James Niven, Medical Officer of Health for Manchester, now pronounced, combining his assertion with a renewed demand for better ventilation and less overcrowding.[6] "Tuberculosis is not hereditary in any sense", claimed Dr James A. Gibson, an ardent protagonist of the sanatorium idea.[7] According to Dr Robert Philip, the future high priest of tuberculosis dispensaries, in no more than 23.3 per cent of consumptives in Edinburgh was there a possible family taint,[8] but by the end of the first decade of the twentieth century the corrective trend had begun to falter.

In 1907 Karl Pearson, a gifted publicist though a bad (or unscrupulous) statistician, included among his studies in national deterioration figures which suggested that simple infection could not account for the incidence of consumption in families, "especially when children with two consumptive parents were more likely to develop the disease than children with only one and much more likely than those with neither parent consumptive":[9] to deny the role of heredity showed "a reckless disregard for eugenics and the national welfare". His evidence and that of his subsequent publications – his croak was still being heard in the 1920s – was based on an unstated number of Belfast families, one member of whom had been interviewed by an unstated number of practitioners reporting to Pearson; and yet his limping statistics were widely quoted. At the Destitution Conference of 1911, Sidney and Beatrice Webb warned delegates that there was a "proven family atmosphere" which "nurtured the grand parade of the tuberculous, the syphilitic ... the uncivilised and the undisciplined ... Public money would be better spent on inculcating selective parentage than on building sanatoria".[10] Geoffrey

[5] Jenner, Sir W., *Lancet* (1970), no. 2, 18. Sir William also expressed the view, drawing on his "not inconsiderable personal experience", that offspring were "almost twice as likely to inherit the disease from their father than from their mother".

[6] Niven, J., *British Medical Journal* (1899), no. 2, 181.

[7] Gibson, J. A., *The Nordrach Treatment* (London, 1901), p. 21.

[8] Philip, R., *A Thousand Cases* (Edinburgh, 1891).

[9] Pearson, K., "A First Study in the Statistics of Pulmonary Tuberculosis", in *Studies in National Deterioration* (London, 1907), 11.

[10] Webb, Beatrice, in *Proceedings of the National Conference on the Prevention of Destitution* (London, 1911), p. 63.

Drage, an imperialist busybody, advocated restricted farms to house "defective families whose reproduction of drunkenness, consumption, insanity and suicide should be controlled".[11] Dr A. D. Edwards, Schools Medical Officer for Bournemouth, claimed to have investigated 10,000 children before 1914 and to have found proof of the hereditary taint in the fact that ailing children were 40 per cent more likely to have relatives with tuberculosis than non-ailing children.[12] In England and on the Continent these claims never quite carried the day – apart from the crankiness of the assertions doctors had too high a stake in sanatoria – but they lingered on not only in the invincible (and invincibly wrong) popular belief that tuberculosis always ran in families but also in the literature of such pressure groups as the Eugenics Movement. In the 1930s Major Leonard Darwin was still preaching birth control and voluntary sterilisation as a prophylactic remedy for the "undoubted hereditary nature of tuberculosis".[13]

The genetic concept always commanded a greater medical following in the United States. The culmination of the tradition came in 1943 when Kallman and Reismir reported a longitudinal study of twins purporting to reveal an 87.3 per cent tuberculosis morbidity rate among identical twins, compared to 11.9 per cent among half-siblings.[14] These were the palmy days before Sir Cyril Burt's fraudulent twin studies – or rather non-studies – were exposed and these findings were taken very seriously indeed. In addition to statistics there were the case histories of well-known tuberculous families, many of them American. Of course in most of these the familial incidence could be explained by overwhelming cross-infection; but some at least suggested a genuinely familial predisposition.

Thomas Emerson came from England and settled in Ipswich, Massachusetts, in 1638. There was nothing in the first 150 years of the family history to suggest tuberculosis. The first unquestionable case of phthisis occurred in the fifth generation when the Reverend William Emerson died of the disease in 1811 at the age of forty-two. (By then tuberculosis was the most frequent recognised cause of death in New England and especially in Boston.) William's widow, Ruth, was left with five boys and an infant daughter to bring up and no financial resources. A brave and determined woman in the old New England mould, she accepted the challenge of sacrificing physical

---

[11] Drage, G., *The State and the Poor* (London, 1914), p. 60.

[12] Edwards, A. D., *The Child* (London, 1914), p. 156.

[13] Darwin, L., *British Medical Journal* (1928), no. 2, 257.

[14] Puffer, R. R., *Familial Susceptibility in Tuberculosis* (Cambridge, Massachusetts, 1944); Macfarlane Burnet, F., *The Natural History of Infectious Diseases* (2nd edn, Cambridge, 1953), 198.

comforts for high moral and intellectual achievement: better a cold and dark room than a starved mind. The infant daughter and one boy died of unknown causes. The other four boys went to Harvard and, at a cost of great privations, graduated between 1818 and 1828. But all four developed tuberculosis, two dying of galloping phthisis in their twenties. Ralph Waldo Emerson realised that a "mouse was gnawing at his chest" while at Divinity School in Boston; and in 1826, with funds obtained from an uncle, he went south. Even Charleston was too cold for him: he felt "not sick, not well but luke-sick". After a spell in Florida he returned to Boston in better health; but he was never completely cured. Nevertheless, he lived to the age of seventy-nine while tuberculosis continued to claim lives around him.

Ellen, his first wife, was the daughter of a prosperous merchant of Concord, New Hampshire. Her father died almost certainly of tuberculosis at the age of forty-seven. Five years later her brother, George, a medical student, died in Paris from a "horrid cold". When Ralph Waldo married her she was nineteen and already suffering from the disease. They went south to arrest her decline, but even large doses of opium would not control her painful cough. Riding every day in a balmy climate was pronounced to be her best chance of a cure. It was not good enough: she died in 1831, aged twenty-nine. Ralph Waldo married again in 1835 and had four children. Tuberculosis continued to claim his descendants, killing twelve by 1949. When William Emerson, a physician of the eleventh generation, compiled the family history the antibiotic dawn had arrived.[15]

Another ornament of nineteenth-century American letters, Henry David Thoreau, also came from a consumptive family. His grandfather died from consumption in 1801 and his father died after many years' illness during which he had coughed up blood and expectorated a great deal. Henry's brother, John, was probably tuberculous but died of tetanus contracted by accident; his sister, Helen, was consumptive since girlhood and died at twenty-two in 1849. Henry himself developed a severe cold in 1850, probably the beginning of his long, lingering illness. In 1860 he went to Minnesota, then the most popular place for the treatment of consumptives; but he was back in Concord after a few month, no better. For a few more months he held out, stretched on the sofa in his living room, receiving visits from his friends. Many later wrote about his cheerful stoicism unaided by opiates. He was forty-five when he died in 1862.[16]

[15] Emerson, H., "Five Generations of Tuberculosis", in *Selected Papers* (New York, 1949).

[16] Camby, H. S., *Thoreau* (Boston, 1939); Krutch, J. W., *Henry David Thoreau* (New York, 1948).

More difficult to explain and interpret and yet of ongoing importance was the effect of apparently acquired immunity – or the lack of it – on communities and races. The message of such anecdotal evidence as came to the notice of Dr Budd of Bristol in the 1820s was soon reinforced by events better documented and involving greater numbers. The most convincing instances of tuberculosis striking down populations possessing little or no inbred resistance were among the North American Indians. The descriptions left by Jesuit Fathers who explored the Great Lakes in the seventeenth century suggest that there may have been a few cases of glandular and pulmonary tuberculosis among the natives; but they were so rare that the Fathers assumed that the disease had been imported by European settlers.[17] In 1880 two thousand Sioux were made prisoners of war by the United States Army; none at the time were noticed to suffer from ill-health. They were moved into barracks in a prison camp; and within a month Army Surgeon Washington Billings, an admirable doctor, diagnosed several cases of tuberculosis in its most fulminating form. None of his first patients lived longer than a month; and by the time they died there were dozens of new cases. At Billings' insistence the prisoners were resettled in widely scattered tented accommodation. The spread of the acute outbreak slowed down; but mortality from tuberculosis (confirmed by bacteriological examination in 1902) continued to increase. In 1903 it was then ten times higher than anywhere else in the United States. The last of the inmates – about fifty survivors – were formally released in 1913.[18]

Even more devastating was the epidemic that ran riot among the Indians of the Qu'Appelle Valley Reservation of western Canada. Three decades after they were forced to abandon their nomadic way of life in the prairies, mortality from tuberculosis among them reached the fantastic figure of one in a hundred. The cold and the inhospitable terrain were blamed by the authorities when the facts leaked out. This was universally disbelieved but no one person or body was held responsible; perhaps nobody was. A few years later the fate of the Navaho Indians herded into reservations in Arizona was not much better, despite the dry and sunny climate. Eventually simple public-health measures seemed to check these embarrassing outbreaks. In Minnesota there were sixty-four deaths from tuberculosis among 12,500 Indians in 1937. The figure was reduced to nine among 10,000 in 1949.

[17] It is now generally accepted that tuberculosis existed in America before Columbus: evidence has been found in pre-Columbian Iroquoian ossuaries; and hunchbacks reminiscent of those seen on Egyptian wall-paintings also exist in Mayan and Peruvian art. See Pfeiffer, S., *American Journal of Physiological Anthropology*, 65 (1984), 181.
[18] Dubos, R. and J., *The White Plague: Tuberculosis, Man and Society* (London, 1953), p. 89.

Similar horrors around the globe caused tiny setbacks in the building of great and glorious empires. Between 1803 and 1810 Britain imported 4000 Negro volunteers from Mozambique to Ceylon, today's Sri Lanka, to make up new regiments: Africans, it was predicted, would be well accustomed to the tropical heat and therefore give long and useful service. In contrast to native Sri Lankans, the imported troops had never been exposed to tuberculosis; and by 1820 3640 of them were dead from consumption of a particularly virulent kind. In the light of such wastage, continuation of the scheme was not recommended by Commissioner Foxtown when he reported back to his masters in Leadenhall Street in the City of London.

A hundred years later tuberculosis ran a similarly fulminating course (rarely seen by then in Europe) among the Senegalese troops of the French Army on the Western Front and among the coloured Capetown Boys recruited by Britain: they were the only active units in whom mortality from disease surpassed losses in action.

Less dramatic perhaps, but nearer home and rarely out of mind in England for almost a century, was the high racial susceptibility to tuberculosis of the people of the Celtic Fringe. This meant mainly the Irish, "our great reservoir of consumption", as Sir John Banbury of the Home Office described them in 1912. It was not a new idea. In 1885 in a celebrated treatise, *The Races of Britain*, Dr John Beddoe had already suggested that "the Celtic racial influence [was] the prime cause of tuberculosis in the British Islands".[19] After an abashed lull following Koch's discovery, new evidence fairly bubbled up to support his thesis. Statistics, not all of them inaccurate, were bandied about. While mortality from tuberculosis was falling in England, it was still rising in Ireland, reaching 28 per 10,000 in 1910. (It did not begin to fall – and then very slowly – until 1920, with another upturn between 1942 and 1944.)

Nor did crude mortality figures tell more than a fraction of the story. In the 1920s Ireland had the highest incidence in Europe of non-pulmonary tuberculosis in children under five – around 21 per cent – and probably the highest incidence (with Hungary) of bovine tuberculosis. In 1925 over 8 per cent of milk samples in Dublin contained live tuberculosis bacilli, suggesting that few if any children growing up in the city could escape consuming organisms. (The powerful farmer's lobby saw to it that the Free State Government regularly shelved Clean Milk Bills, let alone compulsory pasteurisation).[20] Not surprisingly, the population at maximum risk remained the fifteen- to twenty-year olds at a time when the transition to an

---

[19] Beddoe, J. H., *The Races of Britain* (London, 1924).
[20] See below, Chapter 29.

older age group was well on the way in England, Scotland and even in Wales.[21] In Hungary too during the interwar years the population group at maximum risk was reckoned to be children in their early teens.

Personal memoirs recalling the period speak as eloquently as statistics.

> Out in the Atlantic Ocean great sheets of rain gathered to drift slowly up the River Shannon and settle forever in Limerick. The rain dampened the city from the Feast of the Circumcision to New Year's Eve. It created a cacophony of hacking coughs, bronchial rattles, asthmatic wheezes, consumptive croaks. It turned noses into fountains, lungs into bacterial sponges. It provoked cures galore; to ease the catarrh you boiled onions in milk blackened with pepper; for the congested passages you made a paste of boiled flour and nettles, wrapped it in a rag and slapped it, sizzling, on the chest.

So begins a memorable evocation of an Irish childhood during the 1930s and 1940s.[22] Poverty and the rain were of course only two of the reasons: alcohol, ignorance, overcrowding and perhaps a certain natural fatalism – or faith in a more merciful and just world hereafter – were some of the others.

For at least one generation the Irish carried their Celtic susceptibility with them wherever they went. In the 1930s Irish and Welsh nurses in English sanatoria were two and a half times more likely to develop signs of the disease than their equally exposed English colleagues;[23] and their lesions were more serious. At least since 1920 the Brompton Hospital in London had tacitly banned Irish applicants from its nursing staff: when in 1941 circumstances – that is lack of applicants – forced the authorities to change their policy, the differential incidence between the English and the Irish recruits was reported to be 900 per cent.[24] as radiography in the 1950s in London showed a difference of 700 per cent between those of Irish and English birth in London. The picture was similar in the United States. First-generation Boston Irish, as defined by the birthplace of the mother, had a three times higher

---

[21] Geary, R. C., *British Medical Journal* (1930), no. 2, 37. Seventy-eight per cent of Irish children were tuberculin positive by the age of twelve in the mid 1920s and the Free State had the highest mortality from tuberculosis in young adults among twenty-four European and North American countries. Not until the mid 1930s did the statistics began to improve. In 1951 a more prosperous Eire still recorded a tuberculosis death rate of twenty-three per 10,000. Streptomycin halved this figure within three years.

[22] McCourt, Frank, *Angela's Ashes* (London, 1977), p. 1.

[23] Smith, F. B., *The Retreat of Tuberculosis, 1850–1950* (London, 1988), p. 221.

[24] *Brompton Hospital Reports*, 13 (London, 1944), 160. Despite the shortage of nurses in many National Health Service hospitals in the United Kingdom after 1947, recruiting in Ireland was strongly discouraged by most health authorities. In one hospital well known to the present writer the tacit ban on Irish recruitment was not lifted till 1968, by which time nurses' pay in the United Kingdom was so abysmal and employment in the Irish Republic so much improved that the campaign turned into an expensive fiasco.

rate of tuberculosis mortality than did the host population and twice that of their neighbours of English or Scottish origin.[25]

In retrospect – though this was hardly envisaged at the time – it is difficult to escape the conclusion that the Celtic and especially the Irish susceptibility to tuberculosis was a replay of the catastrophic upsurge of the disease in England, France and Germany during their respective Industrial Revolutions. It certainly had nothing to do with red hair, beautiful complexions and laughing green eyes. Or not much.

The trouble with the aetiological factors of tuberculosis was that the truth was rarely clear-cut and almost never politically correct. In 1932 F. C. S. Bradbury conducted a searching and unprejudiced investigation of 2963 families and 1033 tuberculous persons in the two towns of Blaydon and Jarrow in County Durham, considering the aetiological significance of poverty, occupation of tenement flats, Irish nationality, undernourishment, bad ventilation, insanitation and number of children. He concluded that "the association of tuberculosis with poverty is of greater importance than any other variable studied". He considered the relationship between the disease and undernourishment to be statistically more significant than that with overcrowding; and, contradicting trendy inanities voiced by sections of the popular press, he insisted that it was poverty which predisposed to tuberculosis, not tuberculosis to poverty. He also commented on the striking difference between Blaydon, a mining town with few Irish immigrants, and Jarrow, a ship-building town with a large Irish population.[26] This was seized upon by the Tyneside Inquiry Committee set up by the National Association for the Prevention of Pulmonary Tuberculosis. "Attention must be directed to the most interesting point in Dr Bradbury's useful report which fully accounts for the disproportionately high mortality from tuberculosis in Jarrow", the committee concluded in their annual report, "viz. the high proportion of persons in Jarrow of Irish origin." Such slanted reporting was calculated to draw the ire of Ellen Wilkinson, "Red Ellen", MP for Jarrow: "There is no mystery and nothing 'interesting' about the high rate of tuberculosis in Jarrow: its cause is poverty, poverty and poverty, not Irishness".[27]

This too was wrong. There was – and there remains – a mystery or a whole complex of mysteries; only it was and is not Irishness.[28] A similar delayed

---

[25] Joyce, J. C., *Tubercle*, 36 (1955), 338.

[26] Bradbury, F. C. S., *Transactions of the NAPT*, 122 (1933), 57.

[27] Wilkinson, Ellen, *The Town that was Murdered: The Life History of Jarrow* (London, 1939), p. 204.

[28] Apart from Irishness and poverty the Depression years provided fertile soil for aetiological speculation, some of it no less blinkered, bigoted and fantastical than the ideas put forward during the century before Koch. The "abnormal stresses, rush and unwholesome excitements"

peak of tuberculosis seems to have occurred in Laënnec's Brittany and, to get away from all suspicions of Celtishness, in Norway and in Hungary. In Hungary too there was surface evidence of a racial factor: the mortality rate throughout the 1920s was at least 50 per cent higher in Hungarian than in ethnic German ("Schwabian") villages of ostensibly the same size and occupational composition. The ethnic German villages were among the most prosperous in Hungary or – as Nazi propaganda would have it – the most industrious. At the other extreme, according to some medical pundits, gipsies were immune to tuberculosis so long as they remained in their shacks at the end of villages in a kind of rural ghetto. How the pundits distilled this wisdom is a mystery: rural gipsies had virtually no access to medical care other than their own wise men and were rarely if ever admitted to hospitals. They were certainly not immune once they had moved to the cities to entertain customers in cafes and restaurants with their fiddles and zithers. The greatest of all gipsy composers, Pista Dankó, died of the disease aged thirty-four in 1912.

Prerevolutionary Russia was both a special case and a prime example of the difficulties of interpreting tuberculosis statistics anywhere.[29] Allowing for the not inconsiderable difficulties of collecting statistical medical data from various nomadic tribes (especially, it seems, from the Khirgiz and the Kamchuks) and from the half-wild races of the Caucasus, Central Asia and Siberia, the total yearly death-rate from tuberculosis in the Empire, as reported by

---

to which modern (i.e., post-1918) urban youth was exposed came in for particular censure: "not surprisingly death rate in country areas is 35 per cent lower than in the cities", L. E. (later Sir Leonard) Hill wrote in *The Science of Ventilation and Open-Air Treatment* in 1930. R. C. Wingfield, medical superintendant of Frimley Sanatorium, opined that "in spite of generations of endurance of the artificialities of civilisation, man is still an animal designed and ordained to live his life in tranquillity in the open air": lack of these were clearly "important factors in the resistance of tuberculosis to medical endeavours to eradicate it". In 1932 Sir Robert Philip saw the chief culprit in the "devitalising influence of restlessness, irregular hours and the general and deplorable misuse of leisure time". In the same year F. R. G. Heaf, later professor of tuberculosis in Cardiff, examined in detail the lives of 120 young adults suffering from tuberculosis and put the chief blame for the disease on the speed of modern life. "The youth of today simply does not lead the peaceful life that it did twenty or thirty years ago." According to N. D. Bardswell, it was no coincidence that the "increase in tuberculosis rates in young women should have been first noticed during a period which has seen the emancipation of women and a profound change in their social habits following their entry into competitive wage earning". All these authorities had a battery of statistics to back up their muscular prejudices.

[29] Meaningful statistics ceased to be published in Russia in 1914. Starry-eyed western travellers (like the Webbs and G. B. Shaw) reported "marvellous progress" and the "virtual eradication of tuberculosis from the rural areas" (Beatrice Webb) in the 1920s and 1930s; but, since millions of starving peasants escaped their notice, they can hardly be regarded as either eagle-eyed or as reliable witnesses.

A. W. Nikolski of the All-Russian League for the Prevention of Tuberculosis in 1910, was 35 per 10,000. This was almost certainly an underestimate. Unlike, moreover, the death-rates in Norway, Hungary and even Ireland, which were beginning to plateau or even hesitantly to decline, the Russian curve was still rising. This was only partly due to the new industrial suburbs springing up around Moscow, Baku and Tiflis, which suffered from social ills not dissimilar from those of Manchester a century and of Lyon half a century earlier. More alarmingly, the death-rate was rising in remote rural areas as well. Ironically, in a country almost inconceivably vast by western European or even by American standards, most of the peasantry lived in conditions of appalling overcrowding. Vladimir Shingaroff's investigation of a hundred houses in two Tartar villages in the Voronesh Region in 1908 showed that

> dwellings that we would barely deem adequate for two people in our towns are inhabited by families of seven or eight in addition to some of their domestic animals ... The inhabitants save wood [in a region covered with dense forests] and close their stoves before the wood is thoroughly burnt: consequently the exhalations which escape into the room poison the air ... Many of the houses have no chimneys.[30]

Shingaroff reckoned that tuberculosis accounted for most deaths in the empire's most backward regions (many the size of several western European countries); and that, far from being a disease of industrialisation, consumption was the scourge of the most technically undeveloped agricultural provinces. Similar evidence, often contradicting received wisdom, could be piled up. Nevertheless, by the end of the interwar years most unprejudiced observers were reluctantly driven to the conclusion that urban and industrial societies tended to breed over a surprisingly short period of time – three or four generations at the most – a population with a rising natural resistance to tuberculosis. The reluctance stemmed not from the conclusion but from the fact that, despite a battery of glib theories, nobody could explain it. It was too late to resurrect Lamarckian ideas about the transmission of acquired characteristics, in this case immunity to tuberculosis: few reputable scientists were prepared to try. The time span, on the other hand, over which the change occurred was far too short for Darwinian selection. It was suggested by some that a rising standard of living in the wake of industrialisation played a part; but it could hardly be the whole answer. Yet other explanations were even more improbable. They still are.[31]

---

[30] Shingaroff, V., quoted by Nikolski, A. W., in Sutherland, H. D. (ed.), *The Control and Eradication of Tuberculosis* (Edinburgh, 1911), p. 346.

[31] Mortality from tuberculosis is not the only biological change which hints at mechanisms still not fully understood or even perhaps envisaged. By what genetic mechanism has the height of the male population of western Europe and even more of the United States been

Veterinary experience sometimes helped to resolve such conundra. In the case of acquired immunity it merely deepened it. S. Lyle Cummins, a colonel in the Royal Army Medical Corps (later first professor of tuberculosis in Cardiff), travelled up and down the Nile many times and vividly recalled

> the joyous colonies of little gray monkeys (*Macaca mulatta*), millions of them, grinning, gesticulating, chattering, leaping from tree to tree, the picture of health. Never once has it been my lot to see a single tuberculous monkey among the thousands brought to Khartoum by natives for sale to British officers or officials, although there were little gray monkey mascots in every mess or club.[32]

At the same time the mortality from tuberculosis among monkeys in the Cairo Zoo was so high that the cages had to be restocked every three months; and similar devastations were experienced from time to time in other zoos. (Some were hushed up by the scientific or commercial bodies running the establishments lest they frighten away visitors. Reports from the director of Cairo Zoo – and perhaps from others placed in a similar position elsewhere – referred to "monkey plague" or "simian virus" as the cause of the epidemic when in fact the disease was almost certainly tuberculosis.) In Philadelphia the mortality began to decline in the early 1900s after the introduction of tuberculin testing, the ruthless culling of all exposed animals (90 per cent) and the non-admission of all tuberculin-positive ones; but paradoxically it did not drop dramatically until the advent of the second or third generation – that is of the zoo-born and zoo-bred – animals most of whom later proved to be tuberculin-*positive.*

It was not only zoo-bred animals which showed a human pattern of changing susceptibility. Guinea-pigs were always regarded as highly suscep-tible to tuberculosis, a knee-jerk reaction to the fact that they were *the* experimental animals in both laboratory research and diagnostic testing. In fact Koch himself wrote that, among the tens of thousands of animals his institute had imported from a variety of guinea-pig breeding farms, they had *never* seen a single case of spontaneous tuberculosis; and that in animal rooms such spontaneous cases did not occur until about a third of the total population had been experimentally infected. After that, unless drastic counter-measures were taken, the entire stock was in danger of rapidly succumbing.

In human societies immunological, social and economic variables were

steadily increasing for at least three generations? More trivially: what evolutionary mechanism can account for the fact that records have been and still are regularly broken in almost every athletic event at every Olympic Game since the modern games were inaugurated in 1896?

[32] Quoted by Francis, J., *Bovine Tuberculosis: Including a Contrast with Human Tuberculosis* (London, 1947), p. 238.

always inextricably mixed; and every argument generated its counter-argument. It was easy to explain the difference in the susceptibility to tuberculosis of European and Oriental Jewish immigrants to Israel: their selective breeding (whatever that meant) had been different over many generations. Yet in the 1920s among first- and second-generation Jewish immigrants in New York City mortality from tuberculosis in the old and congested Gouverneur district was eighty-three per 100,000 in contrast to the fifty-two per 100,000 among ethnically the same mix living in the more affluent Bronx Tremont district. Every country and every society had its own pattern impossible to apply without reservations to other countries and societies. Tuberculosis in China had certainly existed for countless generations but it did not become a scourge of the young and the poor until the sudden growth of the opium-infested cities in the east and their economic misery in the first decades of the twentieth century. In 1932 the Reverend Arthur E. Truman, a missionary doctor in Shanghai and a profound observer of the Chinese scene, reckoned that 90 per cent of young opium addicts died of the disease and that the habit was by far the most important single factor in the spread of the infection. A few years later tuberculosis was rife in Japanese prisoner-of-war camps and tens of thousands died from it, including the Reverend Truman himself, without the support of opium.[33]

Striking examples of the lack of real understanding of the interplay between immunological and social and economic factors (hardly ever discussed in textbooks) are too numerous to attempt to list in full. In South Africa in the early 1920s first-generation South African Bantu working in Johannesburg and other cities had the highest known mortality rate from tuberculosis in the world,[34] and the disease usually pursued a fulminating course rarely seen among the white population. It was the custom among Bantu workers – as it had been for many generations – that those sickening would return to their kraals and die surrounded and comforted by their kin, so it must be assumed that before dying they became massively severe, open sources of infection. Yet, if official statistics are to be believed (and there is no reason to disbelieve this particular one), the Bantu who had never moved out of their villages but were exposed to the bacillus imported by their relations remained as highly resistant to the infection as those migrating to the cities were susceptible.

Chronological age was another aetiological factor whose effect puzzled the generation after Koch and is still unexplained. It was clear by 1900, a time when many babies and young adults were dying of tuberculosis and when

---

[33] Truman, A. E., *A Missionary Life in China* (New York, 1950).
[34] Mortality among North American Indians was by then declining.

the infection itself was beginning to be viewed as almost universal, that mortality from the disease declined sharply around the age of five and remained relatively low till about the age of fifteen. A study over a period of twenty-five years, at the Children's Chest Clinic of the Bellevue Hospital in New York, showed that of infants first diagnosed before the age of six months more than 60 per cent died, as against 28 per cent of those first diagnosed between one and two years and 15 per cent of those first diagnosed between four and fifteen years. Of the survivors 8 per cent developed secondary pulmonary tuberculosis after the age of fifteen, twice as many girls as boys, with a mortality of 70 per cent.[35] It was still true in the 1950s that black school children in the United States rarely developed progressive fatal disease even when living with adults who were openly infected, though many did so after leaving school.[36] In some way this golden age of resistance had to be related to the hormonal and other physiological changes involved in growing up; but how these changes influenced immunity and resistance remained (and remains) obscure.

Lastly, and more often provoking an indulgent smile than serious discussion, were the psychological factors. Sir William Osler said that "if you want the prognosis of a case of tuberculosis it is as important to know what's in the patient's head as what is in his chest". The statement was in the grand tradition of Richard Morton who wrote in his *Phthysiologia* in 1689 that he had often observed that "consumption of the lung had its origin in long and grievous passions of the mind". A century later a celebrated Berlin physician, C. G. Hufeland, listed "a mournful tendency of the soul" second only to an inherited disposition among the causes of scrofula. In his *Inventum novum* Auenbrugger put the chief blame for consumption (almost as a matter of course) on "affections of the mind, particularly [on] ungratified desires the principle of which is nostalgia"; while Laënnec, one of the greatest medical observers and thinkers of any period, wrote about "profound melancholy passions extending over long periods of time" as a potent cause of the disease. These people were not charlatans or naive ignoramuses; and it is odd that, in an age awash with Freudian and pseudo-Freudian lore and professing fervent faith in psychosomatic medicine, their opinions should generally be patronisingly dismissed as archaic vapourings. It is sadly true, however, that in so far as the greatest clinicians of the past were right to detect a link between the soul and the tubercle bacillus, the nature of that link remains as elusive as it was 300 years ago.

[35] Drolet, G. J., *The Epidemiology of Tuberculosis in Clinical Tuberculosis*, edited by B. Goldberg (Davis, California, 1946), 342.

[36] Rich, A. R., *The Pathogenesis of Tuberculosis* (Springfield, Illinois, 1944), 65.

22

Collapse Therapy

The aetiological complexities of tuberculosis were of absorbing interest to academics, pathologists and guardians of the public health; but practising doctors attending medical meetings in the 1920s and 1930s were always more anxious to hear about advances in treatment. Of these there was usually a great deal about – an ominous pointer to their worth. Most authorities agreed that, until something better turned up, the rational management of the disease would have to rest on two pillars. The first was the sanatorium regime, beginning to be questioned and even reviled but still, at its best, something to aim for. The second (which came a little later) was collapse therapy. On the face of it the two were at opposite ends of a spectrum. Sanatoria represented a somewhat ill-defined way of life, an attitude rather than an activity. Collapse therapy was an invasive surgical procedure. Yet they rested on the same underlying principle known and cherished since the days of Hippocrates. To combat active disease – or rather, to let the body combat active disease with all its own resources – the diseased part has to be put to rest. It was therefore appropriate that the two approaches were practised in parallel rather than as alternatives.

The rationale of collapse therapy depended on understanding the basic mechanics of breathing. Central to this mechanism was the elastic recoil of the lung. A rich supply of elastic fibres criss-crosses the walls of the billions of microscopic air sacs or alveoli in which the vital exchange of gases between the blood flowing in the capillaries and the inspired air takes place. Following a simple concentration gradient, carbon dioxide diffuses out of the blood and oxygen diffuses in. But removed from the chest the normal lung would contract into a nearly solid structure smaller than a tennis ball. What prevents this from happening in life, and what allows the expansion and relaxation of the chest-wall and diaphragm to establish the normal rhythm of inspiration and expiration, are the pleural sacs. They are not in fact sacs in the sense that they contain the lungs like shopping bags but rather closed double membranes into which each lung is invaginated. Between the two layers is a potential space. The space is only potential because the pressure between the two layers, referred to in anatomy as the parietal and visceral pleura, is slightly below atmospheric. (This is sometimes inaccurately described as a vacuum.) There is, in other words, no actual pleural space in the normal chest, though lubrication with a few drops of mucus allows the two pleural layers to slide gently over each other. What matters from the point of view of keeping the lungs expanded and making them follow the movements of the chest-wall and diaphragm is that the parietal pleura is firmly tethered to the inner aspect of the chest wall and the upper surface of the diaphragm while the visceral pleura adheres to the lung. Under normal circumstances this is a far more efficient arrangement than if the lung were stuck to the muscles and ribs directly (which theoretically could also achieve regular expansion and relaxation). When the respiratory muscles acting on the rib-cage expand the chest, and the diaphragm contracts and descends, the lung too expands and air is sucked into the alveoli. When the chest wall is allowed to relax and the diaphragm rises, the air (now without the oxygen but loaded with carbon dioxide) is expelled.

Although the two layers of the pleural sacs are held in apposition by the *relatively* negative pressure between them, it is possible to pierce the chest wall and the parietal pleura with a needle and enter the tip of the needle into the potential cavity. Then a measured amount of air (or some other gas) can be injected by connecting the needle to a syringe; or air can simply be allowed to be sucked in. As the air (or gas) enters, the two layers of the pleural sac separate; and the portion of the lung which lies beneath the intrapleural bubble contracts (or "collapses") on itself. If sufficient air is injected, or allowed to be sucked in, a whole lung can be collapsed. Once collapsed, it will no longer expand and relax with the respiratory movements of the chest wall and diaphragm. Because the two pleural sacs enclosing the two lungs do not communicate with each other, one whole lung can be collapsed without affecting the other; and, barring complications, one lung can ensure adequate oxygenation of the blood and the body as a whole. The collapse of one whole lung will inevitably shift the midline structures – known in anatomical parlance as the mediastinum – to the collapsed side; and since these structures include the heart and the great vessels issuing from it, too sudden a shift can be lead to cardiac arrest and death.

When air enters the pleural "space" accidentally – as can happen following a stab wound from the outside or the rupture of an air-filled bubble in the lung substance or a cavity from the inside – the condition is referred to as a spontaneous pneumothorax.[1] There is of course nothing spontaneous either about being stabbed or about an air-bubble rupturing, but the term serves

---

[1] Such air-filled bubbles called *bullae* are not uncommon: they most commonly derive from some temporary obstruction in an air passage building up sufficient pressure to rupture a few thousand (or million) microscopic air sacs and to allow them to merge.

to distinguish an unplanned event from artificial pneumothorax – AP in clinical shortspeak – which is deliberately induced to bring about the collapse of the underlying organ.

Collapse is in fact too passive a term: because of its elasticity, the normal lung actively contracts as soon as it is freed from its bony and muscular cage. But collapse is a fair description if the area contains a tuberculous cavity. As the lung around the cavity contracts, the cavity passively collapses on itself. Ideally, the healing processes around it are then given a chance to obliterate it without having to compete with the elastic pull of the surrounding lung tissue every time the chest expands in inspiration. Other harmful effects of cavitation are also hopefully reversed.[2] The expectoration of caseous material teeming with bacilli stops. Deprived of air – that is oxygen – the tubercle bacilli may die or go into a state of suspended animation. The inflammatory and immune responses of the normal tissues around the lesion are given a chance to arrest their further spread. Scar formation is encouraged. One can draw a parallel between these hoped for happenings and the healing of a broken bone, a similarity that did not escape early advocates of collapse therapy. The broken ends of a bone will never unite while the fragments rub against each other or while they are separated by a mass of soft tissue. Healing and remodelling starts as soon as the bone ends are aligned and immobilised. Eventually the fracture site may become wholly undetectable.[3]

It was not till the 1920s that collapse therapy in the form of artificial pneumothorax became the mainstay of the active treatment of pulmonary tuberculosis; but, like the sanatorium regime with which it was often twinned, it had a long prehistory. It seems that the first time some kind of a direct surgical assault on a diseased lung was advocated (at least in modern times) was in part of a vast medical text by Georgius Baglivi, published in Padua in Italy in 1696:

A phthisick arising from an ulcer in the lungs is commonly branded incurable upon the plea that an internal ulcer in a vital organ cannot be cleansed like external ulcers. But why do surgeons not make it their business to find out the exact situation of the ulcer and make an incision accordingly between the ribs so that proper remedies may be conveyed to it ... About seven years ago when I was in Padua a man received a wound in the right side of his chest which festered for months but which an able surgeon cured by an incision between the ribs to the length of six fingers' breadth. Now practitioners ought to use the same

---

[2] See above, Chapter 19.

[3] The principle was enunciated by Sir Reginald Watson Jones of the London (now the Royal London) Hospital, who, his students claimed, could enclose two billiard balls in one of his superbly moulded plaster of Paris casts and induce them to unite.

boldness and diligence in curing phthisical ulcers in the lungs lest the scroll of incurable diseases should grow too long to the infinite disgrace of the profession.[4]

There is no evidence that Baglivi did more than exhort his colleagues to greater effort or that he understood the role of the pleural cavity; and sporadic references in the eighteenth century to incisions of the chest wall suggest that their purpose was mainly to drain off fluid or pus rather than to induce a pneumothorax. The first clear reference to the therapeutic possibility of collapse was made almost casually by M. Bourru, librarian to the faculty of medicine in Paris, who in 1770 undertook the translation into French of Ebenezer Gilchrist's popular tome, *The Use of Sea Voyages in Medicine: Particularly in Consumption. With Observations on that Disease.* To this now otherwise forgotten treatise – one of many extolling the merits of sea travel – the translator added a lengthy preface of his own. In this he suggested that

> if it were only the movement which is opposed to the healing of the lung ulcer [synonymous in this context with a cavity] one might be able to remedy this by an operation similar to that which one performs in the case of empyema [the accumulation of pus in the pleural cavity]. In this condition an opening is made in the chest to allow the pus to drain. But it is known that as air is introduced into the cavities of the chest the lung on this side collapses and no longer moves on breathing. The other lung carries on respiration. The ulcer is then collapsed and if it is localised may heal by cicatrisation.[5]

Bourru's suggestion excited little comment (as prefaces rarely do) for twenty years, when an eminent Paris doctor, J.-P. Maygrier, came across it by accident and lost no time in damning it: "Such a useless and dangerous operation should never be permitted in our own country or anywhere where the sacred objective of medicine is to save rather than to destroy life".[6] He was clearly under the impression that the idea had emanated from Gilchrist rather than from the translator and wished to protect the purity of French traditions. The interdict did not carry much weight across the Channel.

James Carson (1772–1843) was a Scot and an Edinburgh graduate. Like many of his compatriots he settled in Liverpool, where on the title page of his first publication in 1815, *The Causes of the Motion of the Blood*, he was described as a "Physician to the Workhouse Fever Hospital and the Asylum for Pauper Lunatics and in charge of of the Military Hospital in that Place". Though he built up an extensive private practice, he had an invincibly

---

[4] From *De praxi medica*, summarised by G. N. Balboni in *New England Journal of Medicine* 82 (1935), 1020.

[5] Brown, L., *The Story of Clinical Pulmonary Tuberculosis* (Baltimore, Maryland, 1941), p. 67.

[6] Ibid., p. 70.

inquisitive mind and found time to carry out a series of well-planned experiments. They were designed to explore the physical properties of the lungs and clarify the still largely obscure mechanism of respiration. In this he was remarkably successful: indeed, except for his more vigorous prose and learned classical allusions, the summary in this chapter almost 200 years later could have been written by him.

> Two powers are therefore concerned in regulating the movements in respiration . . . one, the resilience of the lungs, is permanent and equable, the other, the contractile power of the diaphragm and respiratory muscles, variable and exerted at regular intervals. The contractile power of the respiratory muscles is evidently much stronger than its antagonist; but not being subject to exhaustion, takes advantage of the necessary relaxation of the former and, rebounding, like the stone of Sisyphus, recovers its lost ground and renews the toil of its more powerful antagonist.[7]

Carson returned to the subject in a later paper, "On Lesions of the Lung". In this he suggested that the difficulty in the healing of lesions inside the lungs (like cavities) was due to the elasticity which keeps the lungs permanently on the stretch, and that healing could occur or at least be significantly eased if the affected part of the lung was allowed to collapse. "The diseased surfaces would then be brought into close contact [with each other] and allowed to heal as they do in other parts of the body when the part is put to rest." He then turned specifically to tuberculosis:

> It not infrequently and in the early stages perhaps generally happens that this deplorable disease has its seat in one lung only . . . The means we possess of reducing that lung to a state of collapse or of divesting it for a time of its peculiar respiratory function are simple and safe.[8]

Based on his experimental work on rabbits, he emphasised the need to collapse the lung gradually "by admitting only a small quantity of air into the cavity of the chest [meaning the pleural cavity] at a time" and even spoke of establishing successfully a pneumothorax on both sides in the management of bilateral disease.

So far as is known, Carson put his ideas and experimental findings to the test in only two patients, both far gone. He instructed a surgeon to make small incisions between their sixth and sevenths ribs. Neither experiment was successful because of "dense bands" between the two layers of the pleura, an ominous portent. In fact, despite Carson's grasp of the physiology of respiratory movements and the theoretical benefits of a pneumothorax, a successful surgical incision into the pleura in pre-Listerian days would

---

[7] Carson, J., *Essays Physiological and Practical* (Liverpool, 1822), p. 23.
[8] Ibid., p. 58.

probably have been catastrophic: most patients would have died of secondary infection.[9]

Over the sixty-year period between Carson's experiments and Forlanini's first paper there were a few sporadic references to the potential benefits of artificial pneumothorax, some of them fantastical, others less so. More persuasive were cases of spontaneous pneumothorax in which air entered the pleural space through a wound or from a tear in the lung substance. The Irish physician William Stokes, one of a galaxy of medical talent practising in Dublin during the first half of the nineteenth century, wrote that "in many such cases where the pneumothorax becomes chronic we may observe a singular suspension of the usual symptoms of phthisis: the phthisical countenance disappears; the sweats cease; the pulse may become quiet and the patient may gain flesh and strength to a surprising degree".[10] The eminent and popular French clinician, Pierre Charles Edouard Potain, tried pneumothorax on three patients in 1888 with inconclusive results;[11] and his pupil, Emile Toussaint, reported on twenty-four cases for his doctoral thesis.[12]

The man still recognised as the father of the practical therapeutic procedure was the Milanese physician, Carlo Forlanini (1847–1920). As a young man Forlanini interrupted his medical studies to fight in Garibaldi's army, one of the legendary Thousand whose exploits would remain for generations of Italian schoolboys the stuff of patriotic dreams. He then returned to medicine, graduated from the University of Pavia in 1870 and eventually became a professor there; but all his life he remained a Garibaldian: brave, voluble, volatile, pugnacious and generous. His papers, slightly verbose by today's emaciated standards, are full of bold insights and audacious (if usually unfeasible) proposals. He formulated the principles of pneumothorax more clearly than any of his predecessors, predicting that "once the diseased part of the lung is put to rest the micro-organisms which alone sustain the malign process are rendered impotent, dead, eliminated from battle".[13] He also drew

[9] Carson was honoured in his lifetime by being elected a Fellow of the Royal Society in 1837; but his work on the lung was ill-understood and more or less forgotten after his death. His pioneering papers were eventually resurrected in 1909 by a German physician, S. Daus, in an essay, "Historisches und kritisches über dem künstlichen Pneumothorax bei Lungenschwindsucht", *Therapie der Gegenwart*, 1 (1909), 227.

[10] Stokes, W., *A Treatise on the Diagnosis and Treatment of Diseases of the Chest*, i (Dublin, 1837), p. 531.

[11] Professor of Medicine at the Hôpital Necker for forty years, he had the reputation that in a long and distinguished career he never failed a student since, given time, he always answered his own questions to his own entire satisfaction. He died in 1901, aged seventy-seven. He published his two case reports in the *Bulletin de l'académie de medécine*, 19 (1880), 537.

[12] Toussaint, E., "Sur la marche de la tuberculisation pulmonaire", thesis (Paris, 1880).

lessons from the beneficial effects of the occasional spontaneous pneumothorax.

> The lung ... becomes consumptive more often than any other part of the body
> and differently from other viscera. The reason for this is simple: it is the unceasing
> motion of expansion and relaxation or ... to put it differently, it is being con-
> demned never to rest.[14]

Speculations and rumours about a bold new approach to the treatment
of tuberculosis came to a head at the Ninth International Medical Congress
in Rome in 1897. Forlanini, one of the organising committee and effortlessly
a star of any international gathering, described not only two cases of spontaneous pneumothorax (which in his opinion led to the healing of
tuberculosis) but also "a certain number of patients the hopelessness of
whose condition had persuaded [him] to induce an artificial pneumothorax,
using a large hypodermic needle and injecting into the pleura nitrogen gas
rather than air". Most memorably and in greatest detail he described the
case of Maria, a "dear and God-fearing country girl of seventeen with fever,
emaciation, large volumes of foul-smelling sputum laden with tubercle bacilli
and with a large cavity in the right upper lobe". He induced an artificial
pneumothorax in her in October 1894 and by February of the next year her
condition had greatly improved in all respects: her sputum in particular had
become scanty and negative for tubercle bacilli on direct smear. She was sent
on a mountain holiday in the Abruzzi in July 1895 where her progress was
maintained; she then returned to work, being given refills of nitrogen at
six-monthly intervals and – the final coup in the triumphal presentation –
here she was to tell the tale herself.[15]

This was the beginning of the golden half-century of international medical
congresses, self-proclaimed landmarks all in the forward march of mankind.
Tuberculosis was still not treatable, but identification of the cause had made
it scientifically respectable; and congresses devoted to it ranked among the
most prestigious. They also commanded wide interest in the lay as well as
in the professional press, the ramifications of the disease extending from
high-powered laboratory science to homely measures of hygiene and diet
and from burning humanitarian issues to stunningly bold surgical techniques. The delegates met in palaces and were received by Kings and
Presidents. The obligatory *vin d'honneur* on the eve of the inaugural session
would be followed by the Roll Call of the Nations, an orchestra playing the

[13] Lojacono, S., "Forlanini's Original Communications on Artificial Pneumothorax",
Tubercle, 64 (1934), 54.

[14] Ibid., 62.

[15] Forlanini, C., *Gazzetta medicale di Torino*, 46 (1897), 857.

appropriate national anthem as each delegation leader stepped forward to signal his country's presence and sign the register. At the official banquet, attended by the delegates' ladies, full evening dress and decorations were *de rigueur* and tiaras were much in evidence. The after-dinner speeches were long and dwelt eloquently on international co-operation.[16]

In such a setting Forlanini's lecture with its unexpected climax was acclaimed as a *coup de théâtre* just within the bounds of scientific decorum. It also marked the beginning of artificial pneumothorax therapy. This was not immediately apparent. Many felt, as did Professor Béla von Mansfeld of Munich, that the measure was "one of those ingenious operations which required for its success the unfettered enthusiasm of the Latin temperament".[17] The wider acceptance of the procedure owed more to the appearance on the international stage of John Benjamin Murphy of Appleton, Wisconsin. A dominant and domineering personality, Murphy had considerable mechanical skill allied to a useful flair for publicity. When invited to deliver the Surgical Oration at the meeting of the American Medical Association in 1898 he chose as his title "The Surgery of the Lung", a provocation in itself at a time when operating inside the thoracic cavity was regarded as an absurdity, much as operating on the heart would still be fifty years later. Touching briefly on pulmonary tuberculosis, he was scathing about prevailing attitudes which regarded the disease as an exclusively medical condition. "What", he asked rhetorically, "have our physician colleagues achieved?"

> With the exception of a thorough knowledge of its aetiology and pathology, nothing. Yes, nothing. We had hoped and still hope that tuberculosis may be cured, alleviated or curtailed in its destructive effects by products derived from the tubercular bacillus under certain conditions or by some other bacterial poison. The results barely justify the continuation of such hope. Can surgeons stand aside? [18]

[16] The rarity of these congresses – four-yearly intervals were the rule – added importance to the proceedings. Travel was easy but still leisurely and expensive enough to preclude the pitiful spectacle of jet-lagged professorial sheep being shepherded around by smooth professional organisers; or of hordes of expenses-paid hangers on – intent to be seen (or not, as the case may be). The papers read were comparatively few – two or three a day over a period of ten days – but long and weighty; and there was ample chance for delegates to confer informally during leisurely coffee, luncheon, tea and other intermissions (no "breaks" in those days); or in hushed whispers during the louder passages of the string quartets which were often played during to the more formal repasts. A gala performance at the opera was inescapable; but after the first act a well-stocked buffet offered another congenial setting for the exchange of compliments, pleasantries and even views. In the fullness of time – never less than two years later but ready for the next congress – the proceedings were published in lavishly bound commemorative volumes and sent to each delegate. Judged by their pristine state in medical libraries, they must rank among the most unread medical publications ever.

[17] Mansfeld, B. von, *Münchner medizinische Wochenschrift*, 48 (1897), 63.

Whatever was true of surgeons in general, John Benjamin Murphy, by now chief of surgery at the Mercy Hospital in Chicago, could not. Reiterating (knowingly or not) Carson's speculations, he vigorously set out the underlying principles of collapse therapy:

> The pathology of repair of pulmonary tubercular cavities involves certain physical conditions which are peculiar to the chest ... namely the constant resistance of the bony framework against contraction, the effort of expansion of the cavity in each respiratory act ... Allow the wall of an abscess to collapse having emptied it thoroughly, it will heal. This must surely be the keynote to the successful treatment of pulmonary cavities ... Primary tuberculosis too might surely be conquered by prolonged, enforced rest.[19]

Murphy went beyond Carson and artificial pneumothorax. He envisaged not only introducing gas into the pleural cavity but also allowing the lung to collapse by separating the parietal pleura from the chest wall (later to be known as extrapleural pneumothorax) and even by removing part of the bony cage of the chest (the future thoracoplasty). Nor was Murphy a man to waste time on protracted preliminary experiments. He devised a simple apparatus of movable bottles attached to a trocar, worked out a simple (and, with hindsight, exceedingly dangerous) technique and proceeded to introduce staggering volumes of nitrogen (up to three litres) into the pleural cavity of seven patients. His only guide as to when to stop was watching the patient, who became increasingly short of breath and eventually turned blue, and intermittently percussing and auscultating the chest to see how far the midline had shifted. In two of his seven cases the procedure was abandoned because adhesions prevented the gas from diffusing, but in five it was adjudged to have been either a success or a complete success. (The difference between the two results was never spelt out.) No follow-up was ever reported and refills were not apparently carried out or even contemplated.

Murphy's later claim to having invented artificial pneumothorax cannot be sustained, especially as he himself soon abandoned thoracic surgery for new fields to conquer (passing that side of his vast practice to his faithful disciple, A. F. Lemke); but his international celebrity and his gift for simplifying problems and offering technically feasible (if not always beneficial) solutions assured his teaching wide publicity. In particular, it inspired Ludolph Brauer of Marburg in Germany, a generally cautious and conservative operator, to try artificial pneumothorax in two patients. Both survived

[18] Murphy, J. B., *Journal of the American Medical Association*, 31 (1898), 151.

[19] Murphy's eponymous fame rested for a long time on Murphy's button, an ingenious device which helped to suture cut ends of the small intestine end-to-end. He died in 1916, aged sixty-six.

and he followed up the initial procedure with regular refills. Reporting his results to the Marburg Medical Society,[20] he stressed the importance of the operator knowing where the tip of the needle was and, unlike Murphy, listed a number of possible complications. The fact that he described the treatment as "*nach* Murphy" galvanised Forlanini both into reclaiming priority and into publishing a new series of eight cases in German and in a scientifically more respectable format than his previous communications.[21]

Artificial pneumothorax can still provide a blueprint of how therapeutic innovations fare in modern medicine. It was a brilliant conception and a valuable contribution to the treatment of pulmonary tuberculosis, but it was fraught with unforeseen difficulties and subject to strict practical limitations. Its progression was the story of ups, downs and sideways; of the interplay of gains, risks, triumphs and complications; of the impact of professional publicity and the influence of the mass media; of private and national jealousy as well as of impressive intellectual achievement and generosity. In Denmark Christian Saugman had had some initial failures when in 1906 he read Forlanini's paper and immediately ordered the apparatus described in it. Even before trying the contraption he saw the danger – or one of the dangers – of the Forlanini procedure. Putting the hollow needle connected to a nitrogen gas cylinder into what was assumed to be the pleural space, the operator could be sure of being in the right place only by the sudden start of the gas flow. The blindness of the manoeuvre explained the episodes of pleural eclampsy which, in the language of Forlanini, meant anything from minor and transient attacks of dizziness, breathlessness and cyanosis to convulsions and sudden death. Saugman and several of his colleagues thought (almost certainly rightly) that most of these were caused by minute gas-bubbles – so-called air *emboli* – being forced or sucked into the blood stream and being carried to the brain. Forlanini would have none of this. Like many other bold innovators, he strenuously resisted any further bold innovations. Bubbles were inconceivable and, insofar as they were conceivable, of no risk whatever. Or perhaps – he was nothing if not open-minded – a minimal risk. Minimal or not, it was not a risk Saugman was prepared to take. To do so seemed the more irrational since the introduction of a simple water manometer, which allowed the monitoring of the pressure in the needle, could largely eliminate it. Like many such apparently minor improvements, it also made the operation safe – or relatively safe – in untutored hands.[22]

[20] Brauer, L., *Münchner medizinische Wochenschrift*, 53 (106), 337.
[21] Forlanini, C., *Deutsche medizinische Wochenschrift*, 32 (106), 101.

Many such hands were now itching to try it. In France the treatment was introduced by a Forlanini pupil, F. Dumarest,[23] and adopted and improved by G. Küss of Agincourt;[24] but its best-known practitioner was Edouard Rist of the Hôpital Laënnec in Paris, the first to publish a balanced and critical review of the procedure in English.[25] In the United States, after Murphy had lost interest in tuberculosis (to pursue his career as a general surgeon), the method was reinvented and popularised by Mary Lapham,[26] S. Robinson and Cleveland Floyd.[27] The unwitting pioneer in England – other than those long dead – was Claude Lillingston who was himself tuberculous and who had had his first artificial pneumothorax induced at Mesnalian Sanatorium in Norway. On returning to England he went to work at Mundesley Sanatorium in Norfolk where, with the help of his wife and the sanatorium carpenter, he gave himself the first refill. Such boy-scout exploits could not fail to fire the enthusiasm of Englishmen and the method was quickly adopted by leading chest physicians.

Forlanini's self-appointed role as high priest of orthodoxy delayed for some years another important development. He had expressed the opinion that the full benefits of collapse therapy could be obtained only if the lung was kept in a condition of complete collapse for a prolonged period. The doctrine was challenged in 1912 by his compatriot Maurizio Ascoli, who had found that sufficient relaxation could be achieved by slightly below atmospheric pressure.[28] Apart from increased safety and less discomfort, this also made it possible to induce a pneumothorax in both lungs. A similar idea occurred to W. Parry Morgan, who noted in 1913 that if only a small volume of gas was introduced into the pleural space the bubble tended to localise over the diseased – that is the least expansile – area of the lung.[29] Soon selective collapse virtually replaced the original Forlanini procedure.

Growing experience in many centres also focused attention on the single most important limitation to the induction of a pneumothorax. More often than had been realised tuberculosis of the lung reached the pleura and set up a low-grade pleural inflammation. This entailed scarring. Scarring tended to cause the two pleural layers to adhere. When the adhesions became extensive the pleural space was obliterated. Without a pleural space no gas

[22] Saugman, C., *Beiträge zur Klinik der Tuberkulose*, 31 (1914), 571.

[23] Dumarest, F., *Bulletin de médecine*, 2 (1909), 224.

[24] Küss, G., ibid., 3 (1910), 88.

[25] Rist, E., *Quarterly Journal of Medicine*, 1 (1912), 259.

[26] Lapham, M. E., *Southern Medical Journal*, 4 (1911), 742.

[27] Robinson, S., Floyd, C., *Archives of Internal Medicine*, 9 (1911), 452.

[28] Ascoli, M., *Deutsche medizinische Wochenschrift*, 38 (1912), 1782.

[29] Morgan, W. P., *Lancet* (1913), no. 2, 18.

could be introduced. The possibility had been recognised by Carson a hundred years earlier but now became an urgent problem. The first attempt to overcome it was made by P. L. Friedrich of Marburg. He opened the chest and pleural cavity and simply proceeded to divide the adhesions with a scalpel and a pair of scissors.[30] The operation (dignified by the name of thoracoplastic pleuropneumolysis) was extremely dangerous. Even in the patients who survived the surgery it was also usually ineffective. It was soon abandoned.

A more ingenious and acceptable approach was devised by Christian Jacobaeus of Stockholm. More accurately, an ingenious and acceptable but useless technique suddenly found a practical application. Jacobaeus had both an aptitude and a passion for devising clever optical instruments. This led him to invent the endoscope, an instrument not unlike the periscope of a submarine, which allowed the examination of the interior of body cavities. With the peritoneoscope it was possible to look inside the abdomen, an objective whose practical usefulness did not become clear until the advent of keyhole surgery (and, according to some, not very clear even then).[31] The development of the thoracoscope for the exploration of the pleural space providentially coincided with the search for a safe way of dealing with pleural adhesions.[32] Jacobaeus noticed that his illuminated thoracoscope afforded excellent vision of these cord- or membrane-like structures. The idea then struck him that under thoracoscopic vision – that is through a very small incision – it might be possible to divide them, using a fine galvanic electro-cautery. This could easily be introduced through a second channel of the thoracoscope. A small electric bulb would serve as the source of illumination. The procedure would require skill but it was an acceptable challenge. He was encouraged by results published from several sanatoria, especially from Vejlefjord. These demonstrated the strikingly different prognosis in tuberculous patients in whom an artificial pneumothorax was possible from those in whom it was prevented by adhesions. (The alternative explanation, that patients with extensive adhesions had a more advanced disease, does not seem to have been seriously considered.) He made his first successful attempt at dividing adhesions under thoracoscopic vision in 1913, and within the next few years performed fifty such operations. At least two-thirds were successful in allowing the establishment of a pneumothorax. None of his patients died on the operating table or during the immediate postoperative period. His

---

[30] Friedrich, P. L., *Surgery, Gynecology, Obstetrics*, 7 (1908), 632.

[31] These rigid metal scopes were the ancestors of the modern flexible fibreoptic instruments which came into general use in the 1960s.

[32] Jacobaeus, H. C., *Proceedings of the Royal Society of Medicine*, 45 (1922), 78.

results with closed intrapleural pneumonolysis were soon repeated in other centres. With only minor modifications the technique remained an essential adjunct to artificial pneumothorax therapy for the next forty years.

The original artificial pneumothorax was usually performed by physicians (and as time passed often by the most junior doctors on the hospital or sanatorium staff); and it was, compared to the heroic and bloody operations which were to come, properly described as a minor procedure. From the patients' point of view it was never quite so minor as medical papers and textbooks implied. The victims were given morphine and calomel the night before the "gassing" (as the treatment became popularly known in England) and their chest was pierced under local anaesthesia, usually novocaine.[33] In Hungary, Árpád Tóth, the consumptive poet who had the treatment in the early 1930s, wrote that, though the needle prick in the skin did not hurt and the morphine had in any case induced a happily drowsy state, the needle entering the pleura felt like being kicked by a mule: "there was a crunch, a stab and a prayer, O God, let me die quickly".[34] The real pain began a few hours later (after the anaesthetic had worn off and the operator had departed): it was sharp and unresponsive to drugs and kept patients awake. The first refill was often given while the pain was still there, four or five days after the initial procedure; and for the desired degree of collapse three or four injections were usually necessary. After that the treatment protocol generally envisaged refills every six weeks for at least three or four years. Even after the safety measures introduced by Saugmann, pleural shock – from passing faintness to occasional death – remained a real risk. In the 1930s, when in Britain refills were beginning to be administered in tuberculosis dispensaries, a Ministry of Health memorandum on the design of such premises emphasised the need for a separate exit from the operating room for the emergency evacuation of unconscious patients without the need for traversing the waiting area. (Where to? The hospital? The municipal mortuary? The memorandum did not specify.) More common was low-grade pleural infection with night sweats and often severe discomfort. Patients had to learn to live with them.

Nevertheless, by the mid 1920s most sanatorium patients demanded AP: any suggestion that their case was unsuited – and more and more possible contraindications were emerging – was greeted with resentment, despair, sometimes hatred. Nothing perhaps so vividly illustrates the awful futility of sanatorium life than this welcome given to a therapy that was always

---

[33] Subchloride of mercury, a powerful purgative.
[34] Toth, Á., *Levelek* (Budapest, 1939), p. 78.

unpleasant and often painful, whose risks and benefits were sometimes finely balanced.

Pulmonary tuberculosis was, as always, the pace-setter of new therapeutic approaches; but the general principle of resting the diseased part was gaining acceptance in the treatment of other forms of the disease as well. It was difficult or impossible to apply it to many anatomical sites – neither the kidneys nor the small intestine could be put to rest – but it was on the face of it eminently suited to bones and joints. It was in treating tuberculosis of the knee that Hugh Owen Thomas of Liverpool had championed prolonged rest. By the first decade of the century his simple metal splints were being replaced by often immense and elaborate plaster of Paris casts. Patients, usually children, were encased in them for months or years. The flagships of the method were the plaster spicas for tuberculosis of the hip and the double shells for tuberculosis of the spine. It was the ambition of every budding orthopaedic surgeon to have some ingenious new appliance named after him.[35]

The apostle of immobilisation in England, Sir Henry Gauvain, surgeon superintendent of Lord Mayor Treloar's Cripples Home in Hampshire, was also one of the most inventive. For established hunchbacks – that is patients with a collapsed tuberculous vertebra in the thoracic region – he invented a spinal board, on which the patient was placed with a mattress shaped to correct the deformity. Special attires and gadgets were necessary to allow the bowels to open and for regular attention to skin. With lumbar spinal deformities patients were encased in plaster jackets applied (so Gauvain recommended) while they were suspended vertically and after a fortnight's training period to prevent "giddiness and fainting".[36] This was "not only distressing to the patient but also disconcerting to the surgeon". Milk products and vegetables "which tend to induce vomiting while the plaster jacket is applied and for some weeks after" were forbidden during training.[37] Lesions in the cervical region required especially long cases with moulded supports for the chin and forehead. A minimum treatment period of two years was usually envisaged followed by less cumbersome appliances (made from celluloid from the 1920s onward) worn for another three or four years. In 1915, in a review of a thousand cases, Gauvain concluded that the results were good, "under the best conditions: the mortality should not exceed 2 per cent

[35] The Bradford frame, the Phelps box and the Moseley wheel-barrow in particular enjoyed considerable popularity for many years.

[36] Gauvain, Sir H., "Tuberculosis Cripples", in *Defective Children*, edited by T. M. Kelynack (London, 1915), p. 120.

[37] Ibid., p. 140.

and might even be less if patients not previously operated on might be excluded".[38]

Many more cases than those treated at Lord Mayor Treloar's Hospital and a few similar specialised institutions, especially children with infections of the hips or knees, had to be looked after at home. Because of the nursing care needed, plaster beds, spicas and similar appliances were not usually options for working-class families, and much ingenuity went into devising second-best but serviceable alternatives. Even in comparatively comfortable middle-class homes, an immobilised child usually called for the full-time attention of at least one parent. Though terribly prolonged, the treatment was often successful: at any rate, some of the patients recovered. As sometimes happens to children whose childhood is blighted by illness, isolation and suffering, a few of the sufferers also later achieved fame, fortune and perhaps happiness in the arts, literature and public life.

[38] Ibid., p. 142. The battle lines were being drawn on the one hand between orthopaedic surgeons in the United States and to a lesser extent in France who favoured early surgical intervention for draining abscesses, correcting deformities and even internal splinting and, on the other, the far more conservative British school which preferred prolonged immobilisation.

23

Gold Rush

Despite the upbeat if slightly petulant tone of official pronouncements – the cause of tuberculosis was known, it had no business to be hanging about, it would soon be eliminated – neither the melancholy prospect of a sanatorium life nor the pyrotechnics of collapse therapy gave patients what they craved above all: hope for a complete cure *now*. Nor did they satisfy the medical rank-and-file, ordinary doctors who saw beyond the triumphalist utterances of their leaders the misery and despair caused by the illness as it affected ordinary people like themselves. Even though in many countries the incidence of the disease was once again beginning spontaneously but exceedingly slowly to decline in the mid 1920s, pressure to explore new paths – and short-cuts – was increasing. The more outlandish the proposals, the greater was the accompanying razzmatazz.

First among the new remedies were those that were proving effective or at least promising in other diseases. For many years Paul Ehrlich and his team had been in fanatical pursuit of the holy grail of a magic bullet, a chemical compound that would be lethal to pathogenic organisms without killing the host; and in 1909 they announced the discovery of Compound 606 or Salvarsan. Initially overlooked, it was the 606th in a series of organic arsenicals tested in animals; and for a time it looked as if it might fulfil Ehrlich's hopes in man. It did in fact prove modestly effective, though rarely curative, in syphilis; but, even in its modified forms, it was unpredictably toxic.[1] More a

---

[1] The original search was for a compound active against trypanosomes (the causative agents of sleeping sickness and other tropical diseases). Ehrlich, an insatiable reader of irrelevant scientific literature, then came across a paper in which Fritz Schaudinn, an alcoholic and a visionary, not only identified the *Spirochaeta pallida* as the cause of syphilis but also likened its appearance to that of trypanosomes. (What induced him to do so is a mystery: both are microscopic organisms but there the similarity ends.) Ehrlich promptly switched his search for a useful role for his arsenical compounds to spirochetes and found Compound 606. (It had in fact been available for some time but had been written off by an incompetent assistant – of whom Ehrlich had many – as having no effect.) It was highly active in animals against Schaudinn's spirochete and soon shown to be active in man as well. However, in its original form it was extremely dangerous even to manufacture and very unstable: prolonged contact with air could convert it into a deadly poison. A later modification, known as Neosalvarsan, was safer but it was superseded in the 1940s by penicillin and is never used today.

hopeful trailer than an actual advance, it was nevertheless taken up by workers in tuberculosis research and had extensive trials in Germany and England. It soon became apparent that neither in the test-tube nor in animals was the drug (or any of its numerous arsenic-based analogues) active against the tuberculosis bacillus. It was also agreed that it was not without risk.

Of greater promise and of immense benefit to mankind was the discovery by Gerhard Domagk of the sulphonomides in the 1930s. The first of the synthetic wonder drugs, they were life-saving in many acute bacterial infections;[2] and for a time one of Domagk's early preparations, Prontosil, raised high hopes that it might be effective in tuberculosis.[3] It did indeed prove useful in containing secondary infections, an ever-present danger in patients who needed surgery to drain their tuberculous abscesses; but against the tuberculosis bacillus itself it was powerless.[4]

Sun-lamps of varying elaboration were widely used either on their own or in acclimatising courses before exposing patients to genuine sun-rays. X-ray therapy was tried for no better reason than that X-rays were available. Patients lost their hair and became sick; and in 1924 Dr R. A. Young of the Brompton Hospital described "some initial benefits".[5] But there was never any experimental evidence to suggest that Koch's bacillus was particularly sensitive to X-rays; and Young was reduced to speculating about unspecified and nebulous tissue defence reactions. Whatever the mechanism, the initial benefits, if any, were not sustained.

Inhalations, so popular in the eighteenth and nineteenth centuries, never entirely lost their appeal, only now the various concoctions were usually

[2] The first patient to be treated with them was the six-year-old daughter of the discoverer. She had cut her hand and the cut became septic. Domagk was told that only an amputation could save her life. He refused and gave the girl Prontosil. She recovered. Sulphonomides (originally the by-products of the dye industry) are still widely used, mainly in infections of the urinary tract.

[3] Perhaps because Domagk and his collaborator, Josef Klarer, worked for a large drug company (the Bayerwerke of Eberfeld near Wuppertal) which jealously guarded its patents and may in fact have delayed publication of the discovery, the discoverers never enjoyed the public acclaim accorded ten years later to Fleming, Chain and Florey of penicillin fame. Prontosil did, however, save the life of President Roosevelt's son, Franklin Junior, in January 1937, and in the following year Domagk was duly awarded the last Nobel Prize for medicine before the Second World War. Hitler personally forbade him to accept the honour. Eventually, in 1947, he was given the medal but not the prize money.

[4] It did nevertheless enjoy a vogue for some years both in England and in the United States. The slightly more complex sulphone compounds, especially a preparation marketed as Promin, were also reported as being useful against tuberculosis by W. H. Feldman of the Mayo Clinic and E. M. Medlar and K. T. Sasano of the Bellevue Hospital in New York. They did not fulfil their promise.

[5] Young, R. A., *British Medical Journal* (1924), no. 1, 478.

injected directly into the windpipe.[6] Intratracheal menthol, olive oil, guaiacol, iodides, dyes, creosote, copper cyanurate and pig-spleen extracts (among others) were all reported to give good results by reputable physicians, as did in some hands silica and colloidal preparations of silver, copper, aluminium and antimony. The first issue in 1919 of the leading specialist medical journal of the future, *Tubercle*, contained an article reporting strikingly beneficial effects from "brass digested in a mixture of vegetable oil".

In contrast to such inspirational therapies calcium treatment enjoyed both a semblance of a rationale and several therapeutic trials. The semblance of a rationale was the observation that healed tuberculous lesions often underwent calcification, whereas calcification was conspicuously absent from active sites of the disease. Whether or not influenced by this seductive irrelevance and mistaking effect for cause, a French physician, Louis Renon, reported in 1906 that in the small village of Yonne, a limestone area with many lime-burning furnaces, he had discovered no case of tuberculosis despite the fact that the majority of inhabitants were alcoholics, a well-known predisposing cause.[7] Here, he suggested, was a clue at least to the prevention but perhaps even to the cure of the illness. This was either a stroke of genius or utter nonsense; and clutching at any straw in their constantly losing battle, many otherwise level-headed doctors were prepared to give it the benefit of the doubt.[8] Less than a year after Renon's startling discovery, W. J. B. Selkirk of Edinburgh reported on the apparent excellent health and freedom from tuberculosis enjoyed by workers in lime-kilns near the city, prompting him to suggest that "considerations should be given to the organisation of lime-works as the basis of a curative antituberculous colony".[9] About the same time the Spaniard Eduardo Fisac stated categorically that "all workers in lime and plaster of Paris are immune to tuberculosis in spite of the fact that they live in squalid dwellings and are underfed".[10]

This was purely anecdotal evidence but it was promising enough to prompt Dr Frank Tweddell of Philadelphia to write to all manufacturers of plaster of Paris in the north-eastern states of the United States, enquiring about the incidence of pulmonary tuberculosis among their work-forces. His leading questions would have been ruled out of order in any court of law, but the responses (many of them from company doctors) were all a hopeful heart could desire: in a nutshell tuberculosis was unknown among their employees, even among those working in offices but near the factories. It appeared,

---

[6] This is still a popular route of administration of drugs in some countries, including Russia.
[7] Renon, L., *Bulletin médicale de Paris*, 20 (1906), 294.
[8] Brockbank, W., *Quarterly Journal of Medicine*, 20 (1924), 231.
[9] Selkirk, W. J. B., *British Medical Journal* (1908), no. 2, 1493.
[10] Keers. R. Y., *Pulmonary Tuberculosis: A Journey down the Centuries* (London, 1978), p. 202.

Tweddell concluded, that the continual inhalation of finely divided particles of lime and gypsum confers immunity to tuberculosis, possibly because lime in contact with the moisture in the lungs forms calcium hydroxide which acts as a caustic and antiseptic – the effect being for some reason as specific against tuberculosis as quinine is for malaria.[11]

Several more critical and better designed studies found no evidence to support such an assertion and nothing in fact to suggest that on a normal diet added calcium had any beneficial influence on the course of the illness. Yet the idea had a kind of superficial plausibility (as was true of many wholly ineffective antituberculous remedies): calcium equalled bone and bone symbolised strength. It was also true that in modest doses most calcium preparations on the market did no harm. For whatever reason, in most countries throughout the 1930s patients were given calcium as a useful body-building supplement to whatever other treatment they were having. The trend was not influenced by the demonstration that the only guaranteed effect of most tablets was to make patients mildly sick.

Calcium was at least cheap and in moderation innocuous. Neither could be said about the most loudly trumpeted of the medical advances of the interwar years. Though chemically among the most unreactive and biologically the least interesting of elements, gold had been used in magic potions and alchemists' brews since time immemorial and specifically against consumption at least since the early nineteenth century.[12] Its lack of biological interest does in fact need to be qualified: like other heavy metals (lead or mercury for example), it can block essential enzymic molecular sites and, injected or taken by mouth in large doses, it can be poisonous. Its place in the treatment of human ailments always owed more to its glitter (and to the assumption that what is expensive must be good) than to any experimental evidence. In 1890 Koch gave it a breath of scientific respectability when he reported that gold cyanides (among at least twenty other more active organic metal compounds) slightly inhibited the growth of tubercle bacilli in cultures. Such a pronouncement from Mount Olympus, however cautiously expressed, could not be brushed aside; and the finding was duly followed up by several animal studies in Germany both immediately before and during the First World War. All concluded that in living animals gold in any form promoted rather

---

[11] Tweddell, F., *Medical Records*, 141 (1922), 48.

[12] Gold is biologically uninteresting for the same reasons that make it precious: it is chemically sluggish and it has never been shown to be an essential trace constituent of biological systems (unlike, for example, copper, zinc, cobalt and several other metals).

than inhibited tuberculosis and that, after occasional transient improvement, it tended to shorten rather than lengthen survival.[13]

Whether this humdrum but meticulous work was unknown to or simply ignored by Holger Møllgaard is still not clear. An animal physiologist and professor in the faculty of science of the University of Copenhagen, he announced in 1924 that, having investigated the possible therapeutic useful-ness of numerous metal compounds, he had discovered a complex gold salt, a double thiosulphate of gold and sodium, which had a specific beneficial action in tuberculosis. He christened the compound Sanocrysin. Møllgaard's claim was based on animal experiments; and he always emphasised that he was not a proper doctor but a mere laboratory scientist. To many doctors there was something profound and powerful about his bashful gibberish. "It is a well-known fact", he announced to a rapt audience at the Royal Society of Medicine of London

> that the injection of Sanocrysin into an animal infected with tuberculosis causes a violent reaction which appears clinically as an acute intoxication ... The symp-toms are albuminuria, indicating renal damage, myocarditis and a shock-like fall in temperature. In other cases there is no shock but a high temperature. I regard all these reactions as immune responses to the liberation of toxins from killed and dissolved tubercle bacilli and tuberculous tissue ... This shock-like state can be counterbalanced by the intravenous injection of a specific tuberculous anti-serum made by immunising cattle ... it is possible by prophylactic injection of this serum to remove the animal from the shock-like state induced by Sanocrysin.[14]

Møllgaard's papers – but especially his lectures – suggested a measure of self-delusion rather than any intention to deceive. But they *did* deceive – and for one of the most ancient of reasons. They were so absurd that they had to be true. Within a few months of his initial announcement, his gold-salt treatment was tried in mild observation cases by two Danish doctors, Knud Secher, a Copenhagen physician of high repute, and Knud Faber, professor of clinical medicine in the university. Both confirmed the "sometimes re-markable beneficial and potentially curative" properties of the preparation. Significantly or not, the drug was soon protected by a patent (and therefore to be spelled with a capital S) and in highly profitable commercial production.

Perhaps there was something about the politically and economically grim 1930s which promoted the growth of fairytale fantasies, whether it was Holly-wood glitz, Fascist rallies, Nazi vapourings of blood and soil, or gold treatment in tuberculosis: it is difficult to account for the Sanocrysin success story

---

[13] Anything causing reversible shock can, after recovery, cause a temporary improvement in conditions which involve the immune response (in practice most chronic diseases).

[14] Møllgaard, H., *Proceedings of the Royal Society of Medicine*, 20 (1926), 287.

otherwise. Even in animals Møllgaard's results were terrible. The injections seemed totally to abolish temperature regulation: almost a fifth of his guinea-pigs and rabbits died either of hyperpyrexia or of hypothermic shock. He seemed to regard this as a triumph and attributed the side-effects to toxins released after the "killing and dissolution of the tubercle bacilli". This killing in turn was "clearly due to the unique property of Sanocrysin of penetrating through the organism's fatty capsule". There was not a shred of evidence to support any of these statements. Incredibly, the results were not much better in man. Describing his experience with his first patients, Faber wrote:

> We were of course prepared to see serious consequences follow Sanocrysin in-jections and indeed we had cases in whom the reactions could not be controlled, so that, sadly, some patient succumbed perhaps earlier than they would otherwise have done.[15]

He was nevertheless confident that these teething troubles could be overcome and was in no doubt that "in a certain number of patients the favourable effect was very striking though in many it could not be detected". The madness was widely hailed as a breakthrough.[16]

Not perhaps surprisingly, it was in Scandinavia that enthusiasm for the treatment first began to wane. (Yet, even in Denmark, many doctors felt that, in view of the benefits reported from very small doses, it would be wrong to withhold the drug entirely.) [17] While Sanocrysin was falling out of favour on its home ground, however, the gold rush spread to Spain, France, Eastern Europe and, with slightly attenuated virulence, to England and the United States. The results continued to be frightening: in one early trial out of forty-two patients nine died of shock and prostration and nineteen of the twenty-one severe cases showed no significant improvement. (The remaining two and the less severe cases were eventually "discharged symptom free", presumably after their fever, rash and other evidence of tissue damage had subsided.) [18]

Even in relatively sceptical England this intensely painful and occasionally lethal therapy continued to be prescribed (though with the dosage reduced tenfold or more) by reputable doctors in reputable hospitals. Dr Mary Nannetti of the Papworth Village Settlement claimed highly satisfactory results in "suitable cases", defined as "exudative with nodular caseous pneu-monic force breaking down with cavity formation" (whatever that meant),

[15] Faber, K., *Lancet* (1925), no. 2, 62.
[16] Smith, F. B., *Journal of Contemporary History*, 20 (1985), 733.
[17] Kayne, G. G., *Proceedings of the Royal Society of Medicine*, 28 (1936), 1463.
[18] Amberson, J. B., McMahon, B. T., Pinner, M., *American Review of Tuberculosis*, 24 (1931), 401.

especially when the gold was given together with injections of digitalis and caffeine.[19] She said that her patients' general condition improved, though many still suffered shock, loss of weight and skin eruptions. Dr William Stobie and Dr Sheila Hunter of the Radcliffe Infirmary in Oxford also tried a modification of the treatment and observed "definite improvement" in twenty-five out of forty-five patients, though even those who improved suffered from diarrhoea, vomiting, loss of appetite, rashes and loss of weight during the course. Of the remainder ten discharged themselves and in the rest the treatment was abandoned.[20] Some doctors combined gold with collapse therapy, reporting the usual encouraging results, especially in children.[21]

It might be thought that the exorbitant cost of the proprietary gold salt would have limited if not totally prohibited its use during the Depression; but this was not so. Thomas Osborne of London, an advertisement copy-writer and the father of playwright John Osborne, was fortunate enough to belong to one of the most caring trade insurance societies of his day, the National Advertising Benevolent Society. When in 1938, at the age of thirty-four, he developed pulmonary tuberculosis he was not only dispatched to Menton on the Riviera to recuperate but funds were also made available for him to have a course of the latest and what was generally considered to be the best treatment available. "Your Dad had his bum shot full of gold today, so he's now the most valuable man in Europe", he quipped on a card to his son. "But it was horrible. The nurse who gave me the injection was German: must have been Mrs Hitler." [22] The treatment certainly did him no good: he died less than three years later.

Nowhere in Europe was the charitable antituberculous movement more generously supported or more open-handed than in Holland; and its ben-evolence embraced some of the most bedraggled victims of the First World War. In 1932 the St Elizabeth Sanatorium in Budakeszi near Budapest in Hungary received a large consignment of Sanocrysin from The Hague to be used in early cases of tuberculosis in children. Fortunately the sanatorium at that time only treated adults; and the first recipient of the magic drug was József Egry, a gifted painter and war victim of tuberculosis. Immediately after the first injection he collapsed in a state of shock and recovered only in response to heroic doses of strychnine and extracts of pituitary hormone. The rest of the consignment was then ordered to be destroyed by the

[19] Nannetti, M., *British Medical Journal* (1926), no. 2, 21.
[20] Stobie, W., Hunter, S., ibid. (1929), no. 1, 29.
[21] Ashby, H. T., ibid. (1931), no. 2, 668.
[22] Osborne, J., *A Better Class of Person* (London, 1980), p. 90.

superintendent, Dr O. Országh, except for one course which was tried on the much-loved tuberculous daughter of Hungary's Regent, Paulette Horthy. She survived the treatment but died from the disease two years later.[23]

If cost was no barrier, nothing else seemed to act as a deterrent. Dr Gregory Kayne's discovery and warning in 1935 that Møllgaard had fudged his results in failing to report that his first batch of experimental guinea-pigs had been infected with attenuated bacilli was ignored; suggestions for a controlled trial were resisted; and not much notice was taken even when in 1936 Dr Frank Terrill in the United States showed that there was no substance in the claim that gold salts had any effect on the tuberculosis bacillus even in test-tube cultures.[24] In Britain the craze did not wholly subside until 1940 when, shortly after Dunkirk, an anonymous but eminently sensible Home Office official turned down a medically well-supported application for the import licence of an American substitute drug: it was, he suggested, non-contributory to the war effort.

[23] Recounted to the present writer by Dr O. Országh.

[24] In a retrospective survey in 1946, Dr P. D'Arcy Hart commented: "The astonishing acceptance of a remedy and its subsequent total rejection without any immediate better substitute is only equalled by the earlier dramatic rise and fall of tuberculin. Sanocrysin was too heavily sponsored without any adequate clinical or laboratory groundwork, its toxicity was severely underrated and its clinical benefits were very much overstated". *British Medical Journal* (1946), no. 2, 805.

In many ways the most remarkable fact about gold therapy was its resurrection in the 1960s as an antirheumatoid agent. It was as toxic as before and its benefits, if any, were just as transient.

24

Quacks

The cures peddled by quacks were not more effective than those espoused by doctors, but they were usually less painful and almost always more affordable. After a few decades of relative decline, and reflecting perhaps both the disappointing aftermath of the scientific optimism of the turn of the century and the menacing upsurge of tuberculosis during and after the war, self-diagnosis and home-treatment books enjoyed a renaissance in the 1920s. The authors sported an assortment of qualifications and skilfully drew on standard medical textbooks as well as on the immense literature of herbalism, homeopathy, astrology, divination and other traditional lore. Many of the works were published to promote the writer's own patent medicine and came accompanied by unsolicited letters from grateful patients – or rather ex-patients now fully restored to health.

Though cheap by the standard of Møllgaard's gold treatment, the cost of bottled cures varied. Congreve's acclaimed bright red Balsamic Elixir was not a give-away at £1 2s. 11d. for a family size bottle,[1] but it came with a handsome, sturdy and well-written booklet dispensing sound advice about a balanced diet and the avoidance of stimulants. Although advertised as exclusively herbal, it contained, in addition to innocuous vegetable matter, aromatic sulphuric acid (which may have helped to reduce night sweats), traces of Tolu and Peru balsam (mild antiseptics and stimulants), Virginia prune, a sedative, much sugar and cochineal and over 2.5 per cent by volume of alcohol. Most adults, following the directions to take a teaspoonful three or four times a day, would have found it pleasantly relaxing; and most children between eight and fifteen years, on two-thirds of the adult dose, probably thought it more unpredictably exciting. It was mildly addictive.

In the United States (with busy branches in London and Australia) the firm of Yonkerman prospered. The founder, Dr Derk P. Yonkerman, began his career as a horse doctor in Southern Michigan, the burnt heartland of many healing cults.[2] His book, *Consumption and How it May be Cured*, was

---

[1] The equivalent of at least £25 in purchasing power in 1998.

[2] It also nurtured the Kellogg brothers and Ellen Gould White, founder of Seventh Day Adventism.

issued free to all inquirers and explained why the answer lay in self-control coupled with the "wonderful specific, discovered after twenty years of cease-less research, Tuberculozyne". This substance, of which thirty-two drops were to be taken at specific times every day, possessed what desperate, wasting-away patients wanted above all – "miraculous healing powers ... which had been demonstrated not only in early but also in far-advanced and seemingly hopeless cases".[3] At some length and with great perception, Yon-kerman confirmed patients' disillusionment with orthodox therapies (as well as with innumerable sovereign remedies peddled by other advertisers): "in-travenous injections have proved absolutely ineffective, inoculations with tuberculin (foisted on the public by Koch, a German) frequently hastened death; antimony, prussic acid, emetics, blisters, mercury, digitalis, iron .. all, all have proved useless of worse". By comparison with any of these fraudulent remedies, Yonkerman's Tuberculozyne was benign and not cripp-lingly expensive.

It had to be good if it was to compete with rival nostra: Scott-Henderson & Company's Liquorzone (mostly soap and powerful laxatives); Crimson Cross Fever Powder for the Cure of Consumption; Lung Germaine (whose makers warned patients on the label that "initially the germs being torn mercilessly from their lodgements may induce a feeling of weakness ... but this is the turning point!"); Pastor Felke's Honey Oil; Wewidhaus Liquid; Erben's Healing Inhalation and others.[4] Despite the ceaseless but lukewarm agitation of the great and the good of the medical profession, successive governments refused to legislate against doubtful claims. Who did the doubt-ing? The doctors' leaders. And who doubted the doctors' leaders? Almost everybody – including thousands of ordinary practitioners who saw the exaggerated claims made for new approved remedies and therapeutic regimes disproved in their surgeries every day. There was certainly never any shortage of medical men to recommend patent-medicine bottles. The advertisements were popular with the press – or at least with the press barons – and with the Post Office: in 1914 in the United Kingdom alone the forty-six million

[3] There was always a scientific-sounding rationale. Tuberculozyne, Yonkerman's label on the bottles claimed, "introduces copper into the blood and the consumption germ cannot live in the presence of copper". Bottle No. 1 was a bright red liquid containing 1.5 per cent alcohol with glycerine and potassium bromide with traces of cassia oil, tincture of capsicum, caustic soda and cochineal. Bottle No. 2 held a brown liquid of varying brightness and viscosity: it was 82 per cent water with much burnt sugar and about 16 per cent of glycerine with traces of almond oil, a mild purgative. No copper was ever detected in either preparation, perhaps just as well. The estimated cost of the ingredients was 2½d.: the price (or at least the opening bid) was £2 10s. 0d.

[4] Dr H. H. Crippen, another native of southern Michigan, was associated with at least two of these.

patent items sold (mainly by mail order) represented an income to the Treasury of £3 million.

In contrast to many entrepreneurs of foreign origin, one of the obligatory charges hurled at each other by makers of rival remedies, Major C. H. Stevens, proprietor of the Stevens Consumption Cure, had his headquarters in leafy Wimbledon and was not only a British patriot but also an officer and a gentleman.[5] Born in 1897, he was informed as a boy by the doctor at his boarding school that his lung was weak – "My boy, you're for it!" – and advised as a last resort to try to gain a few years' reprieve in the South African Veldt. "That's a man's world. A healthy world." It was also a world where he was introduced to a Kaffir witch doctor who crushed roots and boiled them and handed them out as a cure for most ailments. Stevens drank the concoction and vomited. He drank it again next day and vomited again. This continued for a week, but he persisted; and after two months he was cured. He returned to England bringing a supply of the wonder drug with him. Its composition allegedly baffled the country's most eminent chemical analysts. He gave away samples to twenty-two patients with advanced consumption. All got better. Many were permanently cured.

The Boer War took him back to South Africa where, serving in the Cape Mounted Police, he rose (according to his authorised but anonymous biography) to the rank of major. He also learnt the Kaffir word for his preparation – *umkaloabo*. His repeated offers to demonstrate its healing powers to the Cape medical fraternity were rebuffed; but between 1903 and 1907 he made a small fortune selling it to grateful consumptives. Unfortunately, he also got embroiled in scandals of a non-scientific nature (instigated, he later alleged, by jealous doctors) which persuaded him to leave South Africa in a hurry. South Africa's loss was England's gain: within a week of his arrival he set up his company, and within a year he was employing fifty people to make, pack and dispatch Umkaloabo to all parts of the world. Though cosmopolitan in his aspirations and indeed success, England remained his bedrock. People responded in their thousands to his advertisements and personal letters. (He encouraged patients to tell him about their regular – failed – practitioner: it enabled him to send the doctor a sample of Umkaloabo to try it himself or to use it experimentally on other

---

[5] Much of the information relating to Major Stevens is derived from an anonymous thirty-two-page booklet, *The Triumph of Major Stevens's Remedy*, published privately in the early 1930s and distributed on request to those subscribing to the course; but his libel case was also reported in *The Times*, 22 July and 28 October 1912. Some of the official files dealing with Stevens and Umkaloabo (PRO, MH 55/1170, 1171) are apparently jealously guarded state secrets and will remain closed until 2002.

patients. He never charged professional colleagues.) His dosage instructions were exact and exacting: and there was never anything furtive about his operation. To satisfy (or circumvent) the law forbidding unregistered practitioners to charge directly for medicines, he issued his famous guarantee bonds. The No. 1 Bond, with its beautifully illuminated capitals and a profusion of small print, guaranteed the refund of the prepayment if after three months the recipient's general practitioner was not satisfied that there has been a substantial improvement. The No. 2 Bond provided that after an unspecified number of further courses there would be a complete cure, again certified by a medical practitioner.

In response to whingeing protests by the British Medical Association questions were asked in Parliament; but Stevens had influential defenders, Colonel Sir Waldron Smithers, Conservative MP for Chislehurst, being a particularly staunch champion. Eventually one of the underpaid and ill-used analysts of the Home Office was instructed to establish the composition of Major Stevens' "liquid remedy" (no civil servant could bring himself to utter the word "Umkaloabo"). He reported that so far as he could tell – but of course he was in no position to identify or exclude any number of possibly important trace constituents – for that both the equipment and the technical staff provided by the Ministry was woefully inadequate – it consisted of 20 per cent proof spirit, 15 per cent glycerol, and a trace of alkali and water. He was roasted for being worse than useless and Stevens went on the offensive. Would a "Representative of the British Medical Association" inoculate him at the Brompton Hospital with "the fiercest tuberculosis germs they could find" and then observe him curing himself with Umkaloabo? The offer was declined as unethical but his sales soared. He also challenged the British Medical Association in the courts and fought two lengthy and expensive libel actions. Proceedings were enlivened by the appearance of specialists summoned from South Africa, Angola and Liberia. They described the widespread and successful use of *umkaloabo* among both natives and expatriates, including titled ladies. A bevy of formerly hopelessly tuberculous but now cured clergymen testified to their recovery. Several more or less registered general practitioners swore that more than one of their far-gone patients had been cured by Major Stevens's medicament. Stevens lost his actions (as he knew he would) but his sales went on soaring. In the 1930s two accounts (by anonymous, allegedly medical authors who happened to share their vigorous turn of phrase with the major) were published, extolling his achievements. Thousands who had suffered relapses after discharge from sanatoria continued to draw courage from his congratulations upon having escaped from these "landslides to the grave".

Stevens's patients came from all walks of life; but the most grateful ones lived on the margins of economic security, too private and too constrained by working hours to become regulars at dispensaries, too poor to pay for specialists, forever fearful of losing their jobs and even more terrified of how the neighbours might react to the very breath of suspicion of tuberculosis. To them, as indeed to many even inside sanatoria, direct-mail sellers of patent medicines (always dispached like birth-control appliances in plain envelopes) were a godsend. They promised the alleviation or cure in which the recipients so fervently wished to believe: often they even induced a soothing sense of well-being. Much of the regime prescribed in the accompanying literature was simple common sense: patients were told to forego alcohol (of which they usually received a sustaining dose in their patent-medicine bottle), to take regular rest, to keep warm and to generally to look after themselves. How much better than being tortured by physicians caught up in the Gold Rush or crippled by surgeons intent on notching up their thousandth thoracoplasty.

Every country, every social group and every cultural tradition had its Major Stevens. Quacks on the Protestant English model never flourished in Ireland, Poland, Hungary or other mainly Catholic countries: there a different breed of charlatans promised miraculous cures by other means. Germany had always been the home of nature cures based on herbs, pine forests, spring-water and elves. In France there was often a philosophical veneer to the promised treatment. Montaigne and Rousseau were quoted together with Hippocrates. Exotic spiritual experiences seemed to appeal to Scandinavians.

Hovering between qualified and unqualified quacks, Dr Serge Manoukhin who practised in a fashionable *faubourg* of Paris, claimed to possess (and perhaps did possess) a medical degree from Russia from before the war; and, though cold-shouldered by the medical establishment, he counted not only several members of the aristocracy but also many of the literary *monde* among his patients. One of the latter consulted him in December 1921. "I have written to M today", Katherine Mansfield wrote to her friend, S. S. Kotelianski, from Montana in Switzerland,

> and whatever he advises that I will do. It is strange – I have faith in him. I am sure he will not have the kind of face one walks away from. Besides – think, oh think of being well again! Health … is as precious as life – no less. Do you know that I have not walked since November 1920? Not more than to a carriage and back. Both my lungs are affected; there is a cavity in one and the other is affected through. My heart is weak too. Can all this be cured? Ah, Kotelianski, wish for me![6]

[6] Mansfield, Katherine, *Letters and Journals*, edited by C. K. Stead (London, 1977), p. 83.

The writer was twenty-nine.[7] She had first noticed vague premonitory signs of ill-health during the summer of 1916 when she and her husband-to-be, the man of letters John Middleton Murry, spent a few months in Cornwall, renting a cottage next to their friends, the D. H. Lawrences.[8] By Christmas she had a "nasty cough" and wrote to Murry:

> Doctor says that there is a loud deafening creak in my left lung but there is a WEE SPOT in my right lung too … so that it's absolutely imperative that I go out of this country and keep out of it all through future winters. It is *évidemment* rather a bad 'un of its kind – at any rate would become one if I didn't fly.[9]

So she flew – that is she took the boat-train from Victoria to the Gare du Nord and then the *Train Bleu* to the South of France – as thousands had done before and would do after her. What distinguished Katherine from the rest was not her cough or the "creak" in her lung but her gift as a writer of letters and of jottings in her diary.

After the choking, killing smog of the London winter, her first impression of the Riviera, the mimosa in blossom and the air balmy with a hundred sweet scents, was one of enchantment: surely, here all would be well. But the first morning

> as I bounded back to bed [after opening the shutters of her room] the bound made me cough – I spat – it tasted strange – it was bright red blood. Since then I've gone on spitting each time I cough … Oh yes, of course I'm frightened. But

[7] She was born in Wellington, New Zealand in 1890, the daughter of Harold (later Sir Harold) Beauchamp, a second-generation colonial and a successful banker. She arrived in England at the age of thirteen to be educated at Queen's College in Harley Street, London. Her first collection of short stories, *In a German Pension*, was published in 1911. Some of her best writings – and at her best her short stories were as good as Chekhov's – were published after her death by her husband, John Middleton Murry.

Her tuberculosis may have been a case of "opportunistic infection" (see above, Chapter 21). Apart from her one-night marriage to her singing teacher, George Bowden, she had had several affairs and at least one miscarriage before she met Murry in 1912. One of her affairs had led to a severe and protracted attack of gonorrhoea complicated by polyarthritis and possibly valvular damage to the heart. She longed to have children by Murry but was almost certainly sterile by the time of their marriage. The intense grief she felt over the loss of her only brother, Leslie Heron Beauchamp, in France in 1915 may also have been a precipitating factor. S. S. Kotelianski (Kot to his friends) was a Russian Jew by birth who became a popular figure in the London literary world in the years just before and after the First World War. He translated many of the works of Dostoievski and other Russian classics.

[8] Murry, a much more slender talent, was two years younger than Katherine. His ceaseless promotion – the editing, publishing and perhaps to some extent the falsifying – of Katherine's literary legacy after her death brought him fame, wealth and much opprobrium. His third wife (the first after Katherine) also died of tuberculosis. He himself died in 1957. Katherine and Murry were witnesses at the Lawrences' wedding on 13 July 1914.

[9] Mansfield, *Letters and Journals*, p. 95.

for two reasons only. I don't want to be ill, I mean seriously ill away from Jack ...
And second, I don't want to find that this is real consumption – what if it starts
to gallop? – and I shan't have my work written.[10]

What did she think it was if it was not "*real* consumption"? The doctor –
there was always an English or, more likely Scottish, doctor wherever English-
speaking consumptives congregated on the Continent – left her in no doubt.
At least, she was seriously enough ill not to return under any circumstances
to England before the summer. She longed for Murry, as tuberculous exiles
everywhere longed for husbands, wives, lovers.

> You mustn't think, as I write this, that I am dreadfully sad. Yes, I am, but you know,
> at the back of it is absolute faith and hope and love. I've only, to be frank like we
> are, had a bit of a fright. See? And I am still "trembling". That just describes it.[11]

She returned to London and in 1918 tried Cornwall again. It was not
a success: there were moments of darkness – terrible fear – and above all, a
constant longing for what she suspected but never admitted was unattainable,
the end of her illness. The iller she got, the more poignantly she could
encapsulate in a paragraph the intensely private experience of millions of
tuberculous.

> I seem to spend half my life arriving at strange hotels and asking if I may go to
> bed immediately ... "And would you mind filling my hot-water bottle? Thank
> you; that is delicious" ... The strange door shuts upon the stranger and I slip
> down waiting for the shadows to come out of the corners and spin their slow,
> slow web over The Ugliest Wallpaper of All.[12]

Like other tuberculous – and perhaps like other disadvantaged minorities
in any society – she developed a sixth sense for recognising fellow victims,
sometimes even across the divide of a hotel wall.

> The man in the next room has the same complaint as I. When I wake in the
> night I hear him turning. Then he coughs. And I cough. And after a silence I
> cough again. And he coughs again. This goes on until I feel we are like two
> roosters calling to each other at false dawn ... at far-away hidden farms.[13]

Instantly she recognised in the young sanatorium doctor in Switzerland that

> of course he has the disease himself. I recognise the smile – just the least shade too
> bright – and his strange joyousness as he came to shake hands – the gleam – the faint
> glitter on the plant that the frost has laid a finger on. He gave a polite little cough.[14]

[10] Ibid., p. 98.
[11] Ibid., p. 128.
[12] Ibid., p. 212.
[13] Ibid., p. 218.
[14] Ibid., p. 226.

A cough was more than a symptom or even a symbol: it became a call.

> I wish I were a crocodile [she wrote to Virginia Woolf]. According to your
> Thomas Browne it is the only creature who does not cough. "Although we read
> much of their Tears, we find nothing of that motion", or so he says; or so you
> say that he says. Thrice happy oviparous quadruped.[15]

She felt the same subtle resonance with the tuberculous writers and poets
of the past – Emily Brontë, Keats and, above all, Chekhov.

> I have re-read "The Steppe". What can one say? It is simply one of the great
> stories of the world ... It has no beginning or end, Chekhov just touched one
> point with his pen and then another point (. – .): enclosed something which
> had, as it were, been there for ever.[16]

In 1920 she was back in Ospideletti on the Italian Riviera, moving later to
Menton. She worked hard on book reviews, short stories, letters, her journal;
but it was a time of suffering and of consuming doubts whether Murry still
loved her. She lacked books and companionship: above all she was terrified
of death, though she clung – as always – to hope.

> 14 January Foster [her doctor] came: says my lung is remarkably better, but
> must rest absolutely for two months and not attempt to walk at all. I have got
> a "bigger chance" then.

> 15 January Bad day. A curious smoky effect over the coast. I crawled and crept
> about in the garden in the afternoon. I feel terribly weak and all the time on the
> verge of breaking down. Afraid. What will happen? Tried to work; could not. At
> six went back to bed. Had a dreadful nightmare. Wrote to Jack.[17]

In May 1921 she was seen by a fashionable Nice quack, appropriately named
Dr Maurice Delaire, self-styled professor of medical climatology, who advised
her that the Riviera was too enervating for her illness. What she needed was
mountain air. Perhaps he was right. Though not significantly better physically, the six months she spent at the Villa Sapin, a small sanatorium in
Montana in Switzerland 5000 feet above sea level, much of it with Murry,
were her last productive and happy time. She loved the mountains and could
laugh at the Swiss sanatorium scene:

> The least postcard or letter penned within view of these mountains is like presenting
> one's true account to one's Maker ... A cart drawn by a cow – I'm sure it is a cow
> – over a little bridge and the boy driver, lying like a drunken bee on his fresh green
> bed, doesn't even try to drive ... It's a perfect windless day. I'm, as you have
> gathered, sitting on the balcony outside my room: the air is just a little too clean ...

[15] Ibid., p. 232.
[16] Ibid., p. 182.
[17] Ibid., p. 250.

> Ah, the cleanliness of Switzerland! Darling, it is frightening. The chastity of my lily-white bed! The waxy pine floors! The huge vase of lilacs in my little salon. Every daisy in the grass below has a starched frill – the very bird-droppings are dazzling.[18]

The fact that briefly she was now enjoying life – she was also getting glowing reviews in England and enthusiastic letters from the literati – and the companionship of Murry made it suddenly even harder to accept her invalid role. On 16 May 1921 she saw Professor Ferdinand Jensen, "the biggest specialist in Switzerland and ... afterwards", she wrote to Anne Estelle Rice, "it was just as if the landscape – everything – had changed a little – had moved a little further off".

> I always expect those doctor men to say: "Get better? Of course you will. We'll put you right in no time. Six months at the very most and you'll be as fit as a fiddle again". But though this man was extremely nice he would not say more than "You still have a chance". That was all. I tried to get him say the word *guéri* just once; but it was no good. All I could wangle out of him was "If your digestion continues good, you still have a chance" ... It's such an infernal nuisance to love life as I do. I seem to love it more as time goes on rather than less. It never becomes a habit to me – it's always a marvel. I do hope I'll be able to keep in it long enough to do some really good work. I'm sick of people dying who promise so well. One doesn't want to join that crowd at all. So I shall go on lapping up *jaunes d'oeufs* and *de la crème* and ...[19]

It was in that week that a fellow patient suggested that she should write to Dr Manoukhin. The Russian, she was told, specialised in "bombarding the spleen *avec des Rayons X*" based on an elaborate theory that the tuberculosis bacilli were dependent for survival on nourishment derived from the spleen. In fact there was no evidence for this any more than there was for the alternative hypothesis that X-rays killed bacilli as they passed through the spleen. But the old idea of a trap – and of a miracle-cure – was taking a grip on even so formidably acute and sceptical a brain as Katherine's. "I have written to M today. Whatever he advises that I will do", she wrote to Ida Baker. "It is strange but I have faith in him." A month later: "M has told me that if I go to Paris he will treat me by his new method and there is the word *guérison* shining in his letter. I believe every word of it; I believe in him implicitly." She arrived in Paris early in 1922, and, staying in a hotel, began treatment. Soon Murry, who had all along opposed her leaving Switzerland, was proved right. Manoukhin's X-rays made her sick and depressed: her faith in its efficacy was fast ebbing away. In the meantime *The Garden Party* was published in London in February. It was an immediate success. In the same

18 Ibid., p. 262.
19 Ibid., p. 278.

month she completed "The Fly", her last short story and the most sombre; also one of her best. Like her beloved Chekhov (never out of her mind), she still also wrote sparkling letters to her friends on literary topics.

After the first course with Manoukhin (never to progress to the projected second), she was back in Switzerland in August 1922. With her last hope of a "scientific" cure for her illness gone, her mind turned to a more transcendental plane – "the attainment of such psychic control as would allow one to ignore one's bodily condition". The message was a remote offshoot of the Theosophical Movement, still popular with many avant-garde artists and writers; and it emanated from the Gurdjieff Institute for the Harmonious Development of Man. The establishment, financed largely by Lady Rothermere, wife of the first Baron, had recently moved to a Romantic but neglected mansion in Fontainbleau-Avon near Paris, once the country retreat of Louis XIV's last mistress and second wife, Mme de Maintenon, later becoming a Carmelite convent. Its new master hailed from Tiflis and was probably a former Tsarist spy, an impressive man with a bald head and black beard who claimed to have instructed the Dalai Lama (or the other way round or perhaps both). He preached inner fulfilment and physical health through work, music, dance, nourishing food, healthy living and contemplation of the universe. There was nothing new about any of this except the magnetism of the man who ran his "colony in the Wilderness" – or *asile*, meaning a madhouse, as the natives of Avon referred to it – with the help of fifty-odd devoted Russian and English helpers. Katherine was admitted on 17 October 1922, having left Switzerland pretending to go for a second course of X-ray treatment. It was to be the last station of her pilgrimage.[20]

In some respects the institute was the ultimate in quackery, faith-healing at its most inspired and most ruthless. Katherine's first weeks were bliss:

> I spend all the sunny time in the garden. Visit the carpenters, the trench diggers. (We are digging for a Turkish bath – not to discover one but to lay pipes.) The soil is very nice here with small whitey pink pebbles in it. Then there are the sheep to inspect and the new pigs that have long golden hair – very mystical pigs. A mass of cosmic rabbits and hens – and goats are on the way ... A dancing hall is being built and the house is still being organised. But the cure has started really. If all this were to end in smoke tomorrow I should have had the most wonderful adventure of my life ... I've learnt more in a week than in years *la-bas*. My wretched sense of order, for instance, which rode me like a witch. Mr Gurdjieff likes me to go into the kitchen in the late afternoon and watch ... Madame Ostrovski, the head cook. She walks about like a queen exactly: she is extremely beautiful ... Nina, a big girl in a black apron – lovely too – pounds things in

[20] The house still stands (though boarded up and derelict in 1994). A street in the village is now named after Katherine and she is buried in the local graveyard.

mortars; another runs in and out with plates and pots, another chops at the table, sings. The dog barks and lies on the floor, worrying a hearth-brush. A little girl comes in with a bouquet of leaves for Olga Ivanovna. Mr Gurdjieff strides in, takes up a handful of shredded cabbage and eats it ... there are at least twenty pots on the stove. And it's so full of life and humour and ease that one wouldn't be anywhere else.[21]

So it continued: wonderful except for the cold which was bitter in Katherine's small, unheated room. She prevailed on Murry to join her for the Russian Christmas celebration on 13 January. He later wrote about the day of his arrival, 9 January 1923:

She seemed happy, transformed as if by love. It was extraordinary. She introduced me to some of her friends and I helped to put up some Christmas decorations. She watched and laughed ... The "theatre" was like a giant nomadic tent in the grounds. Later Katherine and I sat in the Salon: there was no food. About ten she said that she felt tired. As she mounted the steps she was seized by an attack of coughing. Suddenly there was blood welling up all over her. I lay her on her bed. "I think I'm dying", she said. She looked at me imploringly but she could not speak any more. A doctor came, pushed me out of the room. A few minutes later he came to tell me that she was dead.[22]

[21] Mansfield, *Letters and Journals*, p. 312. No extracts from the diaries and letters can do justice to what is the greatest published personal record of tuberculosis in English. Among biographies, Tomalin, C., *Katherine Mansfield: A Secret Life* (London, 1963), is deeply perceptive.

[22] Mantz, Ruth E., Murry, J. M., *The Life of Katherine Mansfield* (London, 1933), p. 302.

25

The Undying Man

Some of the most successful quacks – up to a point – were patients who treated themselves or, with fierce determination, pretended that their illnesses did not exist. Perhaps Katherine Mansfield's affection for D. H. Lawrence was part of that instinctive rapport she (and many other tuberculous writers and artists) felt for fellow artistic and literary victims; but she never actually knew that he too was tuberculous. Yet he had had his first journey to death's door and back as early as 1911, shortly after his first contact with the literary world.[1]

He was twenty-six at the time, a bachelor school-teacher at the Davidson Road School for Boys in Croydon and an exemplary lodger (until his collapse) at Sunnybrea, a semi-detached citadel of respectable lower-middle-class suburbia. One damp November week-end, after staying with the David Garnetts, he caught a cold tramping three miles to the station at Oxted, and was incapable of getting out of bed the next morning. His landlord, the eagle-eyed School Inspector John Jones, "could recognise a hangover when [he] saw one ... and no wonder after carousing with the bigwigs of the literary world – and on the Sabbath too". A doctor was called and diagnosed pneumonia "or worse".

The "worse" was of course tuberculosis; and for the Jones family and for the authorities of the Davidson Road School the very hint of it was enough to make the previously exemplary lodger and dutiful teacher *persona* extremely *non grata*.[2] Indeed, even before his so-called pneumonia, the odious Jones had had his suspicions – or so he now informed the school. "The narrow shoulders, the concave chest, the thin high-pitched voice suggested

---

[1] He was born at Eastwood, Nottingham, in 1885, the son of a miner. His mother had trained as a schoolteacher. He won a scholarship to Nottingham High School and then to the local university college, where he trained as a teacher. His first novel, *The White Peacock*, was published in 1911, the year in which his mother died. Two excellent biographies are Burgess, A., *Flame into Being: The Life and Works of D. H. Lawrence* (London, 1960), and Maddox, Brenda, *The Married Man: The Life of D. H. Lawrence* (London, 1994). His *Selected Letters* were edited by Diana Trilling (New York, 1958).

[2] Only a few months earlier John Burns, MP, had declared at the opening of the Whitechapel Exhibition of Tuberculosis: "Consumption is the child of poverty, the daughter of ignorance, the offspring of drink, the product of carelessness. Our best weapon against it is constant vigilance." Neither Burns nor anyone else clearly explained how that weapon was to be wielded.

bellows too weak to pump the organ": even the faint hint of frenzied sexual activity under the quiet exterior, let alone the mining background "was calculated to arouse the misgivings of a vigilant citizen". It was too late now, though there was no question that Lawrence would have to move as soon as he had recovered from his acute illness – if, that is, he ever did recover; which was doubtful.

Awaiting the results of the repeated sputum tests, he and his sister Ada, who had come from Nottinghamshire to nurse him, were determined to ward off the bad news. They were all too familiar with the fate of many of their Eastwood neighbours and college friends who had contracted the disease. Hilda Shaw, a student-teacher friend, now in the Ransom Sanatorium at Mansfield, had vividly described life in "the San". Only recently a young patient who had received news that her mother was dying was told that she could not go home, "unless she signed papers that she goes against the Doctor's orders and so will be received in no other Sanatorium ...[3] Oh, I can't write more for everyone is crying as we often do". So Bert and Ada conspired like children: with Dr Addey on the alert for spikes of temperature, he consulted a cure-yourself booklet and sucked ice before taking his temperature and before the doctor's visit.[4] He also dosed himself with a "chest balsam", effective without fail in all bronchial ailments. If the thermometer registered above normal, Ada did not record it: Bert would then swallow more balsam and iced water: "then lo, it is normal – a huge joke – the doctor gets so jumpy if I'm high".[5]

Their efforts did not go unrewarded: Dr Addey reported that the sputum tests had proved negative. Of course everybody knew that this was no guarantee of health. The best diagnostic test at the time was a chest X-ray, but that was not available on the insurance and prohibitively expensive privately. Anyway, a firm diagnosis was the last thing Lawrence wanted. As Ada informed Garnett: "The expectoration test is entirely satisfactory. Of course my brother will be liable to consumption if he does not look after his health and the doctors say he will always need great care, and he has to give up school too".[6] It is not certain whether Dr Addey was protecting Lawrence or the pupils and staff of the Davidson Road School: they would certainly have been reluctant to have had him back. Lawrence too wanted to leave: for the first time, with the prospect of having *The Saga of Siegmund* published, he believed he might have a chance of making a living by writing. Dr Addey gave him two other pieces of advice or rather instructions: he must not

---

[3] This was standard practice in all municipal sanatoria.

[4] His family and boyhood friends called him Bert; to others he was David or Lawrence.

[5] Maddox, *The Married Man*, p. 83.

[6] Ibid., p. 90.

overwork and under no circumstances must he marry for many years to come, if ever.

It was the parting of the ways: for the rest of his life Lawrence refused to consult doctors except in dire emergencies; and even in dire emergencies he ignored their instructions. A few months after his brush with death he was paying a courtesy call on Ernest Weekley, professor of modern languages in the University of Nottingham. The professor was late and Mrs Weekley, née Baroness Frieda von Richthoven, opened the door to him. Within twenty minutes she had him in bed with her; by the time Weekley arrived Lawrence was smitten for life.[7] After a protracted and messy divorce they got married.[8] It was a mismatch made in heaven.[9] As for not overworking, even for a fit man his literary output would have been impressive. Yet he was, after the illness in Croydon, never fit. With Frieda alternately leading the way or in tow they tramped round the world in search of a climate that would be kind to his lungs (or, as he insisted, his "bronchi") – to Germany (often), Austria, France, Italy, then further afield to Australia, Mexico, New Mexico. The publication of Sons and Lovers made him famous; and his articles and essays confirmed him as the enfant terrible of English letters. He dosed himself with herbal remedies – he had a particular faith in German herbalists – and from time to time he pursued more elaborate cures recommended by friends, drinking radioactive spring water and inhaling arsenical vapours. Several of these did the trick: at least in warm dry climates he more or less held his own even if during more than one acute episode – always attributed to malaria or the flu – both he and Frieda expected him to die any day.

It was in an hotel in Mexico City in February 1924 that he had his first massive pulmonary haemorrhage, not just streaks of blood in his sputum but a continuous flow like a nose-bleed. For once a doctor was summoned and he happened to be a good one. Sydney Ulfelder, head of surgery at the American Hospital, managed to stop the bleeding (probably simply by calming the patient with large doses of morphine); but he insisted on an X-ray. He did not mince his words: Lawrence had tuberculosis, Stage Three, and had no more than two years to live. He delivered an additional blow: the projected sea voyage back to England was out of the question. Indeed, to chose England over New Mexico with lungs shot to pieces would be suicidal.

---

[7] Frieda and her two sisters were in the vanguard of the fight for sexual liberation, one of the great upper middle-class movements both in England and in Germany during the first decade of the century. (Freud was one of its symptoms, not its progenitor.) She lived up to her principles both before and after marrying Lawrence.

[8] Divorce was still a scandal. Only 514 were granted in England and Wales in 1912.

[9] Brenda Maddox's phrase in The Married Man, p. 2.

They would either have to stay in Mexico City or return to their ranch across the border. They chose the ranch.

The diagnosis was out and inescapable – but it could still be ignored. The shared denial was one of the forces which, despite her infidelities and their volcanic confrontations, bound the marriage together: Frieda's religion, like Lawrence's, was faith in the body's wisdom to know what was best for itself. If their prejudice against doctors needed confirmation, they got it at the frontier on their way back to New Mexico. The United States Emigration Department, never celebrated for the warmth of its welcome to invalids, was in grave doubt whether Lawrence was a fit person to enter the republic and gave him a taste of "their Bolshevist methods … insulting, hateful, filthy with insolence and of the bottom-doggy order". The doctor who examined him was the kind he most dreaded, "an inspector of prisons, not a healer". He was stripped and humiliated and told that he looked like a cadaver. Eventually he was granted a visitor's visa, but only for six months: they would never be allowed to settle.

A few months later they set out for Egypt – or so press agencies reported. In fact they were heading back for England. He swore that he would never leave Europe again: he would have nothing more to do with doctors and emigration officials. There would be no more idiot talk about hospitals, X-rays, sputum tests and sanatoria either. There was fortunately a wide choice of alternative remedies available, requiring no more than common sense and a modest outlay on mail-order subscriptions. Back in his younger sister Emily's house in Nottingham he dosed himself with Regasan Catarrh Jelly and Bumfritt's Incomparable Sputum Softener, the latter a novel and much-recommended preparation which made him feel better, though it did not stop his painful cough. After all their wanderings in foreign lands he was ready, even eager, to be "re-Englished": what a beautiful, green, kindly country it was after all! He resumed his many friendships in the literary and artistic world – with the Eders, the Carswells, John Middleton Murry, Rose Macaulay, the Aldingtons (meaning Aldington and his beautiful mistress Arabella Yorke), Compton and Faith Mackenzie, the Aldous Huxleys, the young novelist William Gerhardie (whom he met for the first time) and others. But some old friends were not readily available, including Mark Gertler, the painter, who had begun to spit blood a few months earlier and was now in Mundesley Sanatorium in Norfolk. It was no good. "If only the climate were not so accursed with a pall of smoke hanging over the perpetual funeral of the sun", he told Emily, "we could have a house in Derbyshire and be jolly. But I always cough – so what's the good?" [10]

[10] Ibid., p. 128.

Above all he had to remain fit enough to write. Like other tuberculous breadwinners engaged in more humdrum occupations, he was haunted by the spectre of the dismal spiral: the weaker he got the more difficult it would be for him to earn a living and yet the more money they would need to survive. So the wandering began again – Germany, Switzerland, Capri, Florence, then back to Germany and Switzerland.

There was one more visit to England. In 1927 he arrived back hopefully, not only in relatively good health but also in a mood of reconciliation. The timing was wrong. It was the aftermath of the General Strike, the miners still holding out, the country at war with itself: "a witches' cauldron of bitterness, hunger, violence and hatred". He was almost equally shocked by the changes in the landscape. Encouraged by successive Conservative administrations, row upon row of semi-detached villas now spread their "ghastly tentacles" out of Eastwood, "great plasterings of brick dwellings on the hopeless countryside".[11] Still, there was the flat bleak North Sea coast, the sweep of sand, sea and sky, where Frieda and he had stayed in a rented bungalow and spent a rapturous fortnight shortly after their first meeting. He also had urgent instructions to give to Ada about their good friend, Gertie Cooper, who was displaying renewed symptoms of tuberculosis. (Five members of her family had already died from the disease.) These were typical of Lawrence but not unique: like many other tuberculous who steadfastly refused to acknowledge their own illness and to accept orthodox treatment, he would not allow any such nonsense when a close friend contracted the disease. Ada must find the best chest specialist in Nottingham for Gertie, demand an X-ray and sputum test. It would of course have to be Mundesley if the diagnosis was confirmed, the best or at least the most expensive sanatorium in England. Somehow or other he would rustle up the funds, no problem. Above all: no quacks and no cheap patent medicines.[12]

Perhaps it was advice he would have done better to direct at himself. He was turning forty-one and he had just discovered a new patent liquid which would clear his chest as if my magic. To Kotelianski he sent a comic seaside

[11] But not everybody thought the new suburbia ugly. Ada and her husband, Eddie Clarke, with whom he was staying in nearby Ripley, were proud of their neat modern home with its tiled hall, profusion of foreign knick-knacks and glass door opening onto a lawn and flower garden: its name, Torestin, was taken from Lawrence's *Kangaroo*.

[12] A few months later – he was back in Florence by then – he was horrified to hear about Gertie's operation. "A horrible business", he wrote to Kotelianski, " ... her left lung removed, six ribs removed, glands in the neck – too horrible – better die. Why not chloroform and the long sleep! ... Why aren't we better at dying, straight dying? ... Why save life in this ghastly way?". Perhaps surprisingly, the operation and the treatment worked: at least they did not kill the patient: born in the same year as Lawrence, Gertie lived on until 1942.

postcard of a woman in striped bathing drawers cavorting on the sands. He apologised for its vulgarity: it was, he wrote, the only paper he could find and the jaunty printed message, "This is how I feel", expressed his own sentiments exactly. Of course it had to end in tears. A month later he and Frieda were back at the Villa Mirenda in Florence, he very weak and coughing badly. Time to start on *Lady Chatterley's Lover*.

Whether or not *Lady Chatterley's Lover* is a great book – it is few people's favourite Lawrence – it was a great bomb: twenty years after its clandestine publication it demolished literary censorship in the English-speaking world.[13] It also kept alive for at least another half-century the ancient myth of *omnis phthisicus alax*, every tuberculous a lecher. "Sadly but truly, perhaps only a dying consumptive could have written such filth", as one prospective expert witness for the prosecution at the *Lady Chatterley* trial suggested.

There was some truth in this – as there was in so much tuberculosis mythology. The illness had claimed over the centuries some of the greatest artists in their creative and procreative prime: and what they could no longer accomplish physically they often expressed in their art. So the consumptive Watteau portrayed himself as the guitar player in *The Lesson of Love*, strumming a melancholy tune to the girl (a little bored perhaps), and in the *Departure from Cythera* painted the ultimate elegiac farewell to physical ecstasy.[14] Beardsley was more explicit in his phantasies: impotent in the terminal stages of his illness, his drawings became increasingly obscene while reaching their peak in elegance and economy. In one of his last he showed himself tethered to Priapus – as he no doubt felt himself to be – and the last sheet of the *Lysistrata* series (drawn between bouts of pulmonary haemorrhage) showing the lady decorating an adoring giant phallus, anticipating the *alfresco* antics of Connie and Mellors. Like *Lady Chatterley's Lover*, it remained unpublishable above the counter until the 1960s.

Lawrence too, by the time he wrote *Lady Chatterley's Lover*, was still Mellors in imagination but closer in reality to the impotent Sir Clifford. Yet the writing of the book was a prodigious physical feat. Like all his novels, he wrote it three times from beginning to end, making it increasingly pornographic. (The first version was tender and the least angry, with comparatively

---

[13] Two legal decisions settled the matter, one hopes forever: the jury verdict in the *Regina v. Penguin Books* in London in 1960 and, in the United States, the Federal Court order a year earlier which allowed the book to be sent through the mail. The first may be said to have launched the permissive sixties or, as Philip Larkin famously put it "Sexual intercourse began / In nineteen sixty three / Between the end of the Chatterley ban / And the Beatles' first LP". It is still a secret bestseller in Asian societies just emerging from sexual repression.

[14] Cythera, today's Cerigo, the most southern of the Ionian Islands, was where mortals were taught the art of love by Venus.

few unprintable words and no sodomy.) Though Frieda was by then having an "away" affair with the dashing Captain Angelo Ravagli,[15] the period was one of rare domesticity. He read to her completed chapters in the evenings under the pine trees. She embroidered and made intelligent suggestions. He praised and ignored them. He also took up painting, which he loved and of which he was inordinately proud;[16] and he churned out a stream of pot-boilers – short stories, essays and book reviews. He then decided – astutely from the commercial point of view but suicidally for his health or what remained of it – that he would publish *Lady Chatterley's Lover* himself.[17]

Early in 1928 they left Florence and the travelling began again – Les Diablerets in Switzerland to visit the Huxleys, Baden-Baden to stay with Lawrence's much-loved *Schwiegermutter*, and to try a new quack cure,[18] then Capri, Sicily then back to Italy, France and Germany. Lawrence felt that both he and *Lady Chatterley* had become contagious objects to be turned back at frontiers and turned out of hotels. Foyles wrote from London to say that the book was not one they could handle in any way and an American critic who reviewed it for the *New York Sun* was banned from ever reviewing for that newspaper again. But, under the counter, the edition printed in Italy and several pirated ones were selling like hot cakes; and while the British popular press was savaging him and his book – "One of the filthiest ever written" (*Sunday Chronicle*), "A Landmark in Evil" (*John Bull*) – they were sending him fat cheques, advances for anything he would care to write for them.

The personal rejection was harder to take. Despite the much-vaunted scientific and medical advances – it was a rare week when the popular press did not report a break-though in tuberculosis (which Lawrence read with studied indifference) – in many parts of Europe the fear of having a consumptive under one's roof had hardly changed. After a particularly tiresome journey through northern Italy and Switzerland Frieda and he, accompanied by their faithful American friends the Brewsters, arrived in Saint-Nizier de

[15] Her third husband to be.

[16] Harold Acton and Osbert Sitwell, both resident in Florence at the time, were the first to see the products: both were horrified, which delighted Lawrence. It is hard to persuade oneself that the paintings have any merit other than being documents about Lawrence in his physical decline and erotic obsession.

[17] It was suggested to Lawrence by Norman Douglas, who had made a great deal of money by having Pino Orioli in Florence print his latest novel and selling it by private subscription. From then on the money rolled in.

[18] He took a deadly-sounding mixture of arsenic and phosphorus twice a day, gave up salt and bread and ate mainly raw fruit, raw vegetables and porridge. "They say I can get quite well in quite a short time on that", he wrote to Enid Hilton in London and promised Orioli, his Italian publisher, that he would live to be a hundred. He stuck the regime for a week.

Pariset in the Savoie and checked into the Hôtel des Touristes. It seemed the discovery of a lifetime: paradise. The air was pure and invigorating, the elevation, 3500 feet, "just right for my bronchi", the view of the Mont Blanc superb, the people simple and friendly. He instantly dashed off a dozen postcards telling family, friends and business associates where they could find him "now and forever". Next morning they were all asked to leave: the coughing that had echoed through the small hours had persuaded the owner to tell them that it was against hotel policy to have consumptive guests. It was also frowned upon by the newly-established *Bureau de Tourisme*: Saint-Nizier de Pariset had no wish to be known as the paradise of the tuberculous. Frieda and the Brewsters tried to hide the truth from Lawrence. They loudly exclaimed to each other how disappointing it was that the hotel they had liked so much the night before had turned out to be dreadful, not to be borne for another minute. Lawrence, "the warthog repellent to society", went along with the game. Another lot of cards were dispatched, telling family, friends and business associates that after all he much preferred Chexbres-sur-Vevey in Switzerland: the hotel in the Savoie had been too high, too raw, too bleak, too comfortless and so badly managed that the idiot staff could not be trusted even with the forwarding of the mail.

In the autumn of 1929 they were installed and seemingly settled at the Hôtel Beau Rivage in Bandol, a pretty little port between Marseille and Toulon where Katherine Mansfield and Murry had also stayed. Then he turned up in Paris on *Lady Chatterley* business and the Huxleys persuaded him to see a bronchial specialist. They even almost prevailed on him to have the X-ray the specialist had recommended. But a few minutes before he was due to leave the hotel, he cancelled the appointment. (An X-ray was hardly necessary, the specialist told Aldous Huxley: just by listening he could tell that one lung had completely gone and the other was three-quarters gone.) For his increasing difficulty in breathing, Lawrence blamed "the stinking petrol fumes: all cities were death-traps". There followed an interlude in Majorca on which he had pinned high hopes; but within a week the Spanish joined many other nations in being summed up by a Lawrentian class libel – "dead-bodied people with ugly faces and and a certain staleness, a bit like city English". So back to Florence.

He was not well enough to travel to London and Frieda represented him with regal aplomb at the opening of the exhibition of his terrible paintings.[19]

[19] At the Warren Gallery in Mayfair owned by Dorothy Warren, a friend of Barbie Weekley, Frieda's daughter, and a niece of Ottoline Morrell. Professional critics were even more appalled than Sitwell and Acton had been (except for the *Nottingham Evening Post*, whose art correspondent loyally applauded the city's more or less native son for his "gift of composition, harmony of colours and delicacy of touch": he or she must have been drunk). Crowds jammed

(It was her first taste of being the famous Mrs D. H. Lawrence, without the encumbrance of his actual presence, and she relished the occasion.) She reported to his friends that he was well but too busy working on another novel to travel. Huxley wrote to the poet Robert Nichols: "It is terribly distressing watching Lawrence gradually approaching dissolution ... especially horrible, because so unnecessary, the result simply of a man's strange obstinacy against professional medicine". To his brother Julian he wrote:

> It's no good, he doesn't want to know how ill he is ... He rationalises the fear in all kinds of ways ... he just wanders about tired and wretched, imagining that the next place and the next quack cure will make him feel better and, when he gets to the next place and has finished the next cure it all starts again ... He's now off to Germany. We have given up trying to persuade him to go to a sanatorium: no one could persuade him except possibly Frieda. But Frieda is worse than he is. We've told her that she is a fool and a criminal but it had no effect on her whatever.[20]

In truth Frieda was as sceptical about professional medical advice as Lawrence, though less abusive: temperamentally, they were more alike than their friends realised.

On his last visit to Germany the word tuberculosis was still taboo but he no longer hid the truth from himself: he knew he was dying. During the day he religiously inhaled the fumes of the newly-discovered radioactive springs in the *Kurhalle*; at night he wrote poetry. A vase of blue flowers by his bed inspired one of his loveliest poems, "Bavarian Gentians":

> Reach me a gentian, give me a torch!
> Let me guide myself with the blue, forked torch of this flower
> down the darker and darker stairs, where blue is darkened on blueness
> even where Persephone goes.[21]

And in the same month he wrote the "Ship of Death":

> Now it is autumn and the falling fruit
> and the long journey toward oblivion ...
> and it is time to go, to bid farewell
> to one's own self, and find an exit
> from the falling self ...
>
> Oh build your ship of death, your little ark

the gallery and the Metropolitan Police took three weeks before obeying mounting public clamour and bursting in on the exhibition. Even then they took away only thirteen of the exhibits, anything showing a penis or pubic hair.

[20] Maddox, *The Married Man*, p. 464.

[21] Lawrence, D. H., "Bavarian Gentians", in *The Complete Poems of D. H. Lawrence*, ed. V. de Sola Pinto and Warren Roberts (London, 1977).

and furnish it with food, with little cakes and wine
for the dark flight down oblivion.[22]

Whatever the Huxleys may have thought of Frieda, in her own way she looked after him with devotion. More precisely, she gave him exactly what he wanted, including playing to him the same three pieces by Schubert on the piano for hours very badly and generally treating him like a child down with a bad cold, not as a dying invalid. They returned to Bandol: he was now racing against time, consciously registering every completed day but also fearful as each day gained was bringing him closer to the last. But it was not only days which he completed. He turned his "Skirmish with Jolly Roger", the introduction to one of the clandestine editions of *Lady Chatterley's Lover*, into a sparkling essay, "A-propos of *Lady Chatterley's Lover*"; produced a 4000-word introduction to Kotelianski's translation of Dostoievski's *The Grand Inquisitor*; and sketched out another novel. The titles of some of his last and best short stories hinted at his innermost thoughts – "A Dream of Life" and, above all, "The Undying Man".

In the meantime his London friends arranged for an English chest specialist, Dr Andrew Morland, to go to Bandol to examine him. Lawrence remonstrated: it was "a total waste of time to talk to a lung specialist when my trouble is all bronchial". On Christmas Eve he got up to make lemon tarts and he celebrated his last New Year's Day by walking to the village at snail's pace to lunch with friends. Morland did arrive in mid January and insisted that he must go to a sanatorium at least 600 feet above sea level.[23] At last he surrendered – or seemed to: there was nothing else to do. "I have decided to go to a sanatorium for acute bronchitis aggravated by the lungs", he wrote to Ada. Encouraged by Frieda he was studying ship time-tables, planning to go to New Mexico later in the summer, by-passing "hateful New York", or further afield, perhaps to Sarawak. Waiting for his transfer to Vence where a sanatorium had been found at an altitude approved of by Morland, he wrote to Elsie: "I would do anything to get better ... anything, I mean, except stop working". Of that there was no question. Too weak to get up, sleepless and driven to distraction by cramps in his calves, he was working on book reviews. Illness had not mellowed him. "Mr Gill is not a born writer: he is crude and crass", began his review of Eric Gill's latest collection of essays. Eventually he was taken by private train from Toulon to Antibes and then by car to the sanatorium, a medium-sized chalet picturesquely perched 1000 feet above the Mediterranean and appropriately

---

[22] Lawrence, D. H., "Ship of Death", in *Complete Poems*.
[23] The height above sea level appropriate for every type of tuberculosis and every individual patient was a matter of intense debate and a vast literature between the world wars.

perhaps named Ad Astra. During the drive, as they passed the cemetery, he turned to Frieda. "You will bury me here." "Oh no", she replied, "it's much too ugly."

Sanatorium life surprised Lawrence by its ordinariness: it was just like a hotel except that there were doctors and nurses milling about ("a little sluggishly") and many rules and regulations which nobody took great pains to enforce. He was taken off milk, which was allegedly bad for his liver ("but surely only Frenchies have livers!"), and he was made to walk down a flight of steps twice a day ostensibly to invigorate his circulation but in fact to save on the nursing. He found the crying of children in other rooms depressing: "it makes one realise how really stupid it is to be ill". He still could not sleep: his cramps improved but his cough was painful and he ached all over. He was not a moaner and quickly disposed of the tablets and foul-smelling liquid restoratives which he was given. "But this place makes one very egoistic ... that's the worst of being sick: you begin to think of nothing but yourself." He longed for Frieda to stay with him – she was lodged at the nearby Hôtel Nouvel – feeling deprived of the comfort he described so well in Sons and Lovers ("Paul loved to sleep with his mother: sleep is still most perfect, in spite of all the hygienists, when it is shared with a beloved"). He had a stream of distinguished visitors: news of his condition had spread around the Riviera and Vence was more accessible than Bandol. H. G. Wells came, as did the Aga Khan and the Duchesse de Caves, who had always wanted to meet the legendary Lawrence of Arabia.

Two weeks was all he could stand. Frieda, her daughter, Barbie Weekley, and the Brewsters were soon scouring Vence for a private villa where the landlord would accept a tuberculous patient. Not many would at any price; but finally they found the Villa Robermond and engaged a local doctor and a nurse to look after him. The Huxleys arrived in their new Bugatti to help with the move. On 1 March, when he left the sanatorium, he was so weak that for the first time he let Frieda put on his shoes for him. At the villa her bed was moved into his room so that he could look at her. He was now too giddy to get up but he went on working in bed, softening his review of Gill's book. Commenting on Gill's statement that a man was free when "what he likes to do is to please God", he put on Gill's Catholicism his own Lawrentian gloss:

> To please God only means happily doing one's best at the job in hand and being lovingly absorbed in an activity which puts one in touch with – with the heart of things; call it God. It is a state which any man or woman achieves when busy and concentrated on a job which calls forth real skill and attention, or devotion.[24]

[24] Review of E. Gill, *Art-Nonsense and Other Essays*, quoted by Brenda Maddox, *The Married Man*, p. 507.

It was the last thing he wrote, the theology a little lame perhaps, but it would do as a tuberculous writer's epitaph.

26

Private Charity: Public Health

The hotel-keeper in Saint-Nizier de Parizet who would not have Lawrence staying in his establishment was not being uncharitable. On the contrary, he was the product of an educational campaign supported by charities and encouraged by governments, the churches, the international socialist movement and, after the First World War, the World Health Organisation, the International Antituberculous League and other impeccably benevolent bodies. Their aim was to enlighten the public about the facts of tuberculosis: the surest way, it was maintained, of containing and eventually of eradicating the disease.[1] Quite how this would work was never explained or even publicly questioned. The benefits of education rarely are. Knowledge of the disease would somehow triumph. Its dissemination was at least a practical possibility, a reassuring sign that something was being done. Two jars filled with formaline were prominently displayed in hundreds of bars, bistros and hostelries like the Hôtel des Touristes in Saint-Nizier. One showed a healthy pink lung, the other a lung grey and ravaged by tuberculosis. The latter fate, the legend informed visitors, could be avoided by avoiding too close a contact with known consumptives, by seeking medical advice at once if one detected ominous symptoms or signs in oneself, and by following the medical instructions devoutly and to the letter.

Many displays were more elaborate. Popular dioramas showed moving illuminated beads against painted backgrounds ranging from the religious to the horrific, each bead representing a soul entering eternity via tuberculosis. Such displays were often combined – especially in schools – with slots

[1] This was enshrined in the founding document of the National Association for the Prevention of Consumption, a title later changed to National Association for the Prevention of Tuberculosis (NAPT), in 1898. The aim of the association – it was to remain Britain's premier charitable antituberculosis organisation for fifty year – was "to carry into every dwelling in the land an elementary knowledge of the mode in which consumption is propagated, and of the means by which its spread may be prevented and thus to strengthen the hands of medical men throughout the country who are dealing with individual cases of the disease". A similar educational purpose was – on paper – the top public-health priority in Commissioner H. M. Biggs's "Contagious Consumption: Rules to be Observed for the Prevention of the Spread of Consumption", issued in New York in 1893.

where a coin could be inserted. As the coin dropped into the bowels of the machine, so the moving beads stopped moving for a second or two, the delay depending on the size of the donation. In some of the more sophisticated automata a window would light up, revealing a tuberculous patient sitting up in bed or getting out of bed or being received with open arms by their families on returning home from a sanatorium fully restored to health. The last image was significant for it showed that public enlightenment, however important, was not the only objective of the charity appealing for support.

For reasons not entirely clear charities always seem to flourish in times and in societies most devoutly dedicated to the pursuit of wealth and power. Charitable foundations on a lavish scale accompanied the bloodiest decades of the religious and dynastic wars. They are blossoming again today in western Europe and North America. But their golden age was the two decades preceding 1914, the end of the Long Peace; and tuberculosis was their principal arena. By the 1890s it was widely, though only tacitly, acknowledged that an upsurge of the disease could in some ill-defined way be a side-effect of technological progress and unfettered capitalism. Nobody could prove or quantify the relationship (or particularly wanted to); but to erase this small blemish from an otherwise perfect system (or a system promising perfection as its attainable goal), society erupted in an orgy of benevolence. Charitable associations, campaigns, societies and leagues dedicated to combating, preventing, treating and eradicating tuberculosis sprang up in five continents. They were no longer the preserve of a few eccentrics or the approved fields of sacrifice of esteemed but sparsely manned (or womanned) and chronically underfunded religious organisations. The new charities raised vast sums of money and carried enormous social prestige. They were secular, unless one regarded royal patronage as semi-divine. Their weak spot – unnoticed at the time as it is once again today – was confusion over the practical means available or, more to the point, *not* available. This was true of charities in general but it applied with especial force to charities directed at tuberculosis. Though the cause of the disease was now known – a reassuring statement which became an incantation – there was no cure; or almost none. Fortunately, the tide of private munificence coincided with the rise of the sanatorium movement. The latter was generally perceived as a momentous advance. It was also expensive. There was a shaming discrepancy between what was available to the few and what was not available to the many. The first task of the new charities was therefore clear. The benefits of sanatorium treatment must be made available to all.

As early as 1890 a Society for the Establishment of Sanatoria for the

Consumptive Poor was established in Austria under the patronage of the Archduchess Maria Pia, the mother of two consumptive Archdukes. In the past such organisations had been a way for the *nouveaux riches* to better themselves and advance in society. This was no longer so. As Prince Felix Lobkowitz a little peevishly observed, donating part of one's hard-earned prize money from the turf became more than a social obligation; it was almost an extortion. In Holland the Queen Mother Emma marked the end of her regency by founding a sanatorium for the poor at Renkum. It was soon followed by similar establishments at Hellendoorn and Hoog-Laren. In Sweden it was the silver jubilee of King Oscar II which inaugurated the national antituberculous sanatorium campaign. With the open-hearted liberality characteristic at all times of British royalty, King Edward VII permitted the use of the royal style to several sanatoria for the poor in Canada, Australia and India. Even in backward Russia Tsar Alexander III came personally to the rescue of the financially floundering sanatorium in Halila in Finland, securing its survival with funds from his private coffers. The example could not be ignored: by 1900 twelve such institutions were supported by private charity in the Crimea, the Caucasus, Russian Poland and even the Irkutsk district of Siberia.

Tuberculous children were an especially urgent and rewarding target. Switzerland regarded her famous mountain resorts in the Grisons as a source of income from foreigners rather than as an amenity for her indigenous poor (who then still existed); but, under the charismatic leadership of Pastor Bion of Zurich, she pioneered summer camps in the mountains for poor consumptive children from the cities. By 1910 the Confederation also had fifteen charity-supported sanatoria in twelve cantons, not places of luxury but all run with exemplary efficiency. Danish charities too began to send youngsters from tuberculous homes for summer breaks to the little fishing village turned holiday camp at Shageback on Bornholm and opened the first poor children's sanatorium in Sjælland in 1901. (A charity-run sanatorium for poor young women, even those who had fallen, was started in Skorping in 1906.) Austrian philanthropists sent their country's consumptive young – a few of them anyway – to the Adriatic; Hungarian industrialists sent their flock to Szent-Endre on the Danube. As could be expected from a country where the sanatorium movement originated (and which was recognised as the standard-bearer of civilised European values), Germany had several charity-supported children's sanatoria by the turn of the century, in addition to holiday camps, convalescent colonies and Europe's first free open-air school in Charlottenburg. The last became the pride and joy of the Dowager Empress who visited it regularly and distributed prizes. Even Italy, a poor country where the Antituberculous League had to be dissolved for lack of funds in

1902,[2] was proud of her marine hospices. The first of those was founded in Viareggio by the energetic Dottore Giuseppe Barellai of the hospital of Santa Maria Nuova in Florence; by the end of the century it had spawned thirty-nine offspring. They were essentially summer camps where deprived children from the new industrial slums could frolic on the beach for three or four weeks in the summer. Unlike tuberculosis, the hospices were closed during the winter.[3]

The antituberculous charities began as an outlet for the generous rich. What transformed them into a worldwide popular movement, unprecedented at the time and more successful than any other since, was the brainchild of a humble employee of the Danish postal service, Einar Holboell. Forty-four years old in 1904, and the head of a large family, Holboell was distressed at reports that young people were still dying of tuberculosis for lack of funds to pay for their treatment in one of the health-restoring sanatoria available to the rich. The thought struck him the more, since he and his family and friends would have been happy to make a modest contribution to prevent such a fate. Of course they could not afford the kind of four-, five- and six-figure donations they read about in the society columns of newspapers; but hundreds, thousands, perhaps – yes, why not? – millions of small sums would amount to a great a deal of money. But how could this be organised without an expensive administrative machinery which would defeat the purpose of the exercise? His inspiration of a lifetime came to him sitting behind the counter at the post office. Of course. It was special stamps! There could be a small surcharge on some of them and nobody would be obliged to buy the surcharged ones in preference to the regular, cheaper issue. But who would not prefer to spend the extra penny or its equivalent?

Denmark was a small country with a high incidence of tuberculosis; and Holboell's idea ascended the hierarchical ladder with remarkable speed. The Post-Master General approved, then the Prime Minister, then King Christian. The first special antituberculosis Christmas issue, showing a likeness of the Queen, was exhibited in Copenhagen at the 1904 International Philatelic Conference and went on sale the following week. It was an instant success.

---

[2] Mediterranean countries like Italy and Spain were not only poor but also traditionally wedded to the idea that charities were the preserve of the church. The fear and stigma of contagion also lingered, but Italy was proud of having pioneered special sanatoria for her prison population, the *Sanatoria Criminale*. The first, established on the island of Pianosa, was reported by Italian delegates at international conferences to be achieving miraculous results, both medically and penologically.

[3] To give unsung pioneers their due, the first state to issue antituberculous stamps was New South Wales in Australia in 1897; but there was no international response. England was a late joiner in 1932.

Within a year Holland followed suit with a memorable, specially designed set showing symbols of healing: the sun for sunlight, a fountain for health-giving waters, an ear of corn for good nutrition. Russia came next with a set of stamped postcards with the portraits of the Tsar's daughters. Then came Belgium, Switzerland, Bavaria, Spain, Portugal, Hungary, Italy, Greece. Many featured spring flowers, symbols of youth and hope but also – unintentionally perhaps – of transience. Some countries issued antituberculous labels or seals which could be added to ordinary stamps on envelopes and postcards. National committees, almost always under royal patronage, took charge of distributing the millions which began to roll in.[4]

Royalty was not available in the United States but the idea was tested in the state of Delaware by Miss Emily Bissel, who managed to raise 3000 dollars for a local antituberculosis project in 1907. Her success led the American Red Cross to experiment with an antituberculosis Christmas seal on a national basis, eliciting a huge response. In 1919 the Red Cross transferred the management of the seal to the National Tuberculosis Association. By then the yearly proceeds amounted to $10 million.

Even the First World War did not entirely extinguish the international relief effort; and after the Armistice the antituberculosis charities were the first to recover momentum. They crossed former enemy lines. Much to the consternation of the boulevard press (squashed by a thunderous intervention from Clemenceau, a former general practitioner),[5] the charter of the Comité National de Défense contre la Tuberculose set up in Paris in 1919 expressed the hope that all countries, including Germany, would join; and in 1920 the plan nearly came to pass. Only Russia was invited but did not become a member.[6] The Antituberculosis Conference in Rome in 1928, hosted with operatic pomp by Il Duce, adopted the red double cross, also known as the Cross of Lorraine, the Apostolic Cross of Hungary or the Cross of Jerusalem, as its emblem. It became one of the best-known logos in the world.[7]

Like many fast-growing charities, the original purpose of the movement – to help poor tuberculous patients to be treated in sanatoria – did not survive

[4] Holland was, per head of population, widely recognised as the most generous.

[5] He had practised in Montmartre, the *arondissement* with the highest incidence of tuberculosis in Paris and therefore France.

[6] The message from Kamenev, Commissar for Health, later a victim of Stalin's purges, stated that tuberculosis barely existed in the Soviet Union and that, insofar as it existed, it did not need international charity. Projecting forwards from figures from before the First World War and backwards from current statistics, Russia at the time probably had the highest incidence of tuberculosis in Europe.

[7] Its association with tuberculosis worried some of General De Gaulle's entourage when it was adopted in London in 1940 to become the emblem of the Free French.

unchanged. The reasons were largely negative. By the 1920s sanatorium was no longer the magical word it had been during the first decade of the century. This was particularly true of England; or perhaps it was expressed in England (where sanatoria had never become a native industry) more openly than in most other countries. As early as 1920 *The Times* gave ponderous voice to widely-felt doubts: "It seems that 54 per cent of patients [supported by the London Country Council] treated in sanatoria are dead at the end of four years ... and of the rest ... all we learn is that they are 'alive'. We are, it seems, neither preventing nor curing the disease."[8] A year later Dr Ernest Ward, Tuberculosis Officer for South Devon, published a much-quoted survey comparing sanatorium-treated with both home-treated and untreated patients all from the poorer classes. Of non-sanatorium-treated Stage I cases 54 per cent were "cured" four yours after the original diagnosis, compared to 34 per cent of sanatorium patients. The corresponding figures for Stage II were 10 per cent of non-sanatorium against 7 per cent of sanatorium patients. Ward went on to reject "graduated labour" as impossible to implement and "absolute rest" as a myth. "A patient", he wrote, "will exert himself more in a simple fit of coughing than by feeding himself rather than being fed four times a day."[9] This was so patently true that it roused the sanatorium establishment to fury. "If sanatorium treatment were not infinitely superior to treatment elsewhere", Dr Thomas Campbell, medical superintendent of the West Riding Sanatorium at Ilkley expostulated a little unwisely, "sanatorium physicians would have to be labelled either crooks or mental defectives".[10] Nobody rose to express shock horror at the thought.

With the advent of collapse therapy the picture changed slightly. Some sanatoria tried to turn themselves into hospitals, combining traditional rest and graduated exercise with more active, some would say more aggressive, surgical intervention. It was rarely a success. In most municipal and charity-supported establishments there was scope for modernisation; but limited resources were often diverted from patient care into building flashy operating theatres, X-ray rooms, sterilising suites and filling stations (for the maintenance of artificial pneumothoraces). Staff costs rocketed in proportion: nursing costs per patient trebled. What was eventually achieved was often admirable – "the days of shack sanatoria are over", Dr P. D. Heffernan, Tuberculosis Officer of Derbyshire, boasted in 1934;[11] but it was the morale of doctors and nurses rather than that of patients which improved.

[8] *The Times*, 21 February 1920.
[9] Ward, E., *Lancet* (1921), no. 1, 53.
[10] Campbell, T., ibid. (1921), no. 1, 83.
[11] Heffernan, P. D., *British Medical Journal* (1934), no. 1, 690.

To patients – at least in the English-speaking world – charity sanatoria remained dread places. They were cold and deliberately, almost aggressively, impersonal. By the 1920s it became axiomatic that under no circumstances and at no level must the staff – especially nurses and doctors – become emotionally involved. But in treating an illness like tuberculosis there is little room between involvement and indifference, compassion and anger. On entering The Pines, Betty MacDonald quickly perceived that there was one characteristic the staff had in common: their hatred of tuberculosis. That was both understandable and admirable, but from hatred of tuberculosis to hatred of the tuberculous was often but a small step.[12]

There would have been more to fuel to criticism if anything else had been on offer. And of course there was: only it was uncertain how effective or preferable the alternatives were – or would be if implemented. The difficulty was that tuberculosis was not only a disease of individuals: it was also a threat to the whole community, a public health problem. Even the most expensive and lavishly equipped sanatoria existed not merely to provide a cure but also to remove and isolate potential sources of infection. While the two objectives were often in hidden conflict, nobody knew how to separate them. Perhaps nobody tried very hard: few wanted to be seen emphasising the quarantine aspect. Yet the healthy, especially children, needed to be protected; and in a democratic society it was the responsibility of the state to do so. On the other hand, in the civilised twentieth century – until the advent of Hitler and Stalin – the sick could not simply be cast off. Nor did doctors ever admit that they were helpless in actually curing the disease. If sanatoria, tuberculin, gold, collapse therapy and vaccines did not work, other means must be found – and surely would be. Nobody knew how and when; but every country had its priorities.

In France it was babies. Even before the First World War French doctors were trying to reduce the death-rate of infants born to tuberculous mothers

---

[12] The widening chasm between patients and nursing staff in sanatoria is enshrined in Betty MacDonald's autobiographical novel, *The Plague and I* (London, 1948). "On January 6th Charge Nurse invited me to the Pines moving picture show, but she handed me the invitation so thickly encased in rules, it was like being given a present wrapped in the Sunday *New York Times*. She said in parting 'You are on the list to go to the movie too Mrs Bard. You may wear make-up if you wish , but you may not talk or laugh. You are to be ready by seven o'clock in your robe and slippers, with your pillow and night blanket. You will be called for by a *male*' – she said '*male*' in a low throbbing voice as if it were some dangerous new sex – 'ambulant patient but you are not to speak to or to laugh with your escort. Your temperature and pulse will be taken as soon as you return to bed and if your temperature or your pulse has increased, you will not be allowed to go to the next moving picture show.' I thanked her, promised not to speak or to pulsate and she left."

in city hospitals. The figures were unreliable and probably exaggerated, but one widely touted statistic maintained that 2000 children were lost through infection from the mother every year in Paris alone.[13] In 1903 a fostering scheme, involving the dispatch of babies to sound Catholic peasant families, was blessed by the government, and, under the title of l'Oeuvre Grancher (after the paediatrician who first proposed it), put into operation.[14] The numbers were initially small; but after the First World War (the country with an already stagnant birth rate had lost 1,300,000 of its young men),[15] the task of saving babies became a national priority, very nearly an obsession. Although the scheme would always remain a private charity, the state now provided a 60 per cent subsidy amounting in 1924 to about six million francs.

In the complete form of the programme the tuberculous mothers were masked and screened during labour and their infants were immediately taken away after delivery. It is difficult to ascertain today how far individual permission was sought and granted: it was required by law but this was never tested in the courts. In official reports the cases were always described as selected, but nobody specified who did the selection and on what grounds. One of the chief advocates of the *Oeuvre*, Dr P. F. Armand-Delille, described its operation to an international conference in 1925:

> The infants remain with their [adoptive] peasant family under the supervision of the country doctor as long as is necessary for the disappearance of the danger of contagion from their own families. Sometimes "disappearance" means a cure: more often, alas, it means the death of the tuberculous parent. That takes on the average three years ... But if the healthy parent after the death of the tuberculous one does not ask for the return home of the child, we leave the children in the country up to the age of thirteen or whenever they have completed their schooling ... We then give the children back to the parent or we place them in the country to earn their living, mainly on farms or in domestic service. The children grow up honest, healthy ... and of good character.[16]

The scheme had several advantages other than the allegedly reduced infant mortality from tuberculosis in the cities. It was cheap, 1200 francs per child in 1920 compared to 7000 francs for a year's sanatorium stay. Since about half of the farmed-out infants remained on the farm where they had been reared, it also helped to stock the French countryside with healthy agricultural

[13] Landouzy, R., in *Revue de médecine*, quoted in the *Lancet* (1888), no. 2, 1921.

[14] Its full official title was *Oeuvre pour la Préservation de l'Enfance contre la Tuberculose*.

[15] The heaviest loss per head of population in the First World War. It seemed to many Frenchman in 1918 that their country had become a land of old men, widows and *mutilés de guerre*.

[16] Armand-Delille, P. F., *Transactions of the Conference of the International Union against Tuberculosis* (Paris, 1925).

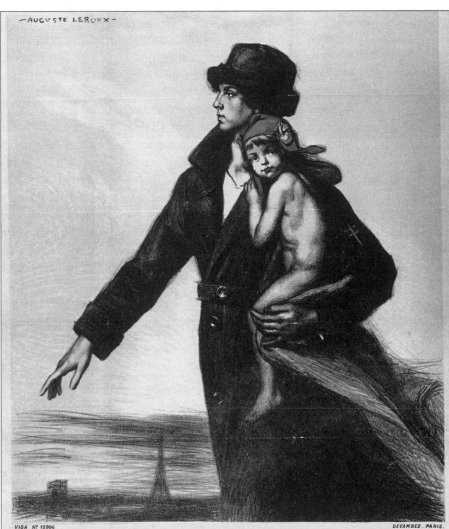

A French health visitor holds a small child. (*Wellcome Institute*)

workers. By 1923 Calmette claimed that it had reduced infant tuberculosis mortality in the Paris maternity wards by 80 per cent.[17] Few outside France believed him.

L'Oeuvre Grancher had a close competitor in the Placement Familial des Tous-Petits, launched by an eminent tuberculosis specialist, E. Rist, in 1920. It was run "with unvarying precision and the separation between tuberculous mothers and babies was absolute".[18] In the rare instances where the doctors deemed it necessary for the mother to nurse her child, this was carried out in an isolation cubicle in the presence of a nurse, the mother wearing a surgical mask, cap and gown. After a BCG vaccination and a Wassermann test (to exclude congenital syphilis), the infants were dispatched as far as possible from home to make it difficult for their parents to visit them. Parents who wished to retrieve their children in less than two years could not be restrained or prosecuted in law; but they were asked to refund the travelling and other expenses of the *placement*. These were formidable or were made to appear so. The organisation liked small farmers and market gardeners or occasionally convents as foster parents: the farmers were "keen to have children ... able to appreciate country pursuits" , while the convents were "good at preventing too frequent parental visits".

Neither the advocates of l'Oeuvre Grancher nor the Placement Familial applied their "absolute precision" to the analysis of their results: indeed between the wars (as was to become obvious during the BCG controversy) French claims couched in statistical terms became something of a byword for creative imagination. Nevertheless, a modified state-sponsored Grancher scheme was adopted in Belgium, Algeria and Quebec and was, according to Armand-Delille, still processing 7000 children in 1955 in France "with (as usual) complete success".[19]

In Britain schemes vaguely based on the French experience were tried in Hastings and Plymouth and in Shropshire; but they lacked official backing and money: as Dr Letitia Fairfield, senior medical officer of the London County Council, lamented in 1931, their operation was always "gravely hampered by lack of cooperation ... from tuberculous parents".[20] The Hastings Tuberculosis Care Committee boarded out older, failing children "with people of their own class" during the summer months between 1925 and 1930; and Plymouth and the London County Council made attempts to copy this. But the numbers were always small, in London about 3 per cent of applicants. In Shropshire Arthur C. Watkin, the county Tuberculosis Officer,

---

[17] Calmette, A., *British Medical Journal* (1925), no. 2, 270.

[18] Bushnell, F. G., ibid. (1929), no. 2, 279.

[19] Armand-Delille, P. F., *Transactions of the NAPT* (1955), p. 57.

[20] Fairfield, L., *Transactions of the NAPT* (1932), p. 32.

launched a scheme in 1933 which placed infants of tuberculous mothers in a county home for babies while the mothers could stay for up to one year in a sanatorium. At the end of that time "the parents were persuaded ... to send their children to relatives or to a public assistance institution".[21] The scheme fizzled out after four years for lack of funds.

The boarding out of infants was never popular in the United States; and American delegates at international gatherings tended to express doubts about the alleged achievements of such schemes. Independent research by and large justified their scepticism. In the 1930s a well-conducted study at the Lymanhurst Health Centre in Minnesota showed that children who remained at home with tuberculous parents had the same chance of developing the disease later as children who were separated. The Americans were not alone in harbouring doubts. In a rare access of plain speaking, Professor Peter Ganzer of Graz in Austria publicly accused Armand-Delille not only of falsifying his figures – that was par for the course – but of sacrificing "like a modern Herod" thousands of innocents to his own glorification. By the end of the decade most doctors in most countries began to realise that the emotional and physical costs of separating children from tuberculous parents outweighed marginal benefits. Addressing a receptive audience at the Royal Society of Medicine of London on the eve of the London Blitz (and the evacuation of schoolchildren on a far larger scale than ever envisaged by workers in tuberculosis), Dr Reginald Lightwood summed up this feeling when he suggested that, terrible as tuberculosis was, "the boarding out of infants at risk might be more dangerous for the future happiness of the child than the disease".[22]

The treatment of the infants of tuberculous mothers was always only a peripheral – though a highly emotional – part of the public-health problem. At its core was the fate of bread-winners and the mothers of large families. Sanatoria were clearly not the answer, at least not the whole answer. Even before the Depression years, never more than a quarter of discharged patients found a job comparable to their previous employment if they found a job at all. Always and everywhere there was also social ostracism. No doubt D. H. Lawrence's obsessive denial of his own illness was rooted in his character; but it was also nurtured by childhood memories. In working-class communities like Eastwood a few families were always shunned: healthy children and their friends would be told by their mothers that – without being in any way impolite – they should avoid becoming friendly with the children of Family X, not go to their house after school or share a meal with

[21] Watkin, A. C., *British Medical Journal* (1935), no. 2, 921.
[22] Lightwood, R., *Proceedings of the Royal Society of Medicine*, 2 (1940), 620.

them, however warmly Mrs X offered her boy's friends cups of cocoa. To young children the exact reason was rarely explained (which added to the pall that hung over the Xs) but, eventually, it would transpire that Mr X or one his brothers or sisters had been treated for tuberculosis in a sanatorium.

By the time Lawrence acquired the disease – or rather, by the time his illness declared itself – the backbone of the public-health effort against tuberculosis in most countries was the specialist tuberculosis dispensary. They varied widely in size per population as well as in name, looks and efficiency; but they pursued the same objective. More accurately, they pursued the same two, not entirely compatible objectives. They existed to look after tuberculous patients (that went without saying); but they were also expected to protect the public against them.

In Britain they took longer to become established beside the old general Poor Law dispensaries than elsewhere. Robert (later Sir Robert) Philip's Victoria Dispensary in Edinburgh, the first specifically designed for the care of the tuberculous, opened in 1887 but remained unique for twenty years.[23] (The founder's commitment to tuberculin injections, increasingly discredited elsewhere, contributed to the delay.) By 1909 both Poor Law authorities and charitable bodies had grasped the main practical advantage of specialised clinics. This had little to do with either the care of patients or the safeguarding of the public: it was their use as marshalling yards. "At a drop of a hat all tuberculous material in the district could be summoned", Dr D. J. Williamson told the Destitution Conference in 1911. Questionnaires could be filled in. Statistics could be compiled. Most importantly, the material could be sorted out. "Early" cases might be put on the waiting list for a sanatorium. "Interesting" cases would be referred to the Brompton or to the local teaching hospital. "Advanced" cases could be handed an instruction sheet, put on the list for home visiting and told to guard their spitting.

---

[23] Sir Robert Philip became one of the leading figures in tuberculosis in Britain and on the international stage. He qualified in the year of Koch's discovery and originally intended to become a gynaecologist. His return journey from postgraduate study in Vienna became his road to Damascus: he saw a vision of a vast new field of therapeutic endeavour opening up in tuberculosis. He was vigorously discouraged by his seniors: he was told (by his own account) that everything that was to be known about tuberculosis was already known and every sensible person realised the hopelessness of even thinking about its prevention and treatment. He refused to be deflected and with the help of a few kind (and wealthy) friends opened the Victoria Dispensary. In 1913 the government-appointed Astor Departmental Committee on Tuberculosis recommended its adoption as the model for a national scheme, and in 1913 it was adopted by the National Association for the Prevention of Tuberculosis. In 1918 Philip was appointed professor of tuberculosis in Edinburgh, the first holder of such a chair in Britain, and received a knighthood in the same year. He died in 1939.

Initially in England tuberculosis dispensaries were staffed almost exclusively by moonlighting young graduates trying to scrape together enough to buy themselves into a practice. The premises opened for three hours twice a week, which could be fitted in with other jobs. (The time officially allotted to each patient was generally three and a half minutes.) Beside the doctor there was also a nurse or volunteer lady health visitor; and after first attendance one of them inspected the patient's dwelling and gave instructions about sleeping arrangements, ventilation, the cleansing of the patient's bedding and eating utensils, the drinking of more milk and the taking of cod-liver oil. (The last was supplied free by most dispensaries together with a bottle of Virol or some other fortifying food-supplement.) She then reported back to the dispensary doctor, who was supposed to conduct a "march-past". This was Sir Robert Philip's great invention. It essence it meant identifying all members of the household who were potential contacts and who were therefore told to report to the dispensary for examination and tests. In Scotland – as in France, Germany and several other continental countries – dispensary officers could legally enter the homes of the tuberculous without permission. While English Local Government Boards were never given such power, doctors and health visitors (like the police) were rarely defied. Yet English officials were generally less intrusive than their Scottish colleagues: Philip chided them for their laziness.

In most of continental Europe tuberculosis became, like scarlet fever, diphtheria, whooping cough, typhoid and cholera, a notifiable disease between 1900 and the outbreak of the First World War.[24] This was hailed both by health reformers and by the literate public as a momentous advance. The few dissenting voices were concerned not with the merits of the case but with the cost. But surely it would be worth it: the dramatic reduction in the prevalence of other infectious fevers after being made notifiable seemed an unanswerable argument in favour of adding tuberculosis to the list. Unfortunately, tuberculosis was unlike all the other fevers: it was not in fact a fever. For many families it was more a way of life – or a way of death. More often than not notification merely made that way more painful.

Attempts were often made to make the unpalatable palatable by false promises. Politicians seeking re-election hinted at the rehousing of the most needy tuberculous families. In execution such promises usually shrank to free sputum cups and paper handkerchiefs. The majority of the unenlightened poor were never taken in and dreaded notification. Soon doctors joined

---

[24] It had been a notable omission from the original Infectious Diseases (Notification) Act of 1889 in Britain. The same was true of similar legislation in most other European countries.

them. Few were prepared to commit themselves if there was the shadow of a doubt about the diagnosis. When in 1912 the law was tightened, they defied both their professional leaders and their political masters and embarked on passive resistance. Some notified but did not give the patient's address (or gave the wrong one) and did not tell the patient. Others only notified if the disease seemed "active" (which was a flexible definition) or if it was "repeatedly sputum positive". The most compassionate ones waited until the case was terminal.

This was a new phenomenon. Doctors were traditionally grumblers against regulations, form-filling and bureaucratic interference; but they were, like most respectable professions, jealous of their powers and privileges and therefore among the most law-abiding citizens. Now their threats of non-co-operation, usually no more than angry splutterings, were put into practice. They knew that the public, especially the poor, avoided keen notifiers. They did not blame them. A notification fee of one shilling and a pat on the back from Sir Robert Philip was no compensation for the loss of their patients' respect and confidence. To most ordinary general practitioners those things still mattered.

In Britain the law was never enforced. The Ministry of Health nagged the profession but never with much conviction or to great effect. In 1918 21 per cent of deaths certified at post-mortem as resulting from tuberculosis had never been notified; and another 27 per cent had been notified less than three months before death.[25] These figures never improved.[26] The picture was not notably different on the Continent. A few German and Scandinavian speakers at international conferences claimed that obstreperous practitioners who consistently defied the law were taken to court and went to prison. Such cases were never identified, are impossible to trace and were probably figments of the imagination. By the late 1920s the high hopes pinned on compulsory notification were widely perceived as having been illusory.

The same was true of tuberculous dispensaries. By the mid 1930s, the grimmest of the Depression years, they were universally disliked. Whatever was true of the leisured classes (among whom tuberculosis never entirely lost its Romantic appeal), among those hardest hit by unemployment the disease no longer aroused great compassion. Many openly resented public money being spent on a system which failed to remove the threat and did the victims no visible good. Local practitioners accused dispensaries (usually wrongly) of stealing their patients. Medical officers of health disliked dispensaries because they were outside their jurisdiction and yet cut into their

[25] Dudfield, R., *British Medical Journal* (1922), no. 2, 869.
[26] Jordan, R., ibid. (1928), no. 1, 692.

budgets. County Tuberculosis Officers preferred dealing with the medically more reputable sanatoria. The result was gross and worsening underfunding.

Most visibly, inadequate budgets meant dingy premises. Some dispensaries, often housed in the basement of buildings which also accommodated the more highly esteemed maternity and school medical services, were so noisy that auscultation could proceed only during breaks in the traffic outside. Transfer to more desirable sites was usually blocked by local residents who feared, not without reason, a drop in property values if the neighbourhood became a den of consumptives. Staffing suffered even more. By the end of the 1920s young moonlighting graduates were no longer allowed to provide medical cover. "Considering the importance of the task their experience is wholly inadequate", the English Anti-Tuberculosis Association stated. Yet recognition of the importance of the task was limited. The role of dispensary medical officers was to diagnose and to keep an eye on their clients, not to treat.[27] Once diagnosed, the patients were to be referred back to their general practitioner. If the case was in any way unusual, he or she was to be referred to a hospital outpatients department. The hospitals never communicated with the dispensaries. Home visiting was time-consuming and unpopular. Not surprisingly, most dispensary doctors regarded themselves as professional failures if not actually the dregs. Some probably were. They were also deliberately kept in their place. When in 1921 the Dispensary Officers' Association pressed for the establishment of a special diploma, then as now the first step towards bettering a speciality's status if not necessarily their performance, the proposal was rejected by the General Medical Council. (The Registrar's reply was witty or sarcastic according to taste: there was, he wrote, nothing to stop the dispensary doctors from examining each other's competence and from conferring diplomas.) The association's plea for affiliation to the existing Tuberculosis Society, the body representing superintendents of sanatoria and medical officers of health, was not even formally considered. When dispensary staff salaries were cut in in 1926, and again in 1931, the protests from the British Medical Association were wholly lacking in holy indignation and of course ineffective.[28]

What was true of doctors was also true of the tuberculosis dispensary nurses. By the 1930s it had become a vicious circle. The jobs were ill-paid and the work arduous. Even in areas of high unemployment the vacancies were therefore difficult to fill. This made the work of the existing staff even harder. Yet many dispensary nurses jealously guarded "their" patients,

[27] The reference in official documents and reports to clients rather than patients in relation to tuberculosis dispensaries is revealing.

[28] Coutts, J. F. H., Memorandum, 27 June 1930, Ministry of Health, PRO, MH 75/l3.

refusing even to allow new doctors to see past notes. When patients moved the notes were never forwarded. Before the First World War, still in the afterglow of Koch's discovery, voluntary work in tuberculosis was generally regarded as socially and morally elevating. After the war, voluntary helpers increasingly pulled out of dispensaries. Eventually the system became the expression not of care but of despair.[29] Beyond a point the course of the disease among the poor was tacitly recognised as being inexorably downhill.

The spirit of dispensary care remains enshrined in thousands of surviving instruction sheets. Printed on cheap paper, they were handed to patients and their relatives in every country with claims to be counted as civilised. Where literacy was low they were embellished by simple line-drawings carrying the appropriate message. Their contents hardly differed and it did not significantly change between 1909 and 1952. "Separate marked utensils ... Spitting only into sputum cups ... Sputum cups to be boiled every day for ten minutes and its contents burned ... Patient's bedclothes to be kept separate and boiled at home ... Dwellings to be fumigated at least once a month ... Dust-gathering corners to be swept up every day ..." But most importantly and therefore usually in bold or capital lettering:

NO FONDLING OR KISSING OF OTHER MEMBERS OF THE
FAMILY, PARTICULARLY NOT OF CHILDREN

MARRIED PARTNERS TO SLEEP IN SEPARATE BEDS
PREFERABLY SEPARATED BY A PARTITION

MOST IMPORTANT: THE SURVIVING HEAD OF THE
HOUSEHOLD IMMEDIATELY TO NOTIFY THE
DISPENSARY OF THE DEATH OF THE PATIENT

[29] It is impossible to recognise the facts, as remembered and recounted in many personal memoirs, in what were almost consistently upbeat official pronouncements; and a large literature based on them ("sterling work", "stirring events". "light at the end of a tunnel"), not only in Britain but in most countries in Europe and North America.

27

A Model Patient

To many tuberculous their illness always remained something external to themselves, an enemy like earthquakes, censors, treacherous friends or corrupt and vengeful bosses. To D. H. Lawrence it was not only external, it was unmentionable. Others came to identify with it to an extent no sufferer ever identified with any other illness: it became the very expression of their being. For years before his ill-health was given a label – almost an accolade – especially during his numerous on-off-on-off relationships with young women, Franz Kafka blamed his delicate health and constitutional frailty for his indecisiveness. There were no external reasons for it. He had been born into a prosperous middle-class Jewish family in Prague in 1883.[1] At twenty-four, after a conventional *Gymnasium* and trouble-free if not particularly distinguished university education, he was gainfully employed and not on the face of it physically ailing. He was liked and even admired by a circle of intellectual friends. He was and would always remain attractive to women. His father, it is true, he later described as a boor and a bully – "all my books were written against him" – and much has been made of this relationship to explain both his inner torments and his creative outpourings. Kafka *père* was in fact probably no worse than many another domineering Victorian paterfamilias, self-made and well satisfied with the outcome of his labours, yet for much of the time the son felt desperately ill at ease in the adult world and, without realising it, in search of a physical cause that would justify his fears.[2] When the disease eventually struck – in 1916 – it therefore seemed

[1] In 1883 Prague was the historic capital of the kingdom of Bohemia, and the seat of the oldest university in central Europe, but no longer one of the official capital cities of the Austro-Hungarian monarchy.

[2] Though his immediate circle appreciated his extraordinary gifts, his most famous works – *The Trial*, *The Castle* and his *Letters* – were not published till after his death and not widely known in English-speaking countries until publicised by W. H. Auden and by the first translators, Edwin and Willa Muir, in the 1930s. But it was the post-war French existentialists to whom he spoke most directly and who coined the term Kafkaesque. As Simone de Beauvoir recalled in *La force de l'âge*: "Our admiration for Kafka was instant and overpowering without quite knowing why we felt that his work concerned us personally. Faulkner and others we admired told us remote stories: Kafka alone spoke to us about ourselves. He revealed to us our own problems confronted by a world without God and in which nonetheless our salvation

not a disaster but an escape, the first station in what Dr Freud of Vienna had recently dubbed *Die Flucht in die Krankheit*.[3] But this would probably have been too simplistic an explanation for Kafka's uncompromisingly tortuous mind. "I am constantly seeking a reason for this disease", he wrote to his closest friend, Max Brod,[4] some years later, "for I did not seek it. Sometimes it seems to me that my brain and lungs came to an agreement without my knowledge. 'Things can't go on this way', said my brain, and after five years the lungs said they were ready to help." Almost to the end, his lungs and his brain maintained their creative alliance.

The year in which Kafka's lungs declared their readiness to help was as doom-laden in Prague as it was in Modigliani's Paris or Kirchner's Berlin. By the end of 1915 most able-bodied men of his age-group had been called up. Half a million had already perished.[5] His work at the Workmen's Accident Insurance Institute exempted him from military service but at his desk he was despairingly trying to cope with tens of thousands of disabled soldiers – blind, limbless, shell-shocked – unceremoniously dumped by the army on the civilian authorities.[6] More than a third of those registered were also suffering from tuberculosis. As in the west, official bulletins reported decisive victories. "Wir siegen uns zo Tode",[7] the wiseacres in the coffee houses were saying. Except that even the coffee houses were beginning to be deserted: they had nothing to offer but dimly lit arctic premises, *Ersatz* coffee and *Galgenhumor*.[8]

was at stake." He was decreed a non-person by Communist ideologues – "a decadent avant-gardist" was George Lukács's verdict – and he was not recognised in his own country as the prophet of twentieth-century alienation until the mid 1960s. He is now one of the tourist attractions of his native city (which he disliked), in the same way as Joyce is of Dublin and Mozart is of his hated Salzburg. Among his biographers, the present writer has found E. Pawel, *The Nightmare of Reason: A Life of Franz Kafka* (London, 1988), particularly illuminating.

  [3] "Flight into the Illness", first mentioned in *Vorlesungen zur Einführung in die Psychoanalyse*, published in Vienna in 1915.

  [4] The writer Max Brod became Kafka's literary executor and ignored his friend's testamentary instruction to destroy all his unpublished works. Their correspondence was published in English in the standard Schocken edition of Kafka's writings.

  [5] In terms of population, the losses of the Austro-Hungarian armies were exceeded only by those of France; and most Czechs were not even fighting for a country they recognised as their own.

  [6] Contrary perhaps to what might be deduced from his novels and correspondence, Kafka was not only a committed but also a highly efficient employee. He was largely responsible for establishing the first hospital dedicated to the care of "shell-shocked" invalids at Rumburk. His superiors regarded him as indispensable and he was in line for a state decoration when he resigned.

  [7] "We are winning ourselves to death."

  [8] Gallows humour.

This was true of all cities of the ramshackle Habsburg monarchy; but Prague was traditionally the seismic centre, registering shock-waves long before the earthquakes. In this fraught atmosphere no section of the city's population felt more threatened than its German-speaking Jews.[9] The death of the old Emperor, Franz Josef, in November 1916, seemed a terrible portent, as was news of the revolution in Russia and the formation of the Czech Legion on Russian soil.[10] By way of precaution Kafka's father, Herrmann, dropped the second "r" from his name: "Hermann", he judged, sounded less Teutonic.

The first big bleed came while Franz was living in two rooms in the Schönborn palace, perhaps the most improbable of his many bizarre residences. Superbly spacious, lavishly stuccoed and with a wonderful view over the baroque rooftops and spires of one of Europe's loveliest cities, the building was damp, drafty, cold, unheatable and without running water.[11] "The blood just kept coming", he later wrote to his then fiancée, Milena Jesenska.[12]

I got so excited, I kept walking around, leant out of the window, sat down on the bed. I wasn't at all unhappy because for some reason I realised that, provided that the haemorrhage stopped, I would be able to sleep for the first time after some three or four almost sleepless years.[13]

The haemorrhage did stop and he did sleep well: nothing in fact could dampen his elation, not even the comment of the maid who came to clear up the mess the next morning: "Well, you're obviously not long for this world, Herr Doktor".[14]

[9] Prague had an "old" Jewish population, mainly goldsmiths and other craftsmen, who spoke Yiddish or Czech; but the Kafkas belonged to the more recent migration from Russia and Poland. Like the emancipated Jews in other parts of the Habsburg Empire, they were among the most loyal subjects of the dynasty – "the only real Austrians" – and spoke German. Franz wrote all his books and the majority of his letters in German, though he was bilingual.

[10] Franz Josef was eighteen when he succeeded his uncle, Ferdinand V (*Der Trottel*), in 1848, and by 1916 he had reigned for sixty-eight years. Despite his personal limitations, even bigotry, his reign spanned the entire period of Jewish emancipation. It was widely (though inaccurately) rumoured that his successor, Charles, was antisemitic. Czechoslovakia, which the Czech Legion helped to establish, became one of the most liberal countries in Europe; but in 1917 this could not be foreseen.

[11] One of the many baroque palaces of Prague built by the Austro-Hungarian aristocracy as their second homes after Vienna. Fully restored and air-conditioned, it is today the United States Embassy.

[12] She was the non-Jewish daughter of an eminent Prague surgeon. After being active in the Czech Resistance, she ended her life in a German concentration camp.

[13] Pawel, *The Nightmare of Reason*, p. 393.

[14] Everybody with a university degree (and many without) was addressed as *Herr Doktor* in central Europe. Kafka had a doctorate in law from Prague University.

Dr Mühlstein, Kafka's kindly general practitioner, was not one to spoil life's little pleasures. After the second major bleed he admitted that there might be some slight pulmonary tuberculous involvement but "half the people in this benighted city are tubercular today; an inflammation of the lung tips isn't all that terrible; nothing a few tuberculin injection will not take care of". Tuberculin injections apart, he was nearly right: in the spring of 1917 half of Prague's youth probably was tuberculous;[15] and not all were doomed to die within six years. But on his personal score Kafka was not fooled or fooling himself. "Let me tell you a secret", he wrote to another of his young women friends, Felicia Bauer,

> which at the moment I myself still don't believe (though the darkness is closing in on me) ... but which nonetheless is bound to be true: I shall never get well again. Just because what we are here dealing with is not tuberculosis that can be nursed back to health in a sanatorium deckchair but a weapon that remains absolutely indispensable as long as I live. It and I cannot go on living together – or apart from each other.[16]

Was Kafka another war victim of tuberculosis? He was certainly living in something approaching squalor and under emotional stress; but looking for aetiological factors there is an embarrassment of riches.[17] Apart from his other fears and inhibitions he was also a food fetishist, not only a vegetarian but also a fanatical believer in the goodness of natural foods. He drank litres of unpasteurised, unboiled milk in a country where the inspection of cattle was compulsory but a joke even in peacetime. He obsessively overworked both at his job and at his writing. In 1919 he was also struck down by the Spanish Flu which killed at least 50,000 people in Prague alone.[18] The illness left him drained of what little physical energy he still had.

In December 1921 he was at last persuaded by his director at the insurance institute (who thought highly of him) to accept the offer of a Dutch anti-tuberculous charity and seek a cure in a sanatorium in Matliary in the High Tatra. This was a very different setting from a Swiss *Zauberberg*, where highbrow intellectuals and a rich cosmopolitan elite exchanged witticisms, indulged in philosophical ruminations, flirted and cultivated brittle gossip. Even the mountain peaks – jagged rocks too treacherous for leisurely walks and gay sleigh-rides – looked dangerous. Although the new country of

[15] This was shown by the first Pirquet skin testing in Prague in 1920.

[16] Pawel, *The Nightmare of Reason*, p. 412.

[17] One of the aetiological factors which did *not* operate in his case was his Jewish origin. Almost certainly as a legacy of their crowded past in ghettoes, the Jewish population in the cities of central and eastern Europe – Prague, Berlin, Vienna, Budapest, Warsaw and others – were significantly *less* prone to tuberculosis than the non-Jewish population.

[18] See above, Chapter 21.

Czechoslovakia of which Kafka was now a citizen was embarking on a twenty-year spell of democracy and prosperity,[19] this was still a region where isolated communities of Hungarians, Slovaks, Poles and ethnic Germans lived in smouldering but implacable hatred, wholly irrational but inextinguishable.[20] Kafka found it highly congenial. Institutions like Frau Forberger's sanatorium amounted to little more than a boarding house, its dining room open to officer patients from the nearby military hospital and to a select few of the local German-speaking intelligentsia. Its patient inmates had mostly been dispatched by international charitable agencies from the starving cities of the former Austro-Hungarian Empire. A doctor – tuberculous himself of course – did however reside on the premises and for a modest retainer saw seriously ill patients like Herr Dr Kafka at least once every day, the hallmark of a sanatorium. Indeed not only saw but also examined them, took their pulse and temperature, and registered their weight before prescribing the requisite amount of milk and cream appropriate for the patient's state of health on that particular day. Dr Strelinger was a specialist who also offered injections of arsenic at twelve kronen per shot and the possibility of a more expensive course of "neo-tuberculin". Kafka declined and Strelinger did not insist: melancholy and wasting away himself, he had modest expectations of medicine's healing powers and put his faith, such as it was, in a diet based on anchovies and eggs. When Kafka, tormented with vegetarian guilt, complained about eating fish the doctor reassured him: "Better you them than they you".[21] More importantly for his future – or what remained of it – it was at Matliary that he met Robert Klopstock, an orphaned Jewish youth from Budapest, a would-be and future medical student, who adopted him as his mentor and would cling to him and then nurse him to the end.[22]

After his return to Prague (neither better nor worse for his six months in a sanatorium), and following his official retirement on health grounds, there

---

[19] It was presided over by Tomáš Masaryk, astute and high-minded philosopher friend of President Woodrow Wilson. Masaryk died in 1937 and his work was undone by Czechoslovakia's western friends in Munich a year later. Among the eventual victims of the betrayal were most of the country's Jews, including Kafka's much-loved sister, Ottla.

[20] The Tatra Mountains, now in the Slovak Republic, were, until 1918, part of the kingdom of Hungary, one of the three hills which support the apostolic double cross on the Hungarian coat of arms.

[21] He was unlikely to have been familiar with Lenin's famous "who whom".

[22] Under the patronage of the Archduchess Augusta (who had lost two brothers from tuberculosis), the International Tuberculosis Relief Agency escaped the rabid spy-fever of 1914 which put an end to the operation of most international agencies in Austria-Hungary (as it did in other belligerent countries). In the immediate post-war years the organisation, financed mainly by Dutch benevolence, saved the lives of thousands of young people without family connections or in many cases – as in Robert Klopstock's – families.

was to be one more important meeting and a last love affair. In the summer of 1923, convalescing from another bout of bleeding at Müritz on the Baltic coast, he met one of the helpers at a nearby summer-camp for refugee Jewish children, the vivacious, brash, ardent and pretty nineteen-year-old Dora Diamant.[23] He must have presented a startling appearance, ensconced in his roofed wicker chair, his dark melancholy eyes watching silently for hours the children building sandcastles by the water's edge; and she was too un-inhibited and inquisitive not to wander over to him and strike up a conversation. Within days her total lack of artifice or reserve overrode his inhibitions and enabled him after only three weeks to risk a step of "death-defying courage, a deed of reckless daring given my condition". He suggested that she should share her life with him. Even then it took another few months of agonising in Prague before he summoned up enough confidence to cancel his other plans and, full of anticipatory guilt and lacerating feelings of self-abasement, set out for Berlin.

There is Kafkaesque irony in the fact that he found, perhaps for the first and certainly for the last time in his life, peace, happiness and even serenity in what was at that time the least peaceful, happy and serene city in the world. Armed gangs of the extreme Right and Left were battling it out nightly in the streets; strikes paralysed the public services; monarchist and other death squads murdered with impunity; and, following the French occupation of the Ruhr, the mark went into free fall. Soon people were carting home their daily wages in wheel-barrows – if they had daily wages, that is, and still possessed a wheel-barrow. When, on 15 November 1923, the inflation ended – a billion old marks could be exchanged for one of the ingenious Dr Schacht's new marks – it precipitated a Depression which ten years later would give Hitler and his thugs (in comfortable prison in 1923 after their failed first *Putsch*) a second chance. But for Dora and Kafka it was magical, a twentieth-century surrealistic replay of *La vie de Bohème*. In their one-room suburban flat the gas and electricity had been cut off, a kerosene lamp serving as light-source, heating and kitchen range: they spent much of their time reading Hebrew and German classics and planning their life together running a restaurant in Tel Aviv.

By the end of the year Kafka's condition had taken a turn for the worse: he ran an almost continuous temperature and began to suffer from a sore throat. They had no money even for a second-class hospital bed or to call a doctor: their landlady and then another gave them notice. Eventually the family in Prague, who had disapproved of his move to Berlin, delegated

---

[23] Kafka's combustible passions were always for younger women. He was forty at the time though, despite his illness, he always looked younger than his age.

Uncle Siegfried Löwy, a country practitioner, to visit him and decide what should be done. There was no doubt about the verdict: Franz needed urgent hospital treatment. A few weeks later Max Brod escorted him back to Prague and in March Dora and Klopstock took him to the Wiener Wald Sanatorium near Vienna. There his worst suspicions were confirmed: the burning sensation in his throat was due to tuberculosis of the larynx. He was first admitted to Professor Hajek's clinic in Vienna, an establishment run with the ruthless efficiency of an army stockade. Dora was horrified by the atmosphere and by Hajek's arrogance; overriding Hajek's objections, she took Kafka to the small Kierling Sanatorium. This was a homely, begabled villa in pleasantly neglected grounds (as were many small sanatoria in the neighbourhood of Vienna) where he had a spacious room and where Dora and Klopstock took charge of him.

They did so with loving care, easing the agony of his final weeks. There were even moments of happiness – the view from the window of the trees in the garden in blossom and then turning green, the scent of lilacs, his favourite flower. Dora, a self-taught cook, invented dishes that were bland and yet tasty enough to coax his appetite. It did not need much coaxing: as long as the pain was bearable, he forced himself to eat. The would-be suicide of the past was now trying his best to stay alive. When a Viennese specialist, one of several whom Dora insisted on consulting, assured him that his throat seemed to be improving, he wept with joy. The specialist was of course being routinely kind and mendacious: privately he agreed with his colleagues that Kafka had at the most a few months to live. They all advised Dora to break off the expensive and useless sanatorium treatment and take him back home, but she refused; to do so would have deprived him of his last hope.

Despite the anaesthetic lozenges and alcohol injections into the laryngeal nerves, the advancing throat lesion soon made speech as well as swallowing difficult. Urged to spare his vocal cords, he began to communicate with his "little family" by means of written notes. Many of these conversation slips were saved by Klopstock; and, more than the usual body of pious oral apocrypha, they document the courage and lucidity with which he faced death; and his love of life. On 11 May Max Brod came for what he knew would be his last visit. He found his friend quietly starving but immersed in the galley proofs of his last short piece, "The Hunger Artist". It was the only writing whose posthumous publication he authorised in his will. Klopstock wrote later:

> Kafka's physical condition at this point ... was truly ghastly. Reading the proofs must have been not only a tremendous emotional strain but also a shattering spiritual encounter with his former self, and when he had finished the tears kept

flowing. It was the first time that I saw him overtly expressing his emotions in this way: he had always shown superhuman self-control.[24]

The erosion of the larynx was now causing such pain that every bite and sip became torture. "I cannot drink this glass of water. But the craving gives me a little satisfaction." He no longer had any illusions. "If it is true – and it seems inescapable – that my present food intake is insufficient then there is no longer any hope." Thirst, though, was worse than hunger: it swamped his mind with hallucinatory recollections of past pleasures – a glass of water, a tankard of beer, a drink of iced lemonade. Yet two day before he died he could still write a long and chatty, almost light-hearted letter to his parents to dissuade them from a visit: "The current heat spell often reminds me of how Father and I used to drink beer together many years ago when he took me to the Municipal Swimming Pool"; and a note about the cut flowers in his room: "How marvellous that lilac is! It's dying but it still goes on drinking, guzzling. How unlike me."

On 2 June he seemed slightly improved and worked on his galley proofs again; but, as the next dawn broke, Dora noticed his laboured breathing. She summoned Klopstock. Kafka was awake and in pain; and croaking he began to rage: "For years you've been promising me morphine at the end. Now you're torturing me ... So be it. I'll die without it." And a few minutes later: "Kill me or else you're worse than a murderer." Klopstock gave him two injections which eased the pain and slowly put an end to his agony.[25] His sanatorium nurse, accustomed as she was to suffering and death, sobbed: "He was so brave. A model patient."

[24] Pawel, *The Nightmare of Reason*, 401.

[25] After Kafka's death Klopstock completed his medical studies in Berlin and escaped the Holocaust by emigrating to the United States. He ended his life as a professor and chief of thoracic services at the Veterans' Administration Hospital in Brooklyn, New York. He died in 1972. Dora Diamant emigrated to Palestine in the 1930s but returned to Italy and was rounded up by the Fascists in 1944 and murdered on the way to a concentration camp.

28

Workshops and Village Settlements

While the declared objectives of tuberculosis care did not change, most countries evolved special schemes, supposedly of wide application but usually tailored to their particular needs. Britain's best-known contribution was the village settlement. An offshoot of Ebenezer Howard's garden city ideal,[1] Papworth, the pioneer venture, was founded in 1915. It was twelve miles outside Cambridge and became the showpiece of the movement. Its aim was to provide tuberculous patients with long-term care in a setting that was medically sound, socially acceptable and financially self-supporting. This was in sharp contrast to what the founder, Dr Pendrill (later Sir Pendrill) Varrier-Jones, described as the short, cruel, expensive and ineffectual regime fostered by sanatoria. Whether or not his scheme ultimately fulfilled its promise, there was much truth in his vigorously expressed criticism of other solutions and therefore in his claim that something better was needed.

> If a man knew that, in the event of his being found tuberculous he would receive immediate treatment, that his family would be supported while he was receiving treatment and that if he was suffering from extensive and permanent damage he would be able to live and work permanently in a village settlement with his family, the whole tuberculosis problem would be revolutionised. Those who thought they had tuberculosis would present themselves for treatment at a very early stage ... and the success rate in treatment would be far better than it is at present.[2]

Like most effective innovators, Varrier-Jones combined enthusiasm and energy with charm; and these qualities, supplemented by the crusading zeal of a few formidable titled and academic lady backers, ensured that his creation flourished. A crucial early coup was his successful claim to the sanatorium benefit provision of the National Insurance Act on the grounds that, though his patients were employed, their employment was part of their treatment. From the start he admitted only patients in Stages One and Two of the disease and initially only for one year. From the hospital section they would

---

[1] It was expounded in Howard's book, *A Peaceful Path to Real Reform* (1894; revised 1902). It inspired the founding of Letchworth and Welwyn Garden City in 1903 and 1919 respectively. Howard, knighted in 1927, a year before he died, remained a great admirer of Varrier-Jones's.
[2] Varrier-Jones, P. C., *British Journal of Tuberculosis*, 24 (1931), 175.

graduate to the sanatorium section (so-called despite Varrier-Jones's efforts
to have it referred to as the "convalescent section"). Then they would start
their industrial training and find employment in one of the village industries.
Eventually they could apply to live in the village settlement with their families
and work at more or less trade union rates of pay. There was also a hostel
for single men and from 1927 one for single women. From its modest
beginning as a small country house surrounded by old oak trees sheltering
a few temporary huts, Papworth reached by 1938 a population of a thousand,
including 360 children, occupying 142 cottages.[3]

The treatment at Papworth was, in Varrier-Jones's phrase, holistic: plenty
of eggs, milk, cocoa, porridge, tuberculin injections, gold, calcium, fresh air,
sunlight (when on offer), exercise and anything else available in the current
antituberculosis arsenal. A psychiatric clinic was established in 1928 to counsel
despairing patients, a move hailed by many as ground-breaking. It proved to
be somewhat disappointing in practice.[4] (The fiasco neither surprised nor
dismayed Varrier-Jones: he never admitted that there were many despairing
patients in Papworth.) The founder had a gift for the ringing phrase, unex-
ceptional in sentiment if not always clear in meaning: "Treat the patient, the
whole patient and his environment as well as his body fluids; and he will
conquer his distemper far more surely than any quantity of medical, surgical
and X-ray apparatus." There was also shrewd practical planning. The site of
Papworth St Everard was deliberately chosen as one remote from the distract-
ions of pubs and the cinema. This was partly for the inmates' sake but also
to pacify local opinion. As in the case of sanatoria, the local population was
hostile or at least apprehensive. And not only the ordinary people. A local
squire, Colonel Sir Mansfield Baker, led the campaign against a diocesan
scheme in 1921 to have the parishes of Papworth St Everard and Papworth St
Agnes, a rural mile and a half from each other, amalgamated. "It would empty
our church as surely as the plague", he wrote to the Bishop of Ely. The scheme
was abandoned. In both Papworths the villagers kept the lungers at arms
length. In 1923 those living along the Papworth-Cambridge bus route lobbied
the local bus company not to stop the buses near the village settlement, at
least on the early morning school-run. That wish too was granted.

The commercial side of the venture began with agriculture and market
gardening but Varrier-Jones soon realised that the returns from these were
too tardy and too low to cover wages and capital outlay. He turned to the

[3] It was last enlarged in 1950, by which time tuberculosis was no longer a long-term
problem. Today it is an internationally renowned centre for cardiac surgery.

[4] It was never clear either to the patients or to the visiting psychiatrists and psychologists
what the clinic was supposed to achieve. Its foundation was something of a knee-jerk reaction
to a case of suicide, the only one in the history Papworth.

IN TRIBUTE TO PAPWORTH.

PAPWORTH has earned so many remarkable tributes that it is impossible to quote them all here. It is possible, however, to record the following:—

HIS MAJESTY THE KING said:—

"IT IS THE MOST PERFECT SCHEME OF ITS KIND THAT I HAVE EVER SEEN."

HER MAJESTY THE QUEEN after her visit in 1918 sent Papworth

£1,000

THE RT. HON. NEVILLE CHAMBERLAIN, M.P., MINISTER OF HEALTH, was reported in "The Times" of 14th July 1926, as having stated in the House of Commons that: *"He desired to bring to the notice of local authorities the success of the experiment which was being carried out by Dr. Varrier-Jones at Papworth in Cambridgeshire. The most remarkable feature of the experiment was that in this village, where every householder was tuberculous,* THE DISEASE WAS UNKNOWN AMONG THE CHILDREN.

SIR WILLIAM THOMPSON, M.D., P.R.C.P.I., REGISTRAR-GENERAL OF IRELAND, after an exhaustive inspection of Papworth, wrote :—*"The visit has impressed me very much and I consider this departure from the ordinary treatment of tuberculosis worthy of support and one that has great future possibilities."*

SIR GEORGE NEWMAN, K.C.B., M.D., CHIEF MEDICAL OFFICER OF THE MINISTRY OF HEALTH AND OF THE BOARD OF EDUCATION, wrote in his Annual Report for 1924:—*"The remarkable success of the Papworth Colony is one of the most encouraging efforts in relation to tuberculosis in this country, and reflects infinite credit upon those responsible for its management."* In his report for 1926 Sir George states: *"No child who was not suffering in a marked degree from tuberculosis before coming to live in the Colony has shown any signs of infection since becoming a resident"*; and in "THE HEALTH OF THE SCHOOL CHILD," his Annual Report for 1926 to the Board of Education, Sir George also states: *"One of the principal contributions of Papworth to its day and generation is the example which it furnishes of the way to deal with children liable to infection. The children in this "tuberculous" village do not get tuberculosis."*

THE RT. HON. SIR ALFRED MOND, BART., a former Minister of Health, thinks that Papworth is *"THE MOST WONDERFUL INSTITUTION OF ITS KIND IN THE WORLD."*

Tributes to Papworth. Under its Medical Director, Sir Pendrill Varrier-Jones, Papworth was conspicuously successful in terms of fund-raising and publicity. (*Cambridgeshire Record Office*)

factory production of travel goods and furniture and to a printery. The travelling cases, emblazoned with the appropriate heraldic beasts, were bought by the royal family, and the furniture (which was cheap and of excellent quality) was purchased by several Cambridge colleges. Turnover rose from £410 in 1918 to £85,000 in 1930 and £100,000 in 1938.

At the personal level Varrier-Jones, assisted by his formidable matron, Miss K. L. Borne, was an unapologetic paternalist. In the interest of the settlement, he vetted the frequency, the length and the character of all entertainments organised by the settlers and all films shown in the village hall; and he rigorously controlled leave passes. A frequently shown film based on Papworth itself, weaving health propaganda into the texture of a romantic story (almost unbearably cloying to modern eyes but well received at the time) was made in 1929, the year when single women were first admitted. Like Trudeau in America (whom he did not otherwise resemble), Varrier-Jones was a superb fund-raiser. The single women's hostel was funded by a strictly anonymous private donation of £20,000; but it was no secret that the donor made a much-appreciated appearance in the next year's Birthday Honours list. The building was sited some distance from the single men's hostel but the authorities also had "a tumulus ... heaped up ... to assist in maintaining the necessary segregation". "Cousining" between the sexes, as practised in many sanatoria on both sides of the Atlantic, was strongly discouraged.[5] Nevertheless several marriages between inmates took place in the 1930s, and, once the projected union was blessed by Miss Borne, widely publicised. An engraved glass vase was the standard and cherished present to the newly-weds from the director.

Eventually Papworth housed between fifty and eighty single woman patients aged between sixteen and twenty-five, predominantly domestic servants from good houses but also former clerks and factory hands. Over half of them had already lost two or more members of their families from tuberculosis. These numbers did not include the nurses, almost all of whom were or had been tuberculous themselves. Generally, even more than sanatoria, Papworth benefited from the influx of trained and mature staff who had lost their jobs before becoming pensionable and before (in the mid 1930s) pension schemes began to admit tuberculosis as a ground for disablement benefit. Tuberculous teachers, secretaries, librarians, clerks, cleaners and cooks were readily available, the last accepted provided they were sputum negative. It made up for the shortage of healthy applicants, put off by the late 1920s by the social stigma of a job in tuberculosis even more than by the fear of infection.

---

[5] The term was coined in the United States around the turn of the century to describe the illicit but widely practised network of sexual liaisons between long-term inmates of sanatoria.

There were of course shadows. The orderly lines of multicoloured shelters conformed to the Garden City ideal, but the benefits derived from their thorough exposure to the elements were seasonal. At the height of winter "false teeth froze to their tumblers and boots froze to the floor", as a disgruntled patient reported to the *Daily Mail* in 1924. But disgruntled patients were few: they tended to be summarily discharged, usually on the grounds that they were in fact unsuitable for training. (What happened to them? Discharges, so far as can be ascertained, were never followed up.) Those who fitted in, especially if they were skilled workers, enjoyed a full communal life: a choice of Protestant denominational worship, a book club, cricket, a horticultural society and tennis. Papworth, as Varrier-Jones explained to Their Majesties when they graced the settlement with a visit in 1918, served well those who were prepared to give more than they got. King George and Queen Mary thoroughly approved of the sentiment, and over luncheon suggested that a Boy Cub pack might be added to the therapeutic amenities.[6] The suggestion was instantly acted upon and two years later Sir Robert Baden-Powell added his signature (and a warm encomium) to the visitor's book.

Even at its best Papworth was not (contrary to what the village newsletter, *The Colonist*, repeatedly claimed) a solution to a world-wide problem. Because it was too uniquely the personal creation of its founder, the London County Council and later other local authorities decided against launching similar enterprises. Indeed, only one other village settlement on the Papworth model was established in England; and for a number of years that served as a warning against expanding the scheme rather than as an encouragement for more.

Preston Hall, near Aylesford in Kent, was founded in 1920 by Dr T. L. Bonar as a private venture primarily (as he was anxious to explain to visitors) for tuberculous ex-service men, an expression of his deeply felt gratitude to the nation's heroes. But by 1921 rumours of corruption began to circulate and the British Legion was forced to investigate. The horror stories were well founded. "Our gallant men" were subsisting on tea, bread, margarine, dripping and herring and the men's canteen welfare fund had mysteriously vanished. Rain entered through the roof and unblockable vents and snow blew in to cover the stretchers on the floor. The workshops had two lavatories for a hundred men: both got blocked every morning. Working conditions on the farm – centred on poultry and pig breeding – were reported by the inspectors as being non-specifically disgraceful.[7]

---

[6] Both the King and Queen were all for public service.

[7] The early ups and downs of Preston Hall, mainly the downs, are coruscatingly described by F. B. Smith in *The Retreat of Tuberculosis, 1850–1950* (London, 1988).

Bonar was not only ruthless and corrupt but also a smooth propagandist. After an excellent meal in honour of visiting journalists, he proudly displayed the prizes won by Preston Hall pigs at local agricultural shows. A tuberculous village settlement which could achieve that could not be all bad. Patients rarely saw him and were frightened of his dog: they dealt mainly with his assistant, formally titled the "Discipline Doctor". Useful men were not allowed to leave while grumblers were expelled before their six months was up. (This meant that they lost their tuberculosis pension because they were deemed to have defaulted on their course of training.) Those who remained were required to work forty-four hours a week for 15s., less 2s. 6d. for lighting and rent. Only men on 100 per cent pensions were allowed to stay and enrol on courses: their pension then went direct to Bonar, who pocketed most of it, together with their national training bonus payable for every forty hours of satisfactory service. The training was desultory at best: the staff were ill-paid and incompetent and the tools in the workshop useless. Eventually, after a horrified Ministry of Health inspector reported that in his view Dr Bonar "entirely lacked the personal touch and organisational skills necessary for the job", the director with his dog was asked to leave. He departed a wealthy man, leaving Preston Hall insolvent.

Sacking Bonar made the Ministry responsible for the scheme. The new medical superintendent, Major Hamilton, formerly of the Royal Army Medical Corps, was instructed to cut costs and raise output. One way of doing this was to stop buying coal and setting inmates to felling trees and splitting logs. (Much of the firewood went on warming the pigs' meals.) One brave former sergeant, A. W. Thomson, who complained to the Ministry about the distance between his dormitory and the nearest washing facilities, had his name passed on to the director. He was promptly discharged on the grounds that he would never make a pig farmer. Hamilton also confided in his Ministry chums that Thomson was a notorious trouble-maker: he had asked for a new set of false teeth when the set provided only a few weeks earlier broke during a fit of coughing.

Yet the colony survived: indeed, so dire was the plight of the tuberculous during the interwar years that its population grew from 165 young men in 1921 to 555 men, women and children in 1928. Hamilton then departed (a Commander of the British Empire) and a new director, Dr J. B. McDougall, took over. McDougall was anxious to establish – or re-establish – the settlement's therapeutic as well as the social and economic credentials. "It is clear to me", he wrote, "that any worthwhile village settlements must always insist that medical principles should take precedence over all others in the life of the community." 8 Whether or not in pursuit of this aim, he discharged two-thirds of the inmates, including all but the most indispensable of the ex-servicemen, as "inefficient", "efficient but temperamentally unsuited to village settlements" or "for disciplinary reasons". He had no difficulty in recruiting younger civilian consumptives who had no fancy ideas about their country owing them anything. Thereafter the colony prospered and, producing high-quality scented soap, fibre suitcases and angora wool, even began to make a profit. When the main building burnt down the British Legion rebuilt it at a cost of £100,000 (unaware perhaps that no more than three old soldiers were still in residence). By the outbreak of the Second World War the settlement had become a miniature garden village, with shops, tea-room, post office, nursery school, church and village hall. With the apple trees in blossom it looked charming in May. It also developed a well-equipped sanatorium with excellent X-ray and surgical facilities.[9] It remained the relatively prosperous haven of about 150 settlers and their families, doctors and nurses until 1952.

Tuberculous village colonies, Papworth in particular, became internationally famous, mainly as a result of Varrier-Jones's eloquence in several languages and generous hospitality to visiting celebrities; and a few settlements based on it were founded outside England. Peamount near Dublin produced chicken coops. The showpiece among several Dutch settlements, Berg-on-Bosch, manufactured luxury toys. Czechoslovakia had a successful settlement near Plzeň, turning out optical instruments. Hungary took pride in its tuberculous market garden and fruit farm near Kecskemét: its apricot brandy became world famous. In Germany the Breslau colony achieved renown under its founder, Dr E. M. Brieger: it specialised in joinery, mainly elaborately carved coffins. It was suppressed by the Nazis and Brieger fled to Papworth, whose not entirely unbiased chronicler he became.

In the United States the emphasis was on workshops rather than on village settlements. The Altro chain founded in New York in 1915 provided garment-making work in hygienic surroundings and under medical supervision. The hours were graduated in accordance with individual needs, the ultimate objective being a seven-hour day. Yet the aim of these establishments was limited: they never pretended to provide sheltered employment for the severely and permanently disabled; nor did they cater for whole families. Within their self-set targets the later results were good: a survey carried out in 1944 showed that 97.8 per cent of the "graduates" were alive five years after discharge.

---

[8] Joint Tuberculosis Council, *Care and After Care Schemes in Tuberculosis: Preston Hall* (London, 1931).

[9] George Orwell spent some time there, see below, Chapter 32.

The advocates of such schemes were always more persuasive at pointing to the shortcomings of other schemes than in making their own very attractive. Western society in the 1930s was not equipped to cope with a disease like tuberculosis any more than it was equipped with coping with the Depression and the hardships and degradations of unemployment.[10] Yet this was not the whole truth. One field offered great rewards at a comparatively low cost. This was widely known. In principle prophylaxis was extolled by every public speaker, medical or non-medical. It was, they intoned, the way forward, the only way forward. Nobody questioned them.[11] Unfortunately, while all agreed on the merits of prevention in theory, only two preventative measures were available in practice. With hindsight either could have saved thousands of young lives. In many countries they did. In Britain they were both strenuously and successfully resisted, and the thousands who could have been saved died. In chronological order they were the eradication of bovine tuberculosis and vaccination.

[10] There was even a small personal link between the two, or at least between tuberculosis and the Great Crash of Wall Street of 1929 which led to the Depression years. In 1927 the Federal Reserve Bank of New York – the Fed – had the power to restrain stock-market credit by raising the interest rate (discount rate) and reducing the reserves. On 27 July it did the exact reverse and the bull market began its fateful ascent into Never-Never Land. In a panic a year later the Fed raised the discount rate; but by then the action had the opposite to the intended effect. Over the second half of 1928 broker's loans increased by another $1.5 billion; and by the end of the year the crash was probably inevitable. Most of the critical decisions leading to the catastrophe were taken by Benjamin Strong, the Governor, a man determined to make his institution the dominant influence in world banking. His private life was touched with tragedy – his first wife committed suicide and his second left him – even before he was diagnosed as suffering from advanced pulmonary and laryngeal tuberculosis. Despite his obviously declining health, he continued to direct affairs through a hectic stream of memoranda (he could barely make himself heard on the telephone) from various sanatoria. In May 1928 he collapsed during a conference in London. By then he realised that his policy had been profoundly misguided, but it was too late. He resigned on his return to New York in August and died six weeks later.

[11] In much the same way, few people dare question the value of prophylactic screening today, however ill conceived or absurd some of its claims.

29

Milk

The diseases caused by the bovine strain of the *Mycobacterium tuberculosis* never achieved the fame of consumption of the lungs;[1] nor have they been given much attention in earlier chapters. Yet at times they accounted for a significant proportion of tuberculous deaths: 15 per cent in Europe around 1900 seems a reasonable guess.[2] The bovine organism entered the body by a different portal from that of the dust- and droplet-borne human bacillus; and, though the clinical pictures overlapped, there were also characteristic differences. Pulmonary tuberculosis was almost always caused by the human bacillus. Intestinal tuberculosis associated with tuberculous peritonitis in children was the typical presentation of the bovine strain. It could be an agonisingly painful illness, a succession of episodes of acute or subacute intestinal obstruction often requiring desperate operations. The operations were desperate because almost inevitably they led to further intra-abdominal scarring leading to further episodes of obstruction. They also tended to leave unhealed wounds and discharging sinuses and fistulae.[3] Few forms of tuberculosis were so lacking in Romantic appeal and were yet

[1] The nomenclature is a little misleading. The human strain of *Mycobacterium tuberculosis* can infect many species other than man (guinea-pigs could not otherwise be used for diagnosis); and the bovine strain is not confined to cattle. Nor is milk the only vehicle of the bovine strain: meat products can be equally infectious though cooking usually destroys the organisms.

[2] According to 1930 Ministry of Health Statistics, 28 per cent of all non-pulmonary tuberculosis deaths (and 2 per cent of pulmonary tuberculosis deaths) in Britain were of bovine origin. Over a thousand children under the age of fifteen died in England and Wales every year from the bovine strain.

[3] The main symptoms were colicky pain, vomiting and constipation (or, occasionally, diarrhoea). The abdomen was distended and hyperresonant. If complete obstruction was not relieved within forty-eight hours, a distended loop of bowel was likely to perforate and set up an acute and almost always fatal peritonitis. Or death could supervene from loss of fluids by vomiting and into the distended intestines. Even in pre-Listerian days the hands of surgeons were often forced.

Sinuses are blind inflammatory tracts leading into the tissues, often chronic abscess cavities, from the skin. Fistulae are abnormal tracts connecting the outside with a hollow organ or two hollow organs with each other.

so heartrending to watch. Death was often due to progressive malnutrition and general debility.[4]

The bovine organism may also have been responsible for nearly half of all cases of tuberculous meningitis, the most rapidly fatal form of the system; and it was probably a frequent cause of tuberculosis of the bones and joints, the genitourinary system, the cervical lymph-nodes and lupus vulgaris. In some parts of the world it was – and still is – the chief killer of babies and young children. It also calls for separate consideration for yet another reason. In contrast to pulmonary tuberculosis and other infections with the human bacillus, infections with the bovine organism were eminently preventable for at least fifty years before the introduction of specific chemotherapy. They continued only in countries where they were not prevented.

Such statements are usually arguable rather than provable, grist to the mill of the if only school of history. Not in this case. With unflinching resolve the United States eliminated bovine tuberculosis within a decade of the scientific evidence and technical means becoming available. This involved around 300 million tuberculin tests on cattle, of which roughly 4 million were positive, and the payment of indemnities to owners amounting to $27 million in a single year (1937). The effectiveness of the measures was never in doubt: nor, indeed, was it ever questioned by those who obstructed similar measures elsewhere. The death-rate in New York from milk-borne tuberculosis decreased by two-thirds between 1910 and 1915 and in Massachusetts by 91 per cent between 1910 and 1932. By 1940, while the bovine disease was still rampant in many European countries, all states of the Union (except, by a small margin, California) were accredited: that is 99 per cent of their milch-cows were attested tuberculosis-free. This was America in pursuit of physical fitness at its determined best.[5]

The same pursuit showed up Britain at its dilatory worst. The need to do something had long been recognised. In 1847 the Lancet reported that it was difficult in London to find samples of milk which did not show some blood or pus on microscopic examination, or even on simple inspection, and percipiently suggested that this might be one of the causes of scrofula.[6] In 1890 Queen Victoria (probably at Lord Salisbury's suggestion: he was a great believer in modern science in the service of mankind) wished to set an example to her subjects and ordered that the dairy cows on the Home Farm at Windsor should be tuberculin tested. It is unlikely that she understood

---

[4] Only a small proportion burnt themselves out and became favoured examination cases, as mentioned in Chapter 2.

[5] This epic achievement is recounted in suitably heroic language (reflected in the title) in Myers, J. A., *Man's Greatest Victory over Tuberculosis* (Baltimore, Maryland, 1940).

[6] Francis, J., *Bovine Tuberculosis* (London, 1947), p. 28.

what the procedure involved. She had regularly visited the establishment (as Prince Albert had done) and its cleanliness and yield of milk and dairy products were bywords at Berkshire agricultural shows. Presumably to her consternation – for once her exact utterances are not recorded – thirty-five of the forty cows were found to be tuberculin positive and even the five negative ones showed suspicious-looking lesions. It might be thought that this would have spurred on public-health authorities to try to eradicate the disease. More probably it subliminally reassured all those who owned or had to deal with tuberculous cattle: if the disease was so prevalent among the cosseted beasts of the Queen, it could surely do no harm to less privileged bovines.

In bovine as in human tuberculosis Koch's discovery was a landmark; but a few years later he caused great confusion about the various strains of his bacillus. At the International Medical Congress in London in 1901, he rightly insisted that the human and bovine strains were morphologically indistinguishable but biologically distinct and that the human strain could not be transmitted to cows; but he was woolly about the reverse transmission and hinted that it was in his opinion equally unlikely.[7] His intended pronouncement was communicated in advance to the English public-health contingent and an eminent and appalled deputation (which included Lord Lister, recently raised to the peerage) pleaded with him to elminate the ambiguous passage from his lecture. He would not budge – it is impossible not to admire his pigheadedness if he thought he was right; only he happened to be wrong – and the British experts had to move quickly. Not only was a Royal Commission set up to explore the question but, in an unprecedented move, it was charged with conducting its own research rather than simply collecting evidence from supposedly independent but usually biased witnesses. This was the high-point of the British effort on behalf of tuberculosis-free milk. The team of Royal Commissioners, Louis Cobbett, Arthur Eastwood, Frederick Griffith and Albert Stanley, were a capable and dedicated group who, in an interim report in 1904, demolished Koch's ambiguities. They showed that the bovine strain of tuberculosis was readily transmitted from cow to man (and to other animals like pigs) both in milk and in meat. They also called for urgent legislation to combat the menace. Shrugging off shrill and personalised criticism, they followed this up with further reports in 1907, 1910, 1913 and 1914, conclusively establishing the links between bovine

---

[7] He did not claim to have investigated the question in any depth, and merely expressed an opinion, but his authority in 1901 (even after the tuberculin fiasco) was such that his guesses were regarded as gospel. A little grudgingly a year later he accepted earlier evidence presented by Theobald Smith, in the *Journal of Experimental* Medicine, 3 (1898), 451,which proved that both the human and the bovine strains could cause disease in man.

tuberculosis, milk transmission and human disease. They emphasised that, in addition to gastrointestinal tuberculosis, the bovine strain was also responsible (at least in Britain) for a high proportion of the so-called surgical forms of the illness, especially for infections of the bones, joints, kidneys and bladder. The date of the last report, March 1914, was probably the last time when resolute government action could have stamped out the threat. It would have been justified not only by the evidence presented by the commission: by then the lessons from several other countries left no room for doubt.

It was not necessary to look to the United States, never a popular exemplar in Britain in matters of public health. (Then as now Americans were regarded by many of the British public health establishment as being besotted with the idea of an unlimited natural life-expectancy.) In Europe Denmark, a haven of common sense, had led the way. In the 1890s the powerful personality of Bernard Bang had bulldozed through Parliament the Danish Tuberculosis Act which provided for the compulsory tuberculin testing of herds and for the slaughter, against reasonable compensation by the state, of all tuberculous animals.[8] Remote Finland was next to act, then Saxony in Germany. Austria-Hungary had a pioneer in charge, Baron F. Korányi, and enacted several stringent laws between 1905 and 1910; but in a country where tyranny was traditionally tempered by *Schlamperei*, and where the word of Prince Eszterhazy on his own estate easily overrode any rule promulgated by the jumped-up bureaucrats in Vienna, the regulations were never enforced. Italy carried out an effective programme and Switzerland, home not only of sanatoria but also of the best milk chocolate in the world, could not afford to lag behind. By 1914 Belgium, France, Holland, Norway, Sweden and most states in Germany had more or less strict rules, as did, outside Europe, South Africa, New Zealand and most Canadian provinces. But not Britain.[9]

Perhaps legislation was doomed from the start. The opposition to preventative measures – most particularly to the elimination of the disease at source – did not have to collect scientific evidence. Of that there was none. What it needed was sound and fury. That it possessed in abundance. Bovine tuberculosis was so widespread and rural representation in both the main political parties so great and so overwhelmingly against legislation that a

[8] The Act left a small loop-hole. Cattle only "doubtfully" affected could be exported rather than slaughtered. It was widely rumoured in later years that British farmers took advantage of this and purchased many such animals at bargain prices.

[9] Only the Irish Free State in western Europe was to continue with a record as dismal as Britain's. There, under pressure from the farming lobby, even the least ambitious Clean Milk Bills were almost automatically shelved throughout the 1920s and 1930s.

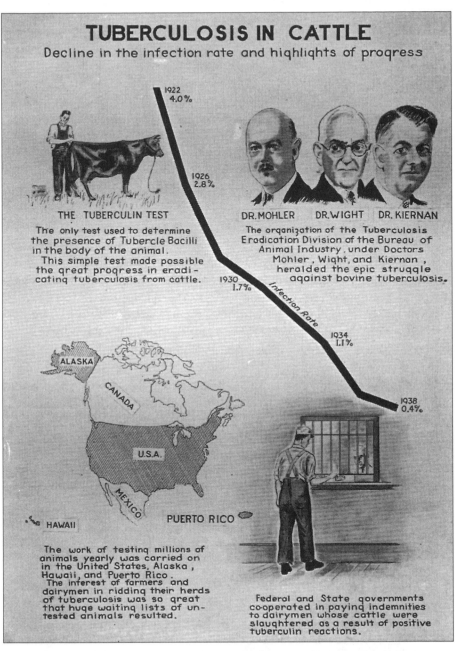

Tuberculosis in Cattle: A Success Story. Poster issued by the United States Federal Department of Health in 1939. The curve over the period 1922 to 1938 in Britain would have shown a steady *upward* rise.

change in policy would have been difficult to bring about. At the least it would have needed political skill and moral courage. Both were lacking. On the other side, every successful stalling operation increased the confidence of the farming lobby. There were successive Acts of Parliament designed to curb the transmission of contagious diseases of animal origin and the sale of infected meat and milk. All expressly excluded tuberculosis. Nobody asked why. The catchword was "voluntaryism", meaning nothing. When in Paisley in 1887, during a particularly virulent outbreak, some cattle owners voluntarily acceded to pleas from the local council to restrict the marketing of milk from obviously diseased animals, others lost no time in capturing the market with products from cows no less severely affected.[10]

The campaign for prevention was further weakened by divisions within the professions. By the turn of the century most academic veterinarians supported compulsory inspection, culling, pasteurisation and any other steps necessary to eliminate the disease; but in councils and committees they were regularly outvoted by veterinary surgeons in the field whose living depended on the goodwill and custom of farmers. Some influential medical voices were also raised in opposition to any kind of government action. Dr R. D. Powell, a textbook writer and pillar of wisdom at the Brompton Hospital, told the Royal Commission that there was no scientific *proof* that children acquired tuberculosis from drinking infected milk;[11] and Dr J. E. Goodhart of Guy's Hospital stated that his hospital never thought it necessary to take any special precautions about tuberculous milk, and never would so long as he had any say in the matter.[12] (Nobody could envisage a time when he would not.) Most bizarre was the calculation of Dr John Tatham of the Registrar-General's Office which purported to show that, although milk sellers in England and Wales had a significantly higher death-rate than other generally occupied males, they had a 10 per cent lower mortality from pulmonary phthisis (which was well known *not* to be caused by the milk-borne infection).[13] Buoyed up by the failure of the interventionists, the veterinary and farming lobby went on the offensive. It was spread around that doctors in Austria (never to be named) had shown that small doses of tubercle bacilli introduced in milk in infancy might actually enhance the resistance of babies to the more severe adolescent and adult infection.[14]

[10] Smith, F. B., *The Retreat of Tuberculosis, 1850–1950* (London, 1988), 178.

[11] Powell, R. D., Royal Commission Evidence (1904), vol. 46. He was asked (Question 1135) but did not deign to answer how such proof might be obtained.

[12] Goodhart, J. E., ibid. (Question 1405).

[13] Tatham, J., Registrar General Reports, Supplement to Volume 55 (1897), 45.

[14] Dr Clive Riviere in England was the chief advocate of the drinking of "slightly" tuberculous milk as a prophylactic, Riviere, C., *Tuberculosis and How to Avoid It* (London, 1917). Despite

By 1914 it was possible to buy certified milk in many of the more prosperous suburbs of the big cities of England; but a pint was 1d. (nearly 25 per cent) dearer than ordinary grocer's milk and its sales in terms of overall milk consumption remained negligible. The 1913 Tuberculosis Order had compelled dairy farmers to keep milk from tuberculous and non-tuberculous cattle separately; but there was nothing to stop them from selling both. The more stringent Milk and Dairies Bill of 1915, which would have given local authorities some control over notification and labelling, was passed without much debate but was immediately suspended. It was withdrawn in 1917 in view of wartime stringencies. In the same year Lord Astor, true perhaps to his partly-American ancestry, founded the National Clean Milk Society and started a campaign in his newspaper, the *Observer*, for a Milk Act. When the unpatriotic nature of such a campaign was pointed out to him, he correctly responded that the number of infant deaths at home in 1914/15 was twice as high as the number of those killed in action at the Front. The argument cut no ice and, even in a good cause, did not perhaps deserve to.

What made the milk saga even more indefensible than failure to legislate against tuberculous meat and meat products was the availability of pasteurisation. The heating of milk to between 60–80 degrees centigrade for about twenty minutes followed by quick cooling was named in honour of Pasteur in the 1890s – he had used a somewhat similar procedure in the course of his work on fermentation – and was not the whole or even the principal answer to bovine tuberculosis.[15] It was nevertheless better than nothing and, combined with other preventative measures, *much* better than nothing. It might be thought that the war would have made it popular since, coincidentally to its action on organisms, pasteurisation also helped to preserve milk. The war had in fact the opposite effect. Rebellious miners and restive factory workers were headaches enough; the government had no taste for taking on the farmers as well. The overriding aim of farmers themselves was to ward off, for as long as possible, all government interference and regulation. Nor were farmers alone in their opposition. Dr R. Stenhouse Williams, Research Professor of Dairy Bacteriology at Reading University, expressed his grave concern that pasteurisation would diminish the social standing of

official denials, he had a sizeable following, big enough to prompt the Tuberculin Committee of the Medical Research Council to write to the Ministry of Health as late as 1926, deprecating the suggestion "current in some quarters" that children who drank milk containing tubercle bacilli benefited in some way by developing immunity.

[15] The essential idea was to heat liquids to below their boiling point for a sufficient length of time to kill bacteria without destroying the liquid's appearance, flavour and nutritive value. Quick cooling after the critical period was important mainly to deal with spore-bearing organisms.

veterinarians. He also suggested that it was an ineffective last resort which would abet lazy handlers of dirty milk. His experiments with rats, designed to show that pasteurisation also reduced the nutritive value of milk, were inept and soon demolished;[16] but his argument that "if you pasteurise on a large scale you destroy the whole incentive to produce healthy milk", however fatuous, could not be disproved. Sir Robert Philip, too, was determined in his opposition (as he was by then to all measures not initiated by himself). Not only did he maintain that pasteurisation significantly diminished the nutritive value of milk, but, more importantly, "it would help to whitewash dirtiness and mess and encourage at every turn slackness on the part of the producer".[17]

Such pronouncements by the highest authorities in the land could not but encourage politicians. W. K. Glossop, a farmers' MP, told the House of Commons that it was a scientific fact that the pasteurisation of milk induced rapid tooth decay;[18] and Dr Halliday Sutherland, a tuberculosis specialist, gave his weighty support to Brigadier Sir Arnold Willson who had no doubt that "such typical French meddling with wholesome natural food" threatened British national strength and fertility. The National Association for the Prevention of Tuberculosis, dominated by Philip, discussed the procedure formally only once (in response to one of the rare lay revolts in 1931) and then dismissed it as useless. The editor of the *British Medical Journal* reported that "in the general discussion compulsory pasteurisation made its usual facile and transient appearance".

Not surprisingly, when the thoroughly emasculated Milk Act was finally passed in 1925, it made little difference. Responsibility for reporting tuberculous cattle remained with the farmers and the local veterinary surgeons, and farmers saw no point in ridding themselves of positive reactors early. (There was always something to be gained from waiting: the more emaciated the slaughtered animal, the better value the compensation represented.) The incentives to produce higher-grade milk were also slight. Even to owners of large herds, threepence a gallon extra for Grade A milk barely covered the £8 a year it cost to test a cow; and with herds of less than fifty, the majority in Britain, the proposition made no economic sense. There were always loopholes, perhaps deliberate, and often wilful sabotage in Whitehall and Westminster. A wheeze British farmers learnt from their French *confrères* was to inject valuable cows with tuberculin shortly before the arrival of the officially appointed tester: properly timed this was guaranteed to render the

---

[16] Which it does not (as had been abundantly shown), though it may affect some micronutrients like vitamins.

[17] Philip, R., *Edinburgh Medical Journal*, 22 (1925), 100.

[18] Glossop, C. W. K., *Parliamentary Debates* (1932), vol. 273, col. 906.

animal negative to the subcutaneous test carried out by the official. The practice was well-known and could have been stopped simply by adding tuberculin to the long list of on-prescription-only preparations included in the Therapeutic Substances Act of 1925: this would have made access to it more difficult. But before the Act was passed tuberculin was deleted from the draft. There was no debate and no explanation.

In the late 1920s, when Stanley Griffith began to publish his researches into human tuberculosis, his results relating to the bovine organism were particularly depressing. Not only did the strain account for nearly half of all cases of all human tuberculous lymph-node and skin disease, and about a third of other non-pulmonary forms of the illness, but the proportion was particularly high in children under ten; and while the incidence of pulmonary tuberculosis was by then once again slowly declining, the incidence of in-fections with the bovine strain remained constant.[19] Griffith's findings were described as a slur on the competence of the veterinary profession and he was accused of seeking personal publicity. As late as 1938 the government-sponsored Milk Industry Bill, a relatively modest assortment of preventative measures which would have enabled (not compelled) local authorities to impose pasteurisation, was defeated in the House of Commons at its first reading.

Two social changes, neither related to public concern about prevention, slightly mitigated this disastrous record. As the Depression deepened in the 1930s, children in the worst-hit parts of the country consumed hardly any milk because their families could not afford it. This may have been the explanation for the apparent dip in the incidence of surgical (mostly bone and joint) tuberculosis on Tyneside around 1934–35. With the introduction in 1937 of the school milk scheme – it always used the cheapest surplus milk available – the trend was quickly reversed.

Between the world wars there was also a spectacular increase in the use of dried milk, from about half a kilo per head per year in 1909 to about nine kilos. There were several reasons for this. The powder was relatively cheap, it could be stored, it had a guaranteed nutritive value and it was nearly sterile. (It remained so during reconstitution since it was easiest to use boiling water.) Many general practitioners vigorously promoted it because it was responsible for a fall in the incidence of summer diarrhoea. (Some of course regarded it as the last straw in unnatural practices, akin to incest.) An unintended side-effect of the success of the powder was to frighten the big

---

[19] His findings in fact understated the problem since he carried out most of his surveys in Cambridgeshire. The incidence of bovine tuberculosis in many other parts of Britain, notably in Scotland, was always three or four times higher.

dairy companies – United, Sterilised Milk and ABC among them – into adopting pasteurisation. The object was to give their milk twenty-four-hour life, not to eliminate tuberculosis; nor did it. But it was, to use a cherished civil service cliché, a step in the right direction. The basic requirements of pasteurisation (which involved a considerable outlay in plant as well as a small increase in skilled staff) were not standardised until after the Second World War: 7–10 per cent of "pasteurised" milk sold in London in 1946 still contained live tubercle bacilli.

In 1922 Dr Alex MacLennan told the General Meeting of the British Medical Association what many – probably most – of his colleagues already knew, that the present treatment of milk in Britain was a disgrace. Almost a quarter century later Dr E. R. Boland of Guy's Hospital, known for his tact and moderation, put it only marginally differently:

> It is amazing that this country which claims, and I believe claims rightly, to be a pioneer and a leader in hygiene and preventive medicine should so much lag behind other countries in the enforcement of the life-saving measure of compulsory pasteurisation of all non-tuberculosis-tested milk and indeed of all other preventive measures against milk-borne infection as recommended for years by all experts and medical authorities.[20]

But the record shows that the experts and medical authorities were far from blameless. They rarely are.

[20] Boland, E. R., *British Medical Journal* (1946), no. 2, 16.

30

Vaccines

The battles fought over the second preventative measure of the interwar years were no less fierce; but the rights and wrongs were more evenly balanced. Though the tuberculin debacle had made doctors wary of vaccines,[1] the concept of prophylactic treatment by vaccination remained immensely attractive, and the hope that something better would turn up was never abandoned. Nor was there ever any shortage of candidates. Some were totally innocuous, though without benefit or even aspiring to a rationale. Friedmann Vaccine was prepared from a culture of mycobacteria (remotely related to the *Mycobacterium tuberculosis*) isolated from the turtle. It was exotic and expensive enough to win followers and had particularly strong support in Germany and in Friedmann's native Hungary. In 1934 the *Lancet* exposed the bogus claims made for it;[2] but it was still being sold (and, more remarkably, bought) in the 1950s. In 1920 Carl Spengler of Davos began to advertise his IK – for *Immunkorper* – serum allegedly prepared from the red blood cells of rabbits which had been injected with both human and bovine tuberculosis and which supposedly retained the toxins secreted by the bacilli. (What toxins? None had ever been identified – but that did not worry Spengler.) These, when injected into humans, were supposed to have both a preventative and restorative action. Perhaps it was the magic name of Davos; but IK vaccine had a strong following in England where its devotees, including some fringe medical practitioners, claimed a 100 per cent cure rate in Stages One and Two of the disease.

Other methods were more reputable but also more dangerous. The low

---

[1] Tuberculin was never in fact completely abandoned, though after 1941 it was largely replaced by the safer and more easily standardised Purified Protein Derivative (PPD), prepared by Esmond R. Long and Florence Seibert of Philadelphia. As late as the 1950s this was tried in combination with streptomycin in the treatment of tuberculous meningitis.

For this chapter, as a whole, see Calmette, A., *The Tubercle Bacillus, Infection and Tuberculosis in Man and Animals*, translated by W. B. Soper and G. H. Smith (Baltimore, Maryland, 1925); Calmette, A., *L'infection bacillaire et la tuberculose* (4th edn, Paris, 1936); Irvine, K. N., *BCG Vaccination in Theory and Practice* (Oxford, 1949); Moore, D. F., "The History and Development of BCG", *Practitioner*, 227 (1983), 317; Rosenthal, R. R., *BCG Vaccination* (Boston, 1957).

[2] Young, R. A., *Lancet* (1924), no. 1, 483.

virulence of the human bacillus in cattle suggested that cows might be safely immunised with living human cultures and would thereafter remain immune to the bovine strain as well. Koch himself performed a few experiments along these lines and expressed himself hopeful; and in 1900 Emil von Behring of diphtheria vaccination fame confidently forecast that Bovo Vaccine would entirely eradicate bovine tuberculosis and with it the menace of the milk-borne infection to man. Unfortunately, it was soon – but probably not quite soon enough – discovered that, though human bacilli did not cause tuber-culosis in cattle and might even protect cattle against the bovine organism, the inoculated human bacilli could and did survive for months and perhaps years and could appear in viable and virulent form in the milk of the vaccinated animals.[3]

Attenuation was the aim of Trudeau, who did pioneering work in his primitive laboratory in Saranac Lake which nobody took seriously. (He was too nice a man and too highly regarded as a doctor to be taken seriously as a scientist.) Yet, insofar as there was a right vaccine track, he was on it. The two workers who carried attenuation past the critical divide between bright hope and hard practice were a French bacteriologist, Albert Calmette, and his assistant and later colleague, Camille Guérin, a veterinarian. Like most medical advances, their discovery stemmed from an accidental observation. In 1908, working at the Pasteur Institute in Lille,[4] their daily routine entailed the subculturing of virulent strains of the tuberculosis bacillus. (To keep an organism, as any cell culture, alive it is usually necessary to subculture it at regular intervals.) They were also testing a wide range of different media to see which were the most suitable for keeping the organism virulent during harvesting and transfer.[5] One which was *not* suitable was a glycerin-bile-potato mixture: after every transfer using the medium the bacillus seemed to become slightly less robust. This was unusual. As many of the world's leading bacteriologists were discovering at the time, subculturing tended either to kill the organism or to leave it unchanged.

After some hesitation, Calmette then decided to change the course of his research – easier then than it would be today – and instead of trying to find the best medium for subculturing the organism, a necessary but somewhat humdrum task, he determined to see if repeated subculturing in the unfavourable glycerin-bile-potato mixture might eventually produce a strain

[3] The appearance of human-strain bacilli in the milk of vaccinated cattle was never admitted in print but widely believed and probably true.

[4] They transferred to the Paris Institute in 1919.

[5] One technical problem of working with cultures was the dispersion of the organisms picked up as viscous blobs from the semi-solid culture media into watery saline solutions suitable for injection into experimental animals.

sufficiently attenuated to be considered for use as a vaccine. Fortunately, as he was later to recount, he had no conception of how long this would take or of how many other groups were working toward the same end at the same time. Fortunately, too, every repeated subculture did produce a small but definite attenuation. At the start of the project the organism was so virulent that three milligrammes of a standard suspension injected into a calf would result in the animal's death within thirty days. After seventy subcultures the virulence of the strain was so far diminished that calves would tolerate the injection of a hundred milligrammes without ill-effects. Throughout the First World War, even during the German occupation of Lille, the grind of regular subculturing continued;[6] by 1919, the organism was incapable of producing tuberculosis in guinea-pigs, rabbits, horses and cattle. In 1921 Calmette declared it to be a *virus fixe*, that is a new strain of the tuberculosis bacillus which would breed true to type in all circumstances. He named it Bacille Calmette-Guérin soon abbreviated to BCG.

This was of course only the first step. Not only was it essential that the claim should be confirmed by independent workers, some of them rivals, but it also had to be shown that the new strain, though non-virulent, conferred immunity to the disease. Both the political climate of the postwar years and Calmette's personality promised a stormy passage. In his own country he was immediately hailed as a new Pasteur or, at any rate, a second Villemin – and this time there would be no snatching away of French glory by foreigners. He was well fitted for the role: a native of Nice and a former naval officer, he was intensely patriotic, bearded, excitable, charming, single-minded and hard-working. He was also meticulous where he felt that meticulous work was needed; but, like Pasteur, he was contemptuous of what he considered to be obstructive pedantries. Almost all forms of statistical analysis when applied to medicine qualified under this heading. Nor did he have any patience with abstract ethical concepts, an obsessive preoccupation of Protestant minds: his professional conscience and Catholic faith were adequate guides to what was right and wrong. None of this was calculated to make him universally popular.

Even before his public announcement one of his clinical colleagues,

---

[6] The Germans did not interfere with the working of the institute; but the occupation imposed great hardships. Apart from the physical shortages of fuel, food and chemical reagents, the Calmettes were cut off from their sons who were serving in the French army; and in 1918 Mme Calmette was one of twenty prominent citizens or their spouses who were taken hostages by the German military authorities and transported to an internment camp in Germany. This, by Second World War standards, was luxurious and the inmates were released shortly before the Armistice; but they could not communicate with home and the anxiety experienced by Calmette was acute.

B. Weill-Hallé, implored him to be allowed to administer the oral vaccine to a newborn boy whose mother had died from overwhelming tuberculosis a few days after delivery. The baby was now in the care of a grandmother, also openly tuberculous. (An elder brother and a sister were also affected and at least one sibling had already died of consumption.) No precautions had been taken during the birth, and nobody doubted that the infant would perish within a few weeks. The vaccine was administered and after six months the boy (still in the grandmother's care) was thriving. Largely – according to some entirely – based on this gratifying but as scientific proof astonishingly slender evidence, a major immunisation programme was launched; and by 1928 over 116,000 infants born in France had been given the vaccine.

Outside France enthusiasm was tempered with varying degrees of scepticism. Some of France's political allies, including Romania, accepted Calmette's claims without reservation. Denmark, Sweden, Norway and Italy also embarked on cautious trials. But among *les Anglo-Saxons* (whose approval Calmette valued highly) and especially in Britain the apparent lack of anything that might be described as a controlled trial, and perhaps an almost atavistic mistrust of Gallic fireworks, elicited a chorus of humming and haaing. While of course it was – in the British tradition – a muted chorus, much behind the scenes activity enlivened the 1925 Tuberculosis Conference which hovered a little uneasily on the fringes of the Wembley Empire Exhibition. Public-health representatives from Australia and New Zealand were pressing A. S. (later Sir Arthur) McNalty of the Ministry of Health to give a lead in accepting Calmette's recommendation of mass vaccination.[7] Reluctant to try the French vaccine on their own responsibility, they were nevertheless impressed with recently published claims: no mortality among 2070 newborn babies of tuberculous mothers vaccinated during 1924, compared to a tuberculous death-rate of one in four among an unstated number of unvaccinated infants of a similar background. McNalty, a paragon among medical civil servants, offered to consult the top echelon of Britain's tuberculosis specialists: on a matter of such importance for the future of the Empire nothing but the best would do. The verdict of the authorities was unanimous. They were unsparing in their praise for Professor Calmette's enthusiasm. In case the Australians and New Zealanders missed the significance of this, McNalty spelt it out in a private memorandum. The recommendation of the top echelon was an indefinite wait-and-see policy.[8]

---

[7] McNalty, A. S., Draft to High Commissioner for New Zealand, 7 April 1925, PRO, MH55/150.

[8] Both Australia and New Zealand backed off and, like Britain, did not adopt BCG until after the streptomycin revolution of the late 1940s.

They had some grounds for unease. Calmette's dislike of statistics did not stop him from producing calculations of mind-boggling complexity; and the dividing line between fact and expectation was not always drawn with un-compromising rigour.[9] When pressed it soon transpired that of the 2070 infants saved he had actually traced only 423: in the rest he had simply gravely impressed on the mothers the need to report the death of their infants should such a sad event occur. Nor was the death rate of one in four among the unvaccinated above suspicion: as Z. P. Fernandez of Leeds, an authority in the field, pointed out, tuberculosis was difficult enough to diagnose post mortem in infants under twelve months; it was virtually impossible to es-tablish with certainty as the *cause* of death. Calmette riposted with a fresh cataract of figures and several alarming miscalculations. When the latter were pointed out to him, he blamed his foreign postgraduate assistants who had since, he reported, been reprimanded, sent home or taught to add up. A devastating attack on him was then mounted by Major Greenwood, professor of epidemiology in the University of London and statistical assistant to Marcus Paterson of Frimley Sanatorium (one of McNalty's top echelon) and the Ministry of Health. After enumerating a long list of statistical errors in Calmette's paper, he suggested that the author

> having deliberately appealed to the statistical method, has, in my submission, shown himself so grossly defective in that method that no confidence can be placed either in his statistical inferences or in the reliability of the data which he has assembled. Since, moreover, the design of an experiment is as delicate a business as the analysis of the results, a writer who shows so little respect for logic in analysis is not likely to have been been more circumspect in his practical work.[10]

This headmasterly rebuke was no less outrageous than were Calmette's gimcrack statistics: Greenwood had no evidence which could justify him casting aspersions on Calmette's experimental work. That was in fact exem-plary. But as if on cue came another publication, this time from the United States, which seemed to vindicate the doubters. A group of investigators in Trudeau's laboratory in Saranac Lake claimed to have grown virulent variants from three separate cultures of BCG, two of which had been supplied by Calmette himself.[11] This was a bruising allegation, casting doubt on Calmette's claim that his strain was a *virus fixe*. He reacted violently. The leader of the American group, S. A. Petroff, was not only incompetent and a liar, he

[9] Calmette, A., *Lancet* (1931), no. 1, 1299. He and later his disciples never got their statistics right. Even the figures published in the 1936 edition of his book are impenetrable: others are at best implausible.

[10] Greenwood, M., *British Medical Journal* (1928), no. 1, 793.

[11] Petroff, S. A., Branch, A., Steenken, W., *American Review of Tuberculosis*, 19 (1929), 9.

declared to assembled journalists in Paris, but also a defeated rival consumed by envy. On balance he was probably right. Reviewing the evidence in 1949, J. B. McDougall found it impossible to exclude several possible sources of error in the American work; and "many workers who tried to follow exactly the technique of Petroff and his group failed to establish any degree of potential or latent virulence".[12]

By 1928 the debate had blossomed into an international political issue. Under pressure from the French government (in the avuncular shape of Aristide Briand, a friend and admirer of Calmette's) *le BCG* was adopted by the Health Committee of the League of Nations and an international conference was convened for its formal launch. This put Whitehall in a quandary. Officials at the Ministry of Health wanted the United Kingdom to be represented by experts armed with secret statistical evidence to blow the French claims sky-high and approached the Medical Research Council to provide the ammunition. In their tiresome way the Council refused. It was not that they believed Calmette's claims: his statistics, one member stated, were totally up the creek. But so had been Pasteur's; and he had been right despite his miscalculations. Besides, thanks largely to the Ministry's parsimony, the Council had not had the opportunity to investigate the vaccine and produce contrary evidence. At the recommendation of Sir George Buchanan, Chief Medical Officer to the Ministry, the British Government then declined the invitation to attend the meeting on the grounds that all their medical experts were engaged on other, more essential tasks.[13] To the annoyance of Sir Robert Philip, who attended in a purely personal capacity but was cut short in mid-oration, this ensured that the conference was a resounding success. Calmette's claims were endorsed by Alberto Ascoli, a respected public-health figure from Italy, and early results from Scandinavia were encouraging. Of course there were dissenting voices; but the Americans (not members of the League) were surprisingly restrained. In any case bickerings were soon overshadowed by disaster.

Weimar Germany was one of the countries outside France where BCG vaccination was taken up with enthusiasm and where several groups were at work trying to improve it. Such a trial was probably at the root of the tragedy. The details of what happened between February and April 1930, in the Municipal Children's Hospital in Lübeck, are still uncertain, but the main events are stark. Over a two-months period 249 babies in the first ten days of life were given the oral BCG vaccine – or what should have been the oral BCG vaccine. By mid April the babies vaccinated in February began

---

[12] McDougall, J. B., *Tuberculosis: A Global Study in Social Pathology* (Edinburgh, 1950), p. 354.
[13] Buchanan, G., 11 October 1928, PRO, MH 55/150.

to die from overwhelming tuberculosis. By June, despite frantic efforts to save them, sixty-seven were dead and another eighty were gravely ill. There were to be at least another twenty deaths. It is possible that not more than one or two of the babies survived, but on April 30 the government imposed an embargo on further official information. This proved to be a terrible mistake. The continuing deaths could not be denied: silence merely swelled the numbers of those rumoured to have already succumbed. By May the attempted cover-up had begun. One senior physician later admitted that he had destroyed the hospital's vaccine stores. Piles of crucial notes and records suddenly got lost. The fact had transpired early and could not later be denied that some of the medical staff had been engaged in unauthorised research with virulent human bacilli. Authorised or unauthorised by whom? There was at that time no person or body to grant or withhold such authority. The situation was the same in other municipal hospitals in Germany – and probably in other countries.[14]

As the nightmare days dragged on and the death toll mounted, advocates of BCG both in Germany and in France were shattered but also mystified. It had to be a horrible mistake. Enemies of the vaccination programme, a motley bunch, were not slow to proclaim that their apocalyptic predictions had been justified. On 1 May the German government instituted what they promised to be a rigorous enquiry under the chairmanship of two respected experts, Professor Ludwig Lange and Professor Bruno Lange.[15] At the same time they invited other German (but not foreign) scientists and doctors to give evidence about their experience. Despite crass attempts by some of the hospital staff to delay or misdirect the enquiry, the panel quickly exonerated the BCG vaccine as such. Either the hospital supply had been contaminated with highly virulent bacilli or there had been an accidental but actual substitution. Cultures of virulent organisms had been sent to Lübeck apparently for research purposes by the Robert Koch Institute in Kiel, correctly (though not perhaps optimally) labelled and sealed. After arrival the boxes had been opened and vials and plates had been stored in the same incubator as the hospital's store of vaccines. This was such a horrifying breech of elementary safety precautions that several members of the hospital staff were arrested.

The trial of three doctors and a nurse began in the late summer of 1931. It proceeded against a backdrop of mounting political turmoil and violence – and became part of it. The Weimar Republic was tottering: nobody expected it to survive for more than a few months. The only question was who and

---

[14] In Britain ethical committees did not begin to operate in hospitals – and then only on a voluntary basis – until the 1960s.

[15] No relations.

what would take its place. Outside the courthouse Nazi brownshirts and the Communists workers' brigades paraded and clashed. On three successive days the sittings had to be suspended for fear of the building being invaded. To the party presses the case was heaven-sent ammunition. In the Nazi *Stürmer* the French vaccine became the symbol of accursed Versailles. The accused were the scapegoats of a spineless and morally bankrupt system. Ironically, the Communist *Rote Fahne* too was outraged, especially when it transpired that the nurse was the close friend of a prominent Communist deputy. To it the real culprit was International Capitalism, trying to exploit the desperation and hopes of the sick. (Some of the Lübeck research may have been funded by the German pharmaceutical industry, another mystery never cleared up.) What happened inside the courtroom was later described by an American journalist as an Expressionist spectacle. Grieving and crying parents filled the galleries and could not be ejected. Witnesses screamed. Obscure and mysterious Bulgarian and Hungarian experts emerged recounting in vivid detail similar catastrophes in their own countries. These were later authoritatively denied.[16] (But the witnesses were no longer available to be recalled.) Calmette's anguished demands to be heard were rebuffed, apparently on direct orders from Brüning, the embattled Chancellor.[17] If Brüning did give the order, it did him no good: the case became another nail in the coffin of his government.

One of the most depressing aspect of the proceedings – for nothing could bring back the dead babies – was its futility. No new facts came to light about the value, limitations and possible risks of BCG.[18] No lessons were learnt about the dangers of experimentation in hospitals. Another outcome was that, though BCG was officially exonerated, opponents of vaccination now felt justified in demanding its total rejection. They nearly succeeded. All work on it stopped in Germany and later in countries under Germany's

[16] A disaster like the Lübeck one, though on a smaller scale, may have occurred in Chile; and in 1930 there were certainly some deaths following BCG vaccination in Ujpest in Hungary.

[17] In private life Brüning was a high-minded and a devout Catholic and his backstairs intervention seems unlikely; but he was also desperately courting the Nationalist vote, a doomed hope. It is impossible to say how far the trial influenced the outcome of the elections of 1932 – historians of the period, defeated perhaps by the complexities of the case and the lies which still encrust it, barely refer to it. But it is clear from the contemporary German press that it helped to discredit the Weimar regime and fuelled both extreme Nationalist and Communist propaganda. F. B. Smith plausibly suggests, in *The Retreat of Tuberculosis, 1850–1950* (London, 1988), that the full truth about the disaster has still not come to light while many misleading stories continue to be published.

[18] Calmette, A., *Presse médicale*, 2 (1931), 17. His health was broken by the crisis and he died in 1935 at the age of fifty-six. Guérin, his quiet and self-effacing colleague, survived him by twenty-five years to be internationally honoured in his last years.

sway. In Britain considerable pressure was exerted behind the scenes on those who, in the prevailing atmosphere of all too justified despair, might still want to know the truth. The 1931 annual meeting of the National Association for Prevention of Tuberculosis was virtually devoted to its rejection. Top consultants like L. S. T. Burrell explained in spurious scientific detail why the vaccine could not conceivably build up resistance. Sir Robert Philip and his collaborator, Edith McGraw,[19] claimed to have followed the BCG debate with sympathy and to have "sifted the evidence with the utmost care". Alas, they felt constrained to express the view that "there remain grounds for great hesitancy [because] introduction of the vaccine may not always be harmless ... though before this large audience it is unnecessary to go into details". (In the wake of Lübeck one can almost sense the frisson induced by the innuendo.) They preferred the "national communal effort (over which Sir Robert had presided with such distinction over the past thirty years) to continue".[20] Sir Henry Gauvain also preferred his own well-tried regime of prolonged immobilisation, sunlight and vitamins. A Ministry of Health memorandum characteristically praised the undoubted effectiveness of Monsieur Calmette's vaccine *in calves*. Officially the policy remained one of an open mind. In reality, BCG was banned from Britain until 1947. Then, in the face of a nursing crisis which threatened all sanatoria and many hospitals with immediate closure, it was permitted so as "to comfort and give hope to sanatorium nurses".

American rejection was more patchy but in many states even more resolute and longer lasting. Though in tuberculosis-ridden Quebec BCG led to a striking fall in tuberculosis mortality,[21] government bodies both in the United States and in English-speaking Canada turned down repeated suggestions of a controlled trial. Not until after the war – in 1946 – was the vaccine tried on Indian people with impressive results; but an almost obsessive hostility persisted in many centres in the United States till the 1970s.[22]

Fortunately, work on the vaccine continued after Lübeck in some countries. Arvid Wallgren in Gothenburg in Sweden pressed on with the follow-up of a high-risk group of new-born infants and showed that after seven years only one out of 355 had developed tuberculosis. No less important was his establishment of the still current intradermal method of administration: it

---

[19] His future second wife.

[20] *Transactions of the NAPT*, 145 (1931), 8, and 89.

[21] Aronson, J. D., Palmer, C. E., *Public Health Reports: Washington DC*, 61 (1946), 802.

[22] R. Y. Keers recalls, in his book *Pulmonary Tuberculosis: A Journey down the Centuries* (London, 1978), attending a meeting on BCG in a Midwestern state in 1955. The president opened the proceedings by defining the vaccine as "a substance designed to give a false sense of security to a man with an unwarranted fear of tuberculosis".

was more effective than the oral route and less prone than subcutaneous injections to local complications. His results eventually demonstrated that the vaccine gave no absolute immunity but that it significantly increased natural resistance: BCG-vaccinated children developed primary tuberculosis four to ten times less often and pulmonary tuberculosis Stage Three two to three times less often than unvaccinated ones.[23] Neither in his series nor in K. A. Jensen's in Denmark was there a single case of tuberculous meningitis or miliary tuberculosis among the vaccinated children.[24] In Ulleval Hospital in Norway, Johannes Heimbeck reported good results in a small but well-controlled trial on probationer nurses.[25]

The full potential of these studies did not emerge until the end of the Second World War. The fighting had hardly stopped when central and eastern Europe faced an upsurge of tuberculosis more devastating than anything seen before. The disease was erupting not only among the millions of displaced persons living in former concentration camps and army barracks but also in the burnt-out and starving cities. The nightmare scenario never became reality. Relief work was begun by the Danish Red Cross as soon as hostilities had ended: other organisations soon joined in. Between 1945 and 1948 what eventually became the International Tuberculosis Campaign (familiarly known as Joint Enterprises) vaccinated over eight million babies and children in Austria, Czechoslovakia, Finland, Greece, Hungary, Italy, Poland and Yugoslavia. This was not a controlled trial and it is impossible to say how effective the campaign was. Later experience showed that protection by BCG varies widely between populations, depending on past history and the state of immunity as well as the method and dosage of administration. Yet few doubted at the time that hundreds of thousands of young lives were saved.[26]

Partly in the light of the work of Joint Enterprises, witnessed in occupied Germany and Austria by a new and less blinkered generation of doctors completing their wartime or national service, the National Association for Protection against Tuberculosis in Britain took the revolutionary step in 1949 of inviting Scandinavian workers to tell them something about their experience. Wallgren confirmed his published results and concluded: "BCG helps, it is harmless and it is cheap. Why not try it?" Why not indeed? A few months later the first trial sponsored by the Medical Research Council began under the direction of Dr. P. D'Arcy Hart. After four years the panel reported

[23] Wallgren, A., *Transactions of the NAPT* (1949), pp. 249, 267.

[24] Jensen, K. A., ibid., p. 67.

[25] Heimbeck, J., *Tubercle*, 18 (1936), 97.

[26] International Tuberculosis Campaign. Conference on European BCG Programme, Copenhagen, 1949.

on 56,000 children. The unvaccinated showed a pulmonary tuberculosis rate of 1.94 per thousand while in the BCG group the rate was 0.37 per thousand. No child in the BCG group had developed tuberculous meningitis or miliary tuberculosis. Six had in the unvaccinated group.[27] By then even ardent advocates of BCG agreed that much still remained to be unravelled, and that vaccination was not the whole answer to a global problem. The urgency too had been removed by chemotherapy – or so it seemed at the time. The human cost of the lost decades was of course non-returnable. Reviewing "Fifty Years of BCG" in 1971 the editor of *Tubercle* concluded that "future historians will find the story a strange mixture of endeavour, inertia and ineptitude".[28] This was, in the view of one future historian, a charitable understatement.

[27] Medical Research Council Report, *Tubercle*, 37 (1956), 142.
[28] Ibid., 53 (1971), 303.

31

The Surgeon Cometh

In 1921 Sir James Kingston Fowler, a leading authority in British chest medicine (meaning in his day pulmonary tuberculosis), stated that he "had lived to see two real advances in his speciality. One [was] the sanatorium regime. The other [was] the artificial pneumothorax".[1] Twenty-eight years later Gösta Birath of Sweden wrote one of the last comprehensive reviews of the latter. "The pneumothorax needle", he concluded, "was the most dangerous weapon ever placed in the hands of a physician."[2] The two pronouncements signpost the trajectory not only of AP but also of tuberculosis surgery in general.

Typical of the optimism – but also of the confusion – of the early 1920s was a report which the Medical Research Council asked L. S. T. Burrell of the Brompton Hospital and A. S. McNalty of the Ministry of Health to prepare for them. The two-man team interviewed sixteen prominent physicians, all associated with old-established hospitals and sanatoria, about their experience. The experts were unanimous in describing the artificial pneumothorax as a notable advance – but that was the only point on which they agreed. Three saw it solely as a palliative measure for far advanced cases; four would reserve it for early stages (one declaring that no case in his opinion was too early); and the rest assumed more or less intermediate positions. All recognised the problems presented by pleural adhesions but no two agreed on how best to deal with them. Nor could they reach a consensus about the incidence of complications, such as pleural effusions and infection. Perhaps (as often happens in such polls) the most telling point was made not in answer to a question but in an addendum written by Dr Claude Lillingston: "The wide differences in the results achieved at different

---

[1] Quoted by R. Y. Keers, *Pulmonary Tuberculosis: A Journey down the Centuries* (London, 1978), p. 56. For this chapter, as a whole, see Alexander, J., *The Collapse Therapy of Pulmonary Tuberculosis* (Springfield, Illinois, 1937); Burrell, L. S. T., *Artificial Pneumothorax* (3rd edn, London, 1937); Heaf, F. R. G. (ed.), *Symposium on Tuberculosis* (London, 1957); Jones, J. C., *The Surgical Management of Tuberculosis* (Springfield, Illinois, 1957); Packard, E. N., Hayes, J. N., Blanchet, S. F., *The Artificial Pneumothorax* (London, 1940); Sauerbruch, F., *A Surgeon's Life*, translated by G. Renier and A. Cliff (London, 1953).

[2] Birath, G., *Diseases of the Chest*, 35 (1949), 1.

institutions are almost completely to be explained by the differences in the skill and conscientiousness of the physician in charge." [3] Add surgeon to physician and the validity of this point was to become increasingly apparent.

The natural history of surgical advances (and the artificial pneumothorax must be classified as a surgical advance even when carried out by physicians) tends to follow a fairly predictable pattern. There is always an initial period of general doubt, the bolder the proposed intervention, the more forcefully expressed. This may turn into bubbling enthusiasm, the feasibility of the operation suddenly becoming an adequate, indeed often the main, indication for its performance. Lastly, reason may reassert itself and the proper scope of the procedure (if any) may gradually become defined. In the case of surgical collapse therapy the second phase was unusually prolonged.

An important reason for this was the comparatively slow recognition of two facts. First, the division of adhesions, when present, between the pleural layers was an essential precondition of a successful pneumothorax. Secondly, when the adhesions were so widespread that the pleural layers could not be separated, attempts at inducing it were better abandoned. Unfortunately, it was bad enough for a patient's morale to suggest that his or her case was unsuitable for artificial pneumothorax: to attempt and then to abandon the procedure was desolation. Nor was failure readily accepted by professional colleagues. Textbooks hinted that the indivisibility of adhesions often reflected the inexperience or incompetence of the surgeon. Only recognised experts – and there were always too few of them – were allowed to admit defeat.

By the early 1930s artificial pneumothoraces were being performed, often by incompetent operators, in tens of thousands of unsuitable cases; and the results were predictably dismal. Yet the pressure to master the technique continued to grow throughout the decade: as an annual report from Preston Hall, proclaimed "no tuberculosis physician can pose as an expert in the field unless he has at his command the technique of the induction of the artificial pneumothorax". It might be thought that the patients themselves or their families would have rebelled; but the opposite was true. Almost anything active was better than just waiting and hoping. Not altogether surprisingly, when Bloch, Tucker and Adams reviewed 2100 papers published about artificial pneumothorax between 1929 and 1939, they found that only 4.7 per cent were in any way concerned with the results of the treatment.[4]

By 1939 the simple artificial pneumothorax was in any case *vieu jeu*. As

[3] Burrell, L. S. T., McNalty, A. S., *Report on Artificial Pneumothorax*, Medical Research Council Special Reports (London, 1922).

[4] Bloch, R. G., Tucker, W. B., Adams, W. E., *Journal of Thoracic Surgery*, 10 (1941), 310.

long ago as 1891 a French surgeon, Théodore Tuffier, had suggested that, instead of causing the collapse of the lung by filling the pleural space with air, a space could also be created and the underlying lung collapsed by stripping the parietal – that is the outer – pleural layer from the chest wall. The difficulty with such an extrapleural pneumothorax was that, unless the gap between the chest wall and the outer pleura was filled (or unless the underlying lung was hopelessly diseased in which case the procedure should never have been attempted in the first place), it was quickly obliterated by the re-expanding lung. Tuffier himself employed liquid fat as a filler,[5] but in 1913 G. Baer of Munich introduced the plombe, a solid lump of paraffin wax which, after warming, could be moulded into the required shape.[6] This procedure, known as plombage, was popular on the Continent but never liked in Britain or America: British surgeons in particular found the later extrusion of paraffin through a dehiscence of their lovingly sutured incisions a personal affront. From the patient's point of view infection of the extra-pleural space was the main bugbear when air was tried as the filling agent: bleeding into the space (sometimes fatal) was another. After a spell of experimentation with oil as a filler, a procedure known as oleothorax,[7] the final phase of Tuffier's invention was a reversion to the idea of plombage but using small spheres or sponges made of some inert plastic material like lucite.[8] The concept hobbled on till chemotherapy put an end to it not a day too soon.

Operations to paralyse the diaphragm were to play a more prominent and more prolonged therapeutic role. On the face of it the idea was both simple and logical. Much of the expansion of the lungs is due not to the movements of the chest wall but to the contraction of the diaphragm. This causes the muscle sheet to descend in inspiration, the lung expanding to fill the space. Emboldened by the early success of collapse therapy, several anatomically minded doctors suggested that if the diaphragm could be paralysed, more of the lung could be put out of action.[9] The idea seemed the more attractive since (for embryological reasons) the nerves supplying the diaphragm, known as the phrenic nerves, arise in the cervical region of the spinal cord and can easily be located at operation at the base of the neck. Unfortunately, the living body does not always follow the dictates of anatomy textbooks; and the division of the phrenic nerves in the neck revealed the frequent presence

[5] Tuffier, T., *Bulletin de la société des chirurgiens de Paris,* 49 (1923), 1249.

[6] Baer, G., *Münchener medizinische Wochenschrift,* 60 (1913), 1587.

[7] The results were awful: the procedure is worth mentioning only to illustrate the desperate straits to which physicians were reduced trying to make something unworkable work.

[8] Trent, J. C., Moody, J. D., Hiatt, J. S., *Journal of Thoracic Surgeons,* 18 (1951), 173.

[9] Felix, W., *Deutsche Zeitschrift der Chirurgie,* 171 (1922), 283.

of a hitherto unsuspected supplementary nerve-supply issuing from the spinal cord in the lower and more inaccessible regions of the chest. This in turn led to more extensive operations, aimed at cutting or "avulsing" – that is tearing – all the supplementary as well as the main nerves. This was feasible but destroyed the principal merit of the operation, its simplicity. Nevertheless, phrenic crush, the crushing rather than the cutting of the main phrenic nerves in the neck, resulting in at least partial diaphragmatic paralysis lasting for about six months, remained part of more radical operations for many years: it may even on occasions have done some good.[10]

An alternative to diaphragmatic paralysis was suggested by Louis Vajda in 1933. Instead of letting the muscle relax and rise by cutting its nerve supply, it could also be pushed up from below by introducing air into the abdomen.[11] The same idea occurred to A. L. Banyai of Milwaukee after accidentally pumping air into the peritoneal instead of the pleural cavity while attempting an artificial pneumothorax.[12] (Not all accidents in AP lore had such a happy outcome.) The manoeuvre, known as pneumoperitoneum, was moderately effective and remained a popular therapeutic choice for many years in patients considered to be too poor risks for major surgery.

Major surgery could not, however, be long delayed. Surgeons had been onlookers while physicians had been ringing the changes on artificial pneumothorax, phrenic crush, pneumoperitoneum and their numerous modifications; but they had not neglected developing more radical approaches in case the comparatively non-mutilating ones failed. The most spectacular result of their labours was thoracoplasty. This was major surgery with a vengeance, one of the bloodiest operations in the operative canon. (Even in expert hands blood loss and shock were major causes of postoperative deaths.) It consisted of the removal of part of the rigid chest wall – ribs and muscles – allowing that part of the chest to sink in and collapse (relax was the approved expression) the underlying lung. How many of the ribs and which parts of the ribs should be removed and in how many stages became matters of protracted surgical debate; but, whatever the answers, it was an undertaking which demanded highly specialised skills. Indeed, it was soon apparent that what was needed was an entirely new branch of the healing arts.

For much of its rise and fall the apostle – or god in his own and in many other people's estimation – of this new branch, thoracic surgery, was Professor

---

[10] Thorburn, G., Riggins, H. M., *Transactions of the National Tuberculosis Association*, 37 (1941), 146.

[11] Vajda, L., *Zeitschrift der Tuberkulose*, 67 (1933), 371.

[12] Banyai, A. L., *American Journal of Medical Science*, 186 (1933), 513.

Ferdinand Sauerbruch of Berlin. Born in 1875 in Barmen in Saxony, he was the son of the manager of a textile factory who died from tuberculosis when Ferdinand was two. According to his autobiography he had no compelling urge to study medicine but never regretted drifting into it.[13] He qualified in Leipzig in 1901; and, shortly afterwards, apparently influenced by his experience with a patient who had been gored by a bull and suffered a pneumothorax, decided to devote his energies to the exploration of the physical conditions prevailing in the chest. His first and most spectacular contribution to his craft was the development of a low-pressure operating chamber which could accommodate two – later up to five – surgeons (in addition to the patient) and which allowed far more extensive manoeuvres inside the open chest than was possible at atmospheric pressure. The successful removal of an intrathoracic tumour in such a chamber impressed his chief, one of imperial Germany's leading surgeons, Johannes von Mikulicz. Propelled by von Mikulicz's patronage, Sauerbruch found himself occupying the chair of surgery in Zurich at the unusually early age of thirty. Here the proximity of Davos ensured a steady flow of tuberculous patients, many of them rich and famous and often, according to their physicians, in the terminal stages of their illness. For Sauerbruch nobody was terminal: it was simply a matter of devising the right procedure and then carrying it out with intrepidity and skill. He was undoubtedly a brilliant operator, astonishing onlookers by his gentleness and speed as well as by the uncanny precision of his finger-work, "an artist comparable to the greatest instrumental virtuosi in music" as one of his rivals, von Benedek, described him.[14] The similarity was enhanced by the fact that some of his procedures he improvised during operation, leaving his assistants gasping. Sometimes the improvisations worked: at least they sometimes worked in his hands.

After ten years in Zurich he moved first to Munich and then to Berlin to become head of the university department of surgery of La Charité, Prussia's oldest and Germany's most prestigious hospital.[15] Here his ambition to build

---

[13] Many contemporaries felt that Sauerbruch's autobiography, written in the last years of his life, did no justice to his achievements in his prime.

[14] Speed, gentleness and precision in surgery were infinitely more important in the early decades of the century than they are today. Tuberculous patients in particular were not fit to stand a prolonged anaesthetic and any clumsiness on the part of the surgeon which left dead or damaged tissue behind was an invitation to postoperative infection, secondary bleeding and other complications. Because of this, the general level of purely technical – that is operative – competence was almost certainly much higher; and the results of any series of operations reflected the skill of individual surgeons far more clearly than they do today. When asked (in London at the Surgical Thoracic Conference of 1924) how he dealt with postoperative wound infections, Sauerbruch apologised for not being able to answer the question: he had never had to deal with any. Arrogance could go no further.

Europe's leading unit of thoracic surgery was given full rein. To his staff and students he was ruthless, and yet his reputation by the 1920s was such that even well-established and experienced surgeons flocked to his department. His ward rounds, described in numerous memoirs, were imperial progressions. After one of his acolytes presented the patient's symptoms and another demonstrated the physical signs (and woe betide those who missed even a minor feature), he addressed the sufferer briefly but decisively, pronouncing on his or her future management. Only the elect were allowed to speak to him directly; but the elect soon included some of the most famous and powerful men on the Continent. (He also had many celebrated women patients; but he did not think much of women.) Attending the dying President, Field Marshal von Hindenburg, he berated the old man for not putting on a dressing gown when receiving him. "But I am a simple soldier, *Herr Geheimrat*, I never in my life possessed a dressing gown", the Field Marshal expostulated. "In that case you will acquire your first one today", Sauerbruch snarled. Even in the depth of the Depression his unit was given all he ever asked for; and he always asked for the latest, the best and the most expensive. The tomograph, an important radiological development, soon to be regarded as indispensable, was only one of many technical innovations first tried out under his aegis.[16] He also insisted that his staff should engage in scientific research and publish a steady flow of papers. "You have all the hours between midnight and 6 a.m. at your disposal", he snapped at one of his minions who pleaded pressure of work. All manuscripts he corrected personally, with caustic (but mostly pertinent) annotations: nothing shoddy ever emanated from La Charité. (Of course nothing truly ground-breaking emanated from it either: real advances in medicine and surgery are incompatible with the *Führerprinzip*.) Above all, he operated almost every day from seven in the morning, rarely for less than eight hours. Total silence reigned during these marathons (though the two tiers of galleries in the operating theatre were always packed), except for his own barked commands.

Hitler and the Nazis came and accepted Sauerbruch as a prestige asset, even though he did not join the Party, nor was he ever seen giving or acknowledging the Nazi salute; and throughout the war, in the huge underground bunker of La Charité (rivalling, it was said, the bunker of the Reich

[15] It was originally founded by Frederick William I of Prussia as a school of anatomy; Frederick II (the Great) had it enlarged into a hospital. Its chief at the end of the eighteenth century was Ludwig Hufeland, one of the celebrated physicians of his day, who counted Goethe, Schiller and Wieland among his patients. Sauerbruch was professor of surgery there from 1927 to 1950.

[16] It allowed the focusing on thin sections of the lung, permitting the localisation of cavities with greater accuracy.

Chancellery), he continued to bark and operate.[17] His labours were only briefly interrupted by the entry of the Red Army. Instructed by the Russians to take charge of ruined Berlin's formidable public health problems, he accepted on condition that his son Peter, a prisoner of war in Siberia, was promptly returned. He was. Only in his last few years, struggling to the end to maintain his position and influence, did his faculties begin to decline. When he died in 1951, an ornament of the German Democratic Republic, as he had been to the Second and Third Reichs and to the Weimar Republic, he was given a state funeral.

Sauerbruch was the best known but not the only pioneer of thoracic surgery. In the United States John Alexander was held in high esteem and affection. He had served in France in 1917 with the United States Medical Corps before joining Léon Bérard's department in Lyon, at that time the most advanced centre of tuberculosis surgery in France. Returning to the United States he was appointed assistant professor of surgery at the University of Michigan but was himself struck down with spinal tuberculosis. He spent two years lying on his back in a plaster cast at Saranac Lake. The setback revealed great hidden reserves of courage and energy. He used much of his enforced idleness to design ingenious devices to help immobilised patients to read, write and draw; and he himself wrote his first textbook, *The Surgery of Pulmonary Tuberculosis*. After his return to Michigan in 1926 he devoted himself entirely to the new speciality and in 1937 published what was to become a classic, *The Collapse Therapy of Pulmonary Tuberculosis*. He was a gifted teacher as well as a compassionate doctor. Until his death in 1954, he trained more thoracic surgeons than anyone else in the English-speaking world.

In Britain Hugh Morriston Davies returned to London from the 1910 Surgical Congress in Berlin fired with enthusiasm by the papers on thoracic surgery read by Brauer, Friedrich and the young Sauerbruch. He managed to obtain a disused broom-cupboard in a turret at University College Hospital, London, where he pursued his obsession with pulmonary disease. (Useless and generally unusable spaces were the glory of Victorian Gothic, the obligatory style in Britain for schools and hospitals during the latter half of the Queen's reign.) Assured by his seniors that X-rays were useless in the diagnosis of chest disease, he made radiology his first speciality. By 1915 he had also carried out his first three thoracoplasties. Almost miraculously all his three patients survived and his reputation soared. Then disaster struck. In the course of a rib resection for empyema, a bone splinter pierced his skin and set up a virulent infection. Amputation was avoided – just – but

---

[17] He may have been marginally involved in the July 1944 plot against Hitler.

his right hand became deformed and useless. Resigning his surgical appointment, but still attracted to diseases of the chest, he purchased a small
sanatorium in the Vale of Clwyd in North Wales and set out to become a
chest physician. But the lure of surgery proved too strong: he learnt to
operate with his left hand, set up a small operating theatre, and by 1924
could report the results of twenty thoracoplasties. Seven patients were relieved of their symptoms and another five improved. In 1935 he went to
America and was persuaded by John Alexander to remodel his operation,
performing a more extensive resection in two or three stages. After that for
some years his sanatorium became a place of pilgrimage for aspirant thoracic
surgeons.[18]

The peak of thoracoplasty was reached by Carl Semb of Oslo, who in 1935
devised a manoeuvre, extrafascial apicolysis, which ensured that the lung
was collapsed not only from the side (by removing the ribs) and below (by
paralysing the diaphragm) but also from above by untethering the upper
lobe from its moorings to the spine and collar bone. It was a procedure
which required considerable skill, but it did produce the desired concentric
relaxation and in fact made it unnecessary to remove as many ribs as had
been obligatory before. Colloquially known as "Semb's Strip", by 1939 it had
superseded most other forms of the operation.[19]

Despite all modifications and improvements, thoracoplasty remained a
horrific operation; and it is not unreasonable to ask how it could have
retained its popularity. Apart from the fact that many patients, despairing
of the unsuccessful artificial pneumothorax, demanded something effective,
it became in many countries the key to both charitable and official funding.
Initially and for several years surgery formed no part of Varrier-Jones's
holistic approach to the treatment of tuberculosis at Papworth: indeed, he
regarded it (according to Miss Borne) as cruel and an obstacle to his ideal
of graduated labour. Yet when he openly opposed it in the 1920s he was
accused by the Health Committee of Cambridgeshire County Council of not
keeping up with advances in treatment;[20] and when a few patients (some
with social connections) began to complain to the Ministry of Health that
at Papworth no treatment in any real sense was given, he decided that the
time had come for an U-turn.[21] He executed it with his usual aplomb. By
1931 his annual report looked forward to the installation of up-to-date surgical
facilities, and the 1933 report boasted that, when the new thoracic surgical

[18] Davies, H. M., *Thorax*, 34 (1948), 198.
[19] Holst, J., Semb, C., Frimann-Dahl, J., *Acta chirurgica Scandinavica*, 76 (1935), supplement,
34–37.
[20] Cambridgeshire County Council, Memorandum, 2 March 1926, PRO, MH 52/5.
[21] Ministry of Pensions, Letter, Nottingham, 13 August 1921, PRO, MH 52/5.

unit was completed, Papworth would have "what is believed to be the most complete scheme for the treatment of tuberculosis anywhere".[22] In 1934 McNalty of the Ministry of Health reported that Varrier-Jones hoped that Papworth would become the centre for the surgical treatment of pulmonary disease for the midlands and all the eastern counties of England. New operating theatres were formally opened two years later.

Growing experience with operations on the chest and the coming of age of the first generation of specialist thoracic surgeons inevitably led to the culmination of tuberculosis surgery, the actual removal of the diseased lobe, lobes or whole lungs. No less inevitably the early results were daunting, a complication rate of 40–70 per cent and a mortality rate between 25 and 40 per cent in centres which troubled to publish statistics. Yet there was, it seemed for some years, no turning back;[23] and the introduction of sulphonamides which controlled secondary infection (often the most intractable postoperative complication), a better understanding of lung anatomy,[24] and a less haphazard selection of patients, had a beneficial effect.[25] By the mid 1940s, the peak period of thoracic surgery, resection was often considered not as a last resort but in preference to other, seemingly less drastic procedures.

The trend in the treatment of the extrapulmonary forms of the disease was along similar lines. Although it was recognised that tuberculosis of the kidney, bladder, the Fallopian tube, the epidydimis or of bones and joints was part of a general infection and that therefore local surgery could not guarantee a permanent cure, it did in practice often relieve patients of their most troublesome symptoms. Uretero-nephrectomy (the removal of an affected kidney and ureter) for urinary-tract disease became a standard and, by and large, successful operation; and epidydimo-orchiectomy for unilateral tuberculous epidydimitis counted as barely more than minor surgery. Diseased joints too began to be excised or "fused" in preference to immobilisation.

The real breakthrough came with the advent of specific antituberculous

[22] *Tubercle* (1962), supplement, 49.

[23] Burrow Hill Colony, administered by the National Association for the Prevention of Tuberculosis, had constant difficulty in filling its beds, mainly because Sir Robert Philip insisted that neither thoracic surgery nor even artificial pneumothorax should be practised there: it was forced to close in 1943. By contrast, Preston Hall, which had experienced great difficulties in filling beds in the early 1930s, suddenly had an upsurge in admissions after the installation of the first tomograph in Britain and the development of thoracic surgery.

[24] R. C. (later Lord) Brock, working at the Brompton Hospital, showed that in planning a resection surgeons should think in terms of bronchial segments rather than of lobes, Brock, R. C., *The Anatomy of the Bronchial Tree* (London, 1946.)

[25] Chamberlain, J. N., Storey, C. F., Klopstock, R., Daniels, C. F., *Journal of Thoracic Surgery*, 26 (1953), 471.

drugs. Under chemotherapeutic cover, as if touched by magic, both the immediate and the long-term results of surgery began to improve dramatically. The terrible postoperative complications – the formation of fistulae, sinuses, abscesses and (most feared of all) miliary spread – became exceptional. Indeed, so successful was surgery under the streptomycin (and later PAS and isoniazid) umbrella that many began to wonder whether the umbrella without the surgery might not be just as effective. And so it proved. At its moment of greatest triumph, surgery suddenly became redundant or at least confined to tidying-up operations like the removal (if necessary) of minor and inactive lesions.

The change took a few years to percolate through the profession. At a conference on tuberculosis in 1960 two eminent London thoracic surgeons, H. D. Teare and Sir Clement Price Thomas, still tried to persuade their audience that there remained a place for operations in the treatment of the disease; and F. C. Edwards, thoracic surgeon to the Liverpool Regional Hospital Board, expressed the view that local factors must always be taken into account. "Because I work in an industrial area with a strong Irish element, my patients are temperamentally undisciplined from the point of view of taking drugs, and they are also racially very susceptible to the disease ... The intelligence of many, often women, who are procreating children at a vast rate, is low, and they have not the time or appetite to take tablets." [26] Despite this novel indication for surgery in preference to chemotherapy, the assembled doctors remained unconvinced; and J. G. Scadding of the Brompton Hospital had no difficulty in persuading them that, in patients on adequate drug treatment, surgery had nothing to offer but misery. When the final report of the National Survey on Major Surgery for Pulmonary Tuberculosis was published, in 1963, it proved to be final in more senses than one.[27] Or so everybody thought at the time.

---

[26] *Tubercle*, 43 (1962), 43, supplement, 49.

[27] It was William C. Fowler in 1956 who summed up three decades of tuberculosis surgery, ibid., 37 (1956), 66: "Let us be grateful to all those human guinea-pigs by whose sufferings and fortitude hope was kept alive which enabled surgeons to step up a ladder runged with blood and sweat and tears ... bereft of many ribs, of phrenic nerves and vertebral transverse processes, padding out their vests to hide their scoliotic figures."

32

Dawn

On 3 November 1943 Peter V., a twenty-one year old medical student, arrived from Hungary in Leysin in Switzerland to be admitted to one of Professor Rollier's famous sanatoria. The son of an eminent surgeon who looked after Regent Horthy's family, it was to this and to his very rich American mother – his parents were divorced – that he owed the privilege of travelling across war-torn Europe to neutral Switzerland. The Sanatorium Beau Soleil had the reputation of being a place where patients with tuberculous joints sometimes got better. Six months earlier Peter's left knee had suddenly swelled up and he had begun to limp. It was odd, since, though a keen footballer, he had not knowingly injured it nor was the swelling or the limp painful. An X-ray, to be on the safe side, was followed by extensive invesigations. Both lungs as well as the knee were found to be affected.

> At home and on the journey [he later wrote] I was not in the least worried. Going to Switzerland seemed a great adventure. My first encounter with death was on the way to the sanatorium. A car picked me up from the station of the funicular. Another lorry had just arrived carrying three coffins. Jean-Pierre, the sanatorium chauffeur, patted one of the boxes with great familiarity. "There, that's one of our customers", he said with a chuckle. And in case I missed the point he took a slightly round-about way to the sanatorium, passing the huge cemetery – huge for a small village that is. "Have a good look at that, Monsieur V. I like to bring new patients this way just to scare them a little. Not too much, you understand: you'll probably be all right. But you must do as the doctors say: they know what's good for you." In my room on my bedside table lay a hefty volume, the sanatorium rule book. It was in fact quite short but printed in at least six languages. (I would later be asked to do a Hungarian translation.) On the last page printed in heavy type was a poem written by a past patient, a well-known Swiss poet apparently. It was jocular in tone, I soon knew it by heart, about "being in a good old fix" but "it was up to me to remain cheerful and to put up a good light and live as long as I could. That was what really mattered." But after a few weeks it wasn't really, not to me.[1]

Although Peter had no choice but to do as the doctors said and spent most of the next eighteen months lying on the balcony of his single room clad in goggles and a loin-cloth soaking up the sun – or the wind – he did

---

[1] Unpublished manuscript in possession of the author.

not get better. His knee, it is true, became less swollen and painful with rest; but his weight continued to drop, he developed an irritating cough and he was soon too tired and breathless to get up for more than the short journey to the bathroom. Then he was no longer able to do even that. He could not exactly remember later when he suddenly realised that he was soon going to die. It threw him into a state of panic and he sobbed and cried for several days. From then on sedatives were added to his regular daily regimen of vitamin pills, calcium, iron and a rather mysterious mixture referred to as Professor's Rollier's special. He suspected that it contained opium as it made him feel more relaxed. He noticed with surprise that any interest he had had in the cataclysmic events that were shaking Europe (even those engulfing his home in Budapest) slowly evaporated: indeed anything outside the sanatorium walls became unreal. What occupied his mind, apart from obsessively registering his own symptoms – a tiny scratching sensation in the throat, a slight delay in starting to pass water, the marginal but frequent increase in the violence of his cough – were the daily events inside the establishment. There were the occasional changes in the nursing and medical staff, a new supper dish, the arrival of new patients. Many of the arrivals were young people like himself and they paid him colonial-style courtesy visits as to an old resident. But it was not just courtesy. They were hungry for information, avid for reassurance. Was Monsieur V. getting better? How long would it take before …? And there were the deaths and the departures, the former always outnumbering the latter but never referred to in the daily exchange of pleasantries with staff and fellow patients. Overriding all else, but a closely guarded secret, there was the totally unreasonable hope of an eventual cure, carefully nurtured daydreams.

> They never left me, not for one moment, though I was not a fool and knew perfectly well that a cure was completely illusory. Doctor D. came to see me every day and the chief, Professor R., once a month. He always examined me carefully, listening to my chest at length. Almost always he ended up with a nod: "Not too bad, not too bad at all, a little clearer than last months I would say". "But I've lost another half a kilo weight." "Have you really? Well, that'll need looking into, won't it?" I knew it was only a ritual. Once every six or seven weeks I also had an X-ray and a sputum test. It was the latter which really mattered; but it took six weeks for the result of the guinea-pig inoculation to come back. We knew that by then our guinea-pigs would always be dead of tuberculosis; but we always counted the days.
>
> I was not afraid of dying – except sometimes at night – but I was terrified that people who knew me in the past would begin and come and visit me when the war was over and be horrified to see me in my ghost-like state. My mother wrote from America to say that she would come as soon as it was possible to travel. I prayed for the war to continue.[2]

2 Ibid.

In August 1946 his best sanatorium friend, a young Swedish musician, died. He was in considerable pain and much distress toward the end. For a few weeks near the end, and as a special privilege, Peter was wheeled into his room and allowed to sit at his bedside and read to him for an hour or two every day. For some reason – he could not later remember whether it was his friend's choice or his own – the book was Dostoievski's *The Idiot* in German. Neither of them would ever finish it. A few months later his mother flew in from America. She was mildly alcoholic and determinedly upbeat. Peter was not to despair: there was a new drug being developed in the States, still very expensive and not on the open market, indeed still a little experimental and hush-hush, but through Mrs Roosevelt, an old family friend, Peter's mother knew somebody who knew somebody else at the Mayo Clinic in Rochester; and dear Eleanor had wangled enough for a few weeks' course.[3] Peter implored her not to press the doctors to give it to him: he had had his fill of new treatments. He would get better without them. He was feeling better that very morning, much much better. To his surprise Professor Rollier had heard of this particular new drug on the medical grapevine and was prepared, even keen, to try it. In fact he had been trying to obtain samples but it was not only scarce but also fearfully expensive. Peter's mother assured the professor that the supply for her son would not dry up. So, in March 1946, Peter began his course of streptomycin and – was it his imagination? It had to be – he began to feel stronger within a week. Suddenly he could sit out of bed. Then slowly and with support he could walk. He tried to convince himself that it was all self-suggestion, in the mind. He was putting on weight: that surely could not be imagination. Ten days after starting the course his temperature remained normal throughout a twenty-four period for the first time since his admission. His sputum definitely diminished in volume: it became almost an effort to cough. He had an out-of-phase chest X-ray. It did not show any change but Dr M. explained that X-ray appearances always lagged behind other changes. It was a small disappointment; but he was still gaining strength. Professor Rollier came to see him between

---

[3] Waksman in his memoirs recalled the anguish caused by this or a similar intervention by Mrs Roosevelt: it was no doubt well intentioned but literally meant the discontinuation of treatment in another patient. Ironically, a few years later Mrs Roosevelt herself died of disseminated tuberculosis: the diagnosis was missed till it was too late because she was on treatment with cortisone for her rheumatoid arthritis (see above, Chapter 21).

For this chapter, as a whole, see Barry, V. C., *Chemotherapy of Tuberculosis* (London, 1964); Grmek, M., *A History of Aids: The Emergence and Origin of a Modern Pandemic* (Princeton NJ, 1990); Lehmann, J., "Twenty Years Afterwards". *American Review of Respiratory Disease*, 90 (1964), 953; Medical Research Council, *British Medical Journal* (1953), no. 1, 435; Ryan, F., *The Greatest Story Never Told* (Bromsgrove, Worcestershire, 1992); Waksman, S. A., *My Life with Microbes* (London, 1958); Watson, J., Gill, O. N., *British Medical Journal*, 300 (1990), 63.

the ritual monthly visits to ask him not to mention the course to other patients: they would all want to try it and there was not enough of this streptomycin to go around. Nor would most of them be able to afford it. Peter protested: how could he even think of telling anybody? Confined to his room and balcony, he hardly ever met other patients any more. In fact, he had been told not to – tactfully of course. Clearly his appearance was bad for morale and his breath unpleasant.

R. hummed and haaed for a while, then informed me that well, there was no reason, if I felt strong enough, why I shouldn't spend some time in the lounge or in the library. Even go for a short walk. And – incredibly – I did feel strong enough. But what about my sputum? R. hesitated. He mustn't raise my hopes but on direct smear there were no bacilli. But of course it was the guinea-pigs which mattered. And so I waited. And a few weeks later, but a few days earlier than usual, he came into my room smiling. I remember thinking that I had not seen him smile before – never ever. I thought at first it was a grimace, almost grotesque. Yet wonderful. I shall certainly never forget it. "Well, you're negative, *mon vieux*." He had never called me that either. "Your guinea-pigs are doing fine. We'll have to repeat the test course; but if another test is negative you can start thinking of going home." [4]

The event which started the revolution which was to save Peter V.'s life took place not in a medical research laboratory, as Trudeau and others had predicted, but in the Department of Soil Microbiology of the Agricultural Experimental Station of Rutgers College, New Jersey. Selman Abraham Waksman who headed the department, a small, podgy man with a bristly moustache and pebble glasses, had been born in Odessa in the Ukraine in 1888 and had emigrated to the United States in 1910. There he studied biology at Rutgers University, obtained his doctorate from the University of California and in 1916 returned to his old college as a lecturer. His main interest, some would say his sole interest in life, lay in the interaction of bacteria and other micro-organisms in the soil, especially in the capacity of some to inhibit others. This inhibition was due to the elaboration of certain chemical substances later to be known as antibiotics. One species of soil-inhabiting micro-organisms were particularly active inhibitors and the small Waksman team were hoping to find a variant which might inhibit pathogenic organisms to humans (which was easy) without actually killing the host (which was difficult). In addition to research the department also had a service commitment to the large local farming community; and in the autumn of 1943 a chicken was presented to the scientists by a farmer who had noticed its difficulty in breathing. He was anxious to ensure that what he had correctly identified as an infection the bird had contracted by picking in the dirt

---

[4] Unpublished manuscript in possession of the author.

should not spread to the rest of his flock. A throat swab was taken from the ailing creature, and in due course yet another soil micro-organism belonging to the family of *Actinomyces* was identified. Once identified, its bacteriocidal properties were routinely investigated. They included inhibition of an unusually wide range of pathogens without marked toxicity to the host. When a few weeks later Dr William Hugh Feldman, professor of comparative pathology at the Mayo Foundation in Rochester, Minnesota, visited Waksman's laboratory.[5] Waksman told him about the new species of mould and the material extracted from it in one of the basement laboratories by Waksman's keen young assistant, Alfred Schatz. The team's first paper on the subject was in fact already in the pipeline.[6]

Feldman was impressed and so was his clinical colleague at the Mayo Clinic, Horton Corwin Hinshaw. They proved to be an efficient team. Before the year was out, they had proved that streptomycin completely suppressed the activity of the tuberculosis bacillus in guinea-pigs without in any way harming the animal.[7] No such powerful and selective effect had been seen before; yet everybody concerned exercised admirable restraint. The memory of tuberculin was still vivid and, in any case, the amount of streptomycin Schatz could produce in his laboratory was tiny. Only one patient was treated outside the strict experimental protocol of the first clinical trial, a twenty-one-year-old woman, Patricia S., in the terminal stages of pulmonary and

[5] Feldman was born William Hugh Gunn in Glasgow in 1892. In 1894 his family emigrated to the United States where his father died. His mother remarried and he took the name of his stepfather. He died in 1971.

[6] Schatz, A., Bugie, B., Waksman, S. A.,"Streptomycin: A Substance Exhibiting Antibiotic Activity against Gram-Positive and Gram-Negative Bacteria", published in *Proceedings of the Society for Experimental and Biological Medicine*, 55 (1944), 66. All the first papers dealing with streptomycin had Alfred Schatz as their first author. Schatz was a young postgraduate student who did most of the actual benchwork in Waksman's department. Waksman thought highly of him – "my best student" – and Schatz initially revered Waksman; but after streptomycin became a success and began to be profitable (though not to Waksman personally) the two became estranged. Schatz eventually accused Waksman of mishandling the profits arising from their joint patent. After an acrimonious law-suit Schatz was awarded a large sum in damages; but the academic establishment closed ranks and the victory blighted his further career in research. An even more bitter dispute erupted when Waksman alone was awarded the Nobel Prize for the discovery of streptomycin. Feldman and Hinshaw shrugged it off but Schatz protested to the Swedish Academy and even to the King of Sweden. It was of no avail. The story is well and sympathetically recounted by Ryan, *The Greatest Story Never Told*. It is never mentioned in hagiographic memoirs that Koch's Nobel Prize, for which he was nominated in the first year of the institution of the award (1901), was similarly beset with acrimony: he did not receive the prize until five years later.

[7] Feldman, W. H., Hinshaw, H. C., *Proceedings of the Staff Meeting of the Mayo Clinic*, 19 (1944), 593.

disseminated tuberculosis. She responded at once – it was like a fairy-tale – and left the hospital cured: she eventually married and became the mother of three children.[8] Otherwise the first guarded preliminary report on thirty-four patients was published by Feldman and Hinshaw in September 1945. It ended with the plea that if the results

> are noticed by lay persons it is ardently hoped that they will be interpreted in the same cautious frame of mind that the scientific investigators have endeavoured to maintain. This unusual suggestion is made for the benefit of the many thousands of patients who have tuberculosis. Morale plays a crucial part in the treatment of this debilitating and chronic disease; and this could be harmed by premature optimistic reports which might not be sustained in practice.[9]

It is true that much still remained to be learnt: the initial dosage was lower than optimal; and occasional toxic effects quickly emerged. But to the insider team it was clear within a year that streptomycin was the first chemo-therapeutic agent in history effective against almost every form of tuberculosis caused by either the human or the bovine strains of the *Mycobacterium* without, in most cases, seriously harming the patient. It was for millions of tuberculous – though still without them being aware of it – the dawn.

Was it in fact the first? After half a century of vain and frustrating effort new drugs now followed each other at an astonishing rate; and one may have been synthesised at the same time as streptomycin and tested on patients a few months earlier. But the world knew nothing about it. Throughout 1943 Jorgen Lehmann, a Dane working at the Sahlgrenska Hospital in Gothenburg in Sweden, had been following up earlier observations which suggested that oxygen uptake by pathogenic strains of the *Mycobacterium tuberculosis*, an indicator of their growth and virulence, was stimulated by two common and simple organic acids, benzoic and salicylic. He conceived the idea that com-pounds which would inhibit the synthesis of these two acids might also retard the growth of the bacillus. Biochemical inhibition is often a function of closely related compounds competing for the same enzyme, and Lehmann soon established that para-aminosalicylic acid, a first cousin of salicylic acid (and of aspirin) soon to be known as PAS, was a powerful inhibitor. Animal experiments were then begun, followed by a small clinical trial involving twenty patients; but it was only in January 1946 that Lehmann reported that the majority had responded favourably with a drop in temperature, weight gain and general improvement.[10]

[8] Riggins, H. M., Hinshaw, H. C., *American Review of Tuberculosis*, 96 (1947), 168.

[9] Feldman, W. H., ibid., 69 (1954), 859.

[10] Lehmann, J., *Lancet* (1946), no. 1, 15. The contrast between streptomycin and PAS provides a striking illustration of the imponderables which determine the fate of medical discoveries

This was welcome news: the more so since the first streptomycin-resistant strains of the tuberculosis bacillus were beginning to emerge. In most western countries the trial of PAS was entrusted to official research bodies (in Britain to a committee of the Medical Research Council), since it was no longer ethical, as it had been at the time of the first streptomycin trials, to use as a control group patients deliberately treated with bed-rest and standard sanatorium regime alone. The trials began in 1948 and most reports were published during 1950. With few reservations, the results showed that PAS not only significantly reduced the risk of resistant strains emerging during streptomycin therapy it also rendered streptomycin more effective.[11]

The advent of the third member of what was to be known for some years as the Triple Therapy marked a change in style. Streptomycin and PAS were the achievements of a few single-minded individuals working on limited budgets in university hospitals and laboratories. Their results sparked off feverish activity in the huge research and development departments of the industrial giants. Once the commercial decision to chase after new antituberculous agents was made, finance was no longer a problem: priority, patenting and marketing was. At least three groups – Hoffmann La Roche, the Squibb

in the modern world. Because all the protagonists in the early streptomycin saga – Waksman, Feldman, Hinshaw and George Merck of the pharmaceutical company Merck & Co. in particular – were in personal sympathy with each other and fuelled by an almost messianic zeal, the path from accidental laboratory observation to clinical use and large-scale manufacture was fast and smooth. By 1946 nobody doubted the value of the drug, though, even manufactured at eight different plants, the amounts produced were inadequate for treating all patients in the United States, let alone worldwide. (The pressure on those in charge of allocating available supplies, in particular on Corwin Hinshaw, was nearly unbearable.) By contrast, the path of PAS was beset with delays and difficulties, none of Lehmann's making. Not only was a sense of urgency lacking at several levels but there was also widespread scepticism. "All work towards finding a chemical cure for tuberculosis is senseless because the bacteria are encapsulated in such a way that they are out of reach of such therapies", one eminent professor of chest diseases declared. The clinician in charge of the preliminary trials was obsessed – not unreasonably perhaps – with the danger of mistaking spontaneous remissions for a positive therapeutic response. Scandinavia had been the starting point of the Sanocrysin fiasco; and the humiliation still cast a shadow. The prospective manufacturers were impatiently counting the cost and issuing thinly-veiled ultimata. There were premature press releases and bitter mutual recriminations. Even after the publication of Lehmann's Preliminary Communication (which caused much bitterness among some of his chemist colleagues who felt that they should have been co-authors), it is doubtful if PAS would have caught the world's attention if Hugh Feldmann of the Mayo Clinic and of streptomycin fame had not acquired streptomycin-resistant tuberculosis. His life was saved by PAS. Many felt that Lehmann should at least have shared the Nobel Prize with Waksman; but he never received the prize. He died in 1989, aged ninety-two. His rival – but they bore each other no personal ill-will – Selman Waksman, died in 1974, aged eighty-five.

[11] Medical Research Council Report, *British Medical Journal* (1953), no. 1, 435.

Institute and Bayer's – came up with a similar compound more or less simultaneously. Negotiations about patent rights and brand names were at an advanced stage when it transpired that the substance had been synthesised in 1912 by two Prague chemists, Hans Meyer and Josef Mally. Neither had any notion of its antituberculous properties: the task of producing iso-nicotinic acid hydrazide, a molecule of modest chemical interest in its own right, was set by their professor for their doctoral thesis in chemistry. Once it was in existence, however, nobody else could patent it. (It was fortunate that the distant past had remained hidden for a year or two: one of the most useful antituberculous drugs would probably never have been developed otherwise.) The new agent soon became known as isnoniazid.

In 1952 Robitzek and Selikoff, after a preliminary clinical trial at the Sea View Hospital in New York, announced that in forty-four consecutive patients "acute, active progressive bilateral caseous tuberculosis, all of them febrile, losing weight and sputum-positive, generally regarded as having a poor prognosis, showed rapid and marked general improvement in response to isonicotinic acid hydrizide".[12] In contrast to the trials of streptomycin and PAS, the launch was accompanied by a full-scale media circus. Reporters and photographers encamped outside Robitzek and Selikoff's unit, offered doctors exclusive contracts, chatted up the nurses, brandished cheque books at relatives and supported their banner headlines with photographs showing patients "before and after"; dying in the "before" and dancing in the wards "after".[13]

Such tasteless exhibitions were endured by the more fastidious because of the obvious merits of the new drug: it was potent, easy to administer, had a lower incidence of toxicity than either streptomycin or PAS and, above all, it was relatively cheap. To millions of tuberculosis sufferers and their doctors around the world this was a historic advance. Eight years after the discovery of streptomycin and PAS the cost of treating the average American for tuberculosis was still a staggering $3500; and in other countries – the drugs were turning up on the black market everywhere, including Communist Moscow – wholly outside the purse of all but a few millionaires, crooks or political bosses. Isoniazid (prepared easily from coal tar) brought the cost down in America to $100 and made treatment at least accessible elsewhere. Yet it was also soon apparent that it would not actually replace either streptomycin or PAS: the emergence of resistant strains was relatively com-mon. Instead, by 1955, a general consensus began to emerge about the best chemotherapeutic combination: streptomycin, PAS and isoniazid.

[12] Robitzek, E. H., Selikoff, I. J., *American Review of Tuberculosis,* 65 (1952), 402.
[13] *Time Magazine,* 3 March 1952, p. 42.

Although on statistical charts tuberculosis had been slowly declining in most of western Europe and in North America (the Second World War rise was reversed more quickly than that which had accompanied and followed the First), there were in 1946 still thousands of sanatoria and specialist hospitals crammed with young people seemingly condemned to an indefinite stay and quite probably to end their lives there. Three years later the sanatoria and specialist hospitals were closing down. In Britain, Papworth was being designated as a centre for heart surgery and Frimley was trying to survive as a specialist hospital for asthmatics. In Switzerland, tuberculosis villages like Davos, Arosa, Leysin and Montana were frantically building ski-lifts and laying on sporting facilities and other *après-ski* amenities to attract the international jet-set or at least the new winter package-holiday trade. (Only the frontage of densely-packed covered balconies of the new grand hotels served as a reminder – or might have done but probably did not – of their original purpose.) In America, establishments which had anything to offer other than a cluster of prefabricated shacks were discovering and promoting as best they could the conference and convention industry: soon they were competing with each other offering not peace, rest and quiet but the latest gadgets in communication technology and scope for expense-account junketing. Warnings were inevitably sounded by a few Cassandras; but in the public perception tuberculosis, the great killer, was on the way to becoming a character in folk memory.

Yet there was a transitional period when patients continued to die, like the young men killed on the Western Front in November 1918 after the signing of the Armistice, and when isolated cases gave a muted forewarning of difficulties to come.

Eric Blair had his first major pulmonary bleed on 8 March 1938. "The bleeding seemed to to go on forever and ... everyone agreed that he must be taken somewhere urgently where really active steps can be taken – an emergency artificial pneumothorax if necessary and a blood transfusion", wrote his wife, Eileen.[14] He was thirty-four, still known only to a small circle of English literati and recently back from fighting, writing and almost getting shot through the head by a sniper in Spain. He was not yet called George Orwell and *Animal Farm* had not yet made him famous. Fortunately Eileen's brother, Laurence O'Shaughnessy, was a visiting surgical consultant at Preston Hall,[15] by then run on conventional sanatorium lines; and this ensured Blair's

[14] Orwell has had several good biographies, including *George Orwell: A Personal Memoir* by T. R. Fywel (London, 1982) and a masterly volume by B. Crick, *George Orwell: A Life* (London, 1988).

[15] He was killed at Dunkirk in 1940.

immediate admission and preferential treatment. He was a good mixer with ordinary people and fellow patients came to accept and like him. He made good progress, characteristically refusing to give up smoking; and in June he and Eileen set out for a convalescent holiday in Morocco. (It was the least expensive place in the sun – Nice and Menton were way beyond their means – and not too far from England in case he had another haemorrhage.)

He then did well for several years, well enough at least to work hard at his writing and to establish his reputation as one of England's leading political thinkers and commentators, the conscience of the left. Eileen and he adopted a little boy, Richard, whom they loved. Then she died unexpectedly under the anaesthetic for what was apparently a routine hysterectomy; and in the same summer of 1947 his own illness re-emerged. This time it was more a general decline than bleeding, weakness and cough while he was finishing *Nineteen Eighty-Four* on the Scottish west coast island of Jura. In December he wrote to a friend:

> I've been in bed for six weeks and was feeling unwell for some time before that. I kept trying to get just well enough to make the journey to London but could not. Finally I saw a chest specialist here. He says I have got to go into a sanatorium, probably for about four months. It's an awful bore, however perhaps its all for the best if they can cure me.[16]

By December 1947 a cure was no longer a pipe-dream. At Hairmyres Hospital, a sanatorium near Glasgow, his treatment began fairly conventionally.

> The treatment they are giving me is to put the left lung out of action, apparently for about six months, which will give it a better chance to heal. They first crushed the phrenic nerve which, I gather, is what makes the lung expand and contract and they pumped air into [in fact below] the diaphragm which I understand is to push the lung into a different position ... I have to have "refills" every few days but later I think it gets down to once a week. For the rest I am still very ill and weak and had lost a stone in weight though they make me eat a tremendous amount and Dick assures me that I'm getting better.[17]

He was not; but Dr Bruce Dick, his doctor, had read about the new drug which was being tried with astonishing success in the United States but was not yet available in Britain outside a preliminary Medical Research Council trial. Dick had also noticed that David Astor, owner of the *Observer* and a rich man, had been among Orwell's first and most concerned visitors. This led to Orwell asking Astor for a rare favour.

[16] Crick, *George Orwell*, p. 538.
[17] Ibid., p. 542.

Dr Dick has said to me that I am getting on quite well but it would speed recovery if one had some streptomycin (STREPTOMYCIN). This is obtainable in the USA but because of dollars the Board of Trade won't normally grant a licence. He suggested that you might with your American connections arrange to buy it and I could pay you. He wants 70 grammes and it costs about £1 a gramme.[18]

Astor leapt at the chance and a cable was instantly dispatched to Astor Estates in New York. He also wrote to Dick impressing on him that money was no problem if any new drug was needed; and he spoke to Nye Bevan, then Minister of Health, to make sure that no obstacles were put in the way of their importation.

The consignment of streptomycin arrived within a month and at first seemed to do its miraculous best. "I have been having this streptomycin and it's evidently doing its stuff ... I am much better in every way", Orwell wrote to his friend, Julian Symonds. Then, however, the side-effects started to appear, and he brought to their description – "it might be useful to have a written record as streptomycin is still a new drug" – the same undramatic precision which characterised his literary essays:

A sort of discoloration appeared at the base of my fingers and toenails; then my face became red and the skin began to flake off and a rash appeared all over my body, especially down my back. After about three weeks I got a severe sore throat which did not go away and was not affected by sucking penicillin lozenges. It was very painful to swallow and I had to have a special diet for some weeks. There was now ulceration with blisters in my throat and the inside of my cheeks and the blood kept coming up in little blisters on my lips. At night these burst and bled considerably, so that in the morning my lips were always stuck together and I had to bathe them before I could open my mouth. Meanwhile my nails had disintegrated and my hair began to come out in patches. It was very unpleasant.[19]

This was almost certainly an exceptionally severe hypersensitivity reaction from which Orwell recovered as soon as the streptomycin was stopped, one of the less common of the occasional complications of the drug. It is probable that a few years later it might have been treated successfully with anti-histamines or steroids; and even at that time at least one other effective antituberculous drug was undergoing a controlled trial, something that neither Dick nor Orwell was aware of.

[18] Ibid., p. 544. The drug was in fact very much more expensive at the time: even when obtainable in Britain, a course cost the equivalent of about £10,000 in 1998 currency.

[19] Ibid., p. 560. The most common and most feared toxic effect was on the eighth cranial nerve supplying the inner ear and the semicircular canals, the organs of equilibrium. It occurred in as many as 10 per cent of cases and the effect was usually irreversible. The reason for this unique selective action is still unknown and it remains one reason why streptomycin is hardly ever used today.

A few months later Orwell seemed to be spontaneously on the mend and the hospital let him have his typewriter back. (But he retained an affection for the biro, another transatlantic postwar wonder.) His sister Avril brought an excited Richard to Glasgow, and for six summer weeks he was at least a long shadow of his former self. It was to be the last such occasion. Though he was able laboriously to finish *Nineteen Eighty-Four* (never to his own satisfaction), the road after that was inexorably downhill. Dick made one more attempt to try streptomycin in a smaller dose; but it caused an immediate rash and the treatment was abandoned. (The cache of drug intended for him, still more precious than gold, was given with his blessing to two desperately ill young woman patients. Both made a complete recovery.) *Nineteen Eighty-Four* was a resounding though controversial success and a money-spinner; and hope remained alive – at least for public consumption. "It looks as if I may have to spend the rest of my life if not actually in bed but at any rate at bath-chair level", he wrote to Anthony Powell, "but that's all right so long as I can work." Sonia Brownell, one-time secretary to Cyril Connolly's literary magazine *Horizon*, was one of his frequent visitors and perhaps the "strong reason why I want to stay alive". They had known each other for many years and he had proposed to her before. She had then declined: now she accepted. He was also seen by a second opinion, Andrew Morland, the kindly Quaker physician who had also attended D. H. Lawrence.[20] Morland declared himself to be reasonably optimistic in the short run; but a relapse was always possible.

In September Orwell moved into his last bed at University College Hospital in Gower Street in London. The flowers and fruit which greeted him in his private room would have embarrassed or wryly amused him a few years earlier; now he was touched. "I'm growing used to the life of an invalid." Morland suggested that a stay in the Alps in France or Switzerland might do the trick: a lowered atmospheric pressure, he explained, would also lower the risk of a haemorrhage. But first there was the wedding to Sonia to be arranged. David Astor obtained the required special licence from the Archbishop of Canterbury to have the celebration in a hospital room and friends were asked to find a smoking jacket: "Even in a hospital one can hardly get married in a dressing gown". "He looked rather grand", Malcolm Muggeridge later recalled, "like an old-style colonial gentleman." The ceremony took place on 13 October, and for some weeks afterwards he seemed to rally. The date of departure was fixed. But on 20 January 1948, in the early hours of the morning, he had another haemorrhage and died within a few hours. He was forty-six.

[20] He survived Orwell by only a year.

There were other deaths like that but a diminishing number.[21] New drugs were removing the spectre of sensitivity reactions and resistance – or so it seemed. Thioacetazone, originally advocated by Gerhard Domagk, discoverer of the sulphonomides,[22] became the centre of renewed interest in the 1960s, especially as it was relatively cheap and therefore, in combination with iso-niazid, suitable for poor countries.[23] Other antibiotics – viomycin, cycloserin capreomycin, pyrazinamide and ethambutol – were joining the list of what were becoming known as the reserve drugs.[24] In 1966 a new family of anti-biotics, the rifomycins, were added, probably the most potent antituberculous drugs so far, though also at the time among the most expensive.[25]

In 1959 an impressive therapeutic trial put the seal on the demise of the sanatorium regime. The Madras Experiment, as it came to be known, was

[21] Among them was that of Mohammed Ali Jinnah, founder of Pakistan. How long he had been tuberculous and how far his illness influenced negotiations leading to the partition of India remain uncertain. He was suffering from severe bronchitis at the time of the second Simla Conference with the British Cabinet Mission in May 1946 and he was on leave with chest trouble between December 1946 and March 1947. The possibility of tuberculosis was never openly admitted before his death. Two years later the journalist and historian, Ian Stephens, was told by Jinnah's doctors that their patient died of galloping consumption. This seemed even at the time unlikely; but, even if true, streptomycin might have been effective. Thirty years later it was semi-officially admitted that a chest X-ray as early as June 1946 had shown extensive cavitation; but this was kept a secret since "it was felt that the leader's imminent death might seriously compromise the negotiations": several of his heirs were less intransigent about a separate Muslim state. Stephens, I., *Pakistan* (London, 1966); L'Etang, H., *Fit to Lead?* (London, 1980).

Among those whose tuberculosis was too far advanced to benefit significantly from chemotherapy was the actress Vivien Leigh: she died in 1967. Albert Camus, the Nobel Prize winning author of *La peste*, translated as *The Plague* by Stuart Gilbert (London, 1960), and an existentialist ikon, fell ill with tuberculosis in 1930 when he was seventeen and suffered recurrent bouts of ill health which improved, but did not cease, on treatment with strepto-mycin and PAS. His medical outlook was poor when he was killed in a car crash in 1960.

[22] Domagk, G., *American Review of Tuberculosis*, 61 (1950), 8.

[23] Hinshaw, H. C., McDermott, W., ibid., 61 (1950), 145.

[24] Miller, A. B., Fox, W., Tall, R., *Tubercle*, 47 (1966), 33. Even then drug resistance, though comparatively rare, was already a problem. "To juggle successfully with a minimum of three potentially toxic drugs required constant and vigilant supervision by the physician, together with maximum cooperation from the patient who in his own interest as well as those of the community had often to be coaxed into persevering with an unpleasant and seemingly endless regimen". See Keers, R. Y., *Pulmonary Tuberculosis: A Journey down the Centuries* (London, 1978).

[25] These were semisynthetic compounds developed in the Lepetit Research Laboratories from *Streptomyces mediterranei*. Initially it was necessary to inject them intravenously but rifamycin AMP, better known as rifampicin, was absorbed when given by mouth. In a comparative review of the new drugs, F. Grumbach concluded in 1969 that "the discovery of Rifampicin opens a new area in antituberculous therapy", *Tubercle*, 50 (1969), 12.

primarily concerned with the effect of diet, accommodation and physical activity on the outcome of antituberculous drug treatment; but no less useful was the light it shed on how far sanatoria protected home contacts from infection.[26] 163 patients were enrolled, all living within an eight kilometre radius of the Tuberculosis Chemotherapy Centre in one of the poorest sections of Madras City. (The fact that this could be done in one morning without any preliminary scouting speaks more eloquently than statistics about the prevalence of the disease.) All were far advanced in their illness, almost all with cavities in the lungs, all with strongly positive sputa. None had received antituberculous treatment of any kind before. At the beginning of the trial all were put on a regime of isoniazid and PAS. They were then divided into two groups. Patients allocated to home treatment took their drugs at home: they were regularly visited by doctors or health visitors and seen at the Health Centre once a week. They also had their urine checked to ensure that they were taking the drugs. (They and their families were liberally bribed to follow the regime by allocations of free milk powder and other sweeteners.)

Those allocated to sanatorium treatment were admitted to the main sanatorium for Madras State, Tamil Nadu, something of a showpiece, with excellent diagnostic and nursing facilities. They were put to bed (with "bed-pan facilities") for three months after which they were allowed up for two and later for four hours a day. After six months they were allowed to visit home for one day once a month. Patients on home treatment were advised to rest but in fact none chose or could afford to do so: women especially went on with their back-breaking daily chores. At least once a week all had to travel to the centre, a walk of up to eight kilometres since few could afford the bus fare. The diet of the two groups was also starkly different: those on home treatment went on with their usual intake, grossly inadequate in first-class proteins, whereas the sanatorium patients had textbook rations. The average floor-space of those treated at home was four and a half square meters: in the sanatorium it was five times greater.

The results were analysed blind by a well-trained team. There were three deaths during the trial (apart from one by accidental electrocution), two in the sanatorium and one in the home-treated group. Those treated in the sanatorium had gained more weight, but radiological progress in terms of cavity size and cavity closure was similar, and the sputa became negative at

---

[26] It was a joint research project organised by the Indian Medical Research Council, the British Medical Research Council, the Government of Madras State and the World Health Organisation. Toman, K., *Tuberculosis: Case-Finding and Chemotherapy*, World Health Organisation (1979); Keers, *Pulmonary Tuberculosis*.

about the same time. The frequency of bacteriological relapse over the next five years was 11 per cent in the sanatorium and 7 per cent in the home-treated patients. Major social problems arose in eight families of the home-treated and in twenty of the sanatorium-treated patients, the latter usually more serious and leading to the disruption of the family in nearly half. Twelve sanatorium patients discharged themselves (though four were later readmitted) against only one drop-out among those treated at home.

The Madras Experiment was widely and deservedly praised for its success as a cooperative effort; but by the end of the exercise its conclusions were somewhat academic. Patients in the Developed World had already voted against sanatoria with their feet; and nobody expected the question of sanatorium versus home treatment in tuberculosis ever to arise again.

33

An Imperfect Civilisation

Tuberculosis has been called the perfect expression of an imperfect civilisation. It is a vague definition but not without an element of truth.[1] As the antibiotic revolution unfolded, and as the tuberculosis saga seemed to draw to a close, that element was often overlooked. Analogies – or pseudoanalogies – were readily available, justifying triumphalist book titles and self-congratulatory endings to chapters in textbooks. Indeed, the chapters would soon shrink to paragraphs and the paragraphs turn into footnotes.

Another historic disease in particular seemed to offer an apt and comforting parallel. Leprosy is caused by the *Mycobacterium leprae*, a bacillus which belongs to the same family as the causative organism of tuberculosis:[2] the two look strikingly alike under the microscope. There are still millions of lepers in the world but the illness has disappeared from Europe. In textbooks and popular manuals it is often referred to as a tropical disease. But it is no more intrinsically tropical than tuberculosis. It was common in every part of Europe for centuries, a dread visitation affecting all age groups including the very young. Like tuberculosis in later centuries, it probably killed mainly the poor but it too could strike across social barriers and fell Popes and Kings.[3] Also like tuberculosis, it spawned a large medical literature, now almost entirely incomprehensible, and inspired gruesome but splendid works of art.[4] It began to decline in Europe in the latter half of the sixteenth century; and, apart from lingering on in a few isolated regions like western Norway and the Danube delta until the early twentieth century, it became for practical purposes extinct.

The reasons are obscure. Changes in the weather, in eating habits, in social conditions and in sanitation have all been canvassed as likely explanations.

---

[1] The writer has been unable to trace the source of this statement.

[2] It was discovered by the Norwegian bacteriologist Armauer Hansen in 1874, twenty years before Koch discovered the tubercle bacillus. Though morphologically the *Mycobacterium tuberculosis* and the *Mycobacterium leprae* are almost indistinguishable, the latter is usually present in vast numbers in leprous lesions. The term is Hippocratic in origin, meaning scaly: the disease was well known to Aretaeus and Celsus.

[3] Like Louis the Great, King of Poland and Hungary, and perhaps Robert the Bruce.

[4] Notably several paintings by Peter Breughel the Elder, showing processions of limbless and eyeless lepers.

None fits all the facts. Treatment there was none, either before or after the decline. The segregation of patients in leprosaria (of which there were thousands in Europe as late as the end of the fifteenth century) has sometimes been given credit for the eradication. Four hundred years later whispered voices even drew parallels with tuberculosis sanatoria which might fulfil a similar salutary role. Yet leprosaria were no more efficient as places of isolation than were the sanatoria. The great medieval epidemics may have killed off many debilitated lepers crowded together in colonies; but leprosy survived the Black Death. It has even been suggested that the repulsive character of leprous lesions may have become a sexual deterrent and a selective eliminator. If true, it is odd that this should have happened within less than a hundred years.

Even more puzzling and perhaps relevant to the conquest of tuberculosis was the behaviour of leprosy when transplanted from one part of the world to another. The disease was introduced into the Upper Mississippi Valley by Norwegian settlers in the early nineteenth century; and the habits and living conditions of the colonists did not change much for at least a generation.[5] Yet, unlike cholera and malaria, both introduced from Europe and both all too readily transplanted, leprosy never became a public-health problem in the United States. Was it the cross-immunity generated by the emergence of tuberculosis which caused the disappearance of the related but less robust disease?[6] It is an intriguing possibility but no more.

Whatever the immunological relation between the two mycobacterial infections, it was widely assumed in the 1970s that in Europe and North America tuberculosis would soon go the way of leprosy (with the pious afterthought that, under the wise guidance of the Developed World, both would eventually disappear from everywhere). Statistics were hardly necessary. The sprawling sanatoria were empty or being put to other, more cheerful uses. Specialists in tuberculosis were now calling themselves allergologists and treating hayfever. Thoracic surgeons were learning to operate on the heart. The tuberculosis charities were petitioning for a change of charter to let them spend their treasure on more contemporary causes. Prestigious tuberculosis research units, some with brilliant records of achievement, were being quietly but briskly phased out.[7] A few dinosaurs maintained that tuberculosis had a habit of staging unexpected comebacks. They were reminded that health resources were finite and new demands mushrooming. The recent craze for hip replacements was a headache enough. Soon millions of the elderly would

[5] Washburn, W. L., *Bulletin of Medical History*, 24 (1950), 123.

[6] Chaussinaud, R., *International Journal of Leprosy*, 16 (1948), 430.

[7] Including the Tuberculosis Research Unit of the Medical Research Council.

be clamouring for new hearts. Science and medicine had to march on: at least scientists and doctors had to.

It was of course known that the disease was still a great killer in the Third World. The Madras Experiment was an eye-opener not only in extinguishing the claims of sanatoria but also in revealing the devastation caused by the illness in the overcrowded cities of Asia. It was true that, as in western Europe a hundred and fifty years earlier, the organism was killing mainly the poor and the young, and of both the supply seemed to be inexhaustible, but the scale of the problem shocked many of the European research teams. Yet, having provided the Third World with the necessary scientific know-how and not inconsiderable financial help, the final eradication of the disease was best left to the Third World countries themselves. In their endeavour they would receive the continued support of such benevolent (if, in Thatcherite parlance, grossly overfunded, dotty and drippingly wet) organisations as the World Health Organisation. As regards the First World, the United States Centers for Disease Control and Prevention, an organisation not given to facile optimism, confidently predicted that, with a derisory annual budget of $35 million, the United States would be a tuberculosis-free zone by 2005. Everything had been taken into account – everything, that is, except what Mr George Bush might have called "that civilisation thing".[8] But that proved to be a serious omission.

Before advancing beyond the triumphalist decades there is, however, one aspect of the conquest – or apparent conquest – of tuberculosis which deserves but rarely gets a mention. A whole group of apparently new clinical entities emerged within a few years of the beginning of specific and successful antituberculous therapy. They can fairly be described as the "successor diseases". The first important feature they had in common is that they were *not* tuberculosis. In a review ostensibly devoted to tuberculosis this might seem an adequate, even compelling reason for ignoring them. But their second common and no less important feature is that for centuries, and until the streptomycin-PAS revolution, they were probably universally misdiagnosed as tuberculosis.

Adrenocortical deficiency due the tuberculous destruction of the cortices of the adrenal glands was described by Thomas Addison of Guy's Hospital in London in the 1840s and still bears his name.[9] A man of powerful intellect

---

[8] Many may recall Mr Bush's reference to "that vision thing" during the 1992 United States Presidential Campaign. Deservedly or not, it did his chances no good.

[9] The son of a grocer in Long Benton near Newcastle, he was born in 1795 and graduated from Edinburgh University in 1815. He became one of a generation of Guy's physicians who had diseases named after them. He described three cases of tuberculous disease of the adrenal glands leading to atrophy of the capsules (now known as the cortices) in a paper read on 15

and an influential teacher, he not only recognised the varied manifestations of the disease as having a common cause but also demonstrated that cause at the post-mortem examination of three of his patients. In life the cardinal symptoms and signs were progressive general weakness, a low blood pressure, a striking darkening of the skin (especially in the creases) with patchy pigmentation inside the mouth.[10] The illness usually ended in a dramatic terminal collapse, later shown to be most commonly due to a fall in blood sugar. The main finding on post-mortem examination was the atrophy of the cortices of adrenal glands which Addison (perhaps rightly in his own cases, perhaps not) attributed to tuberculosis. This could not be proved before the discovery of the tuberculosis bacillus; but several early cases had extensive phthisis of the lungs. It was not unreasonable to assume that this was the primary site of the infection. Since the microscopic appearances too were at least consistent with tuberculosis, until the late 1940s the aetiology was never questioned.[11]

While tuberculosis declined throughout most of the twentieth century, and dramatically after the discovery of streptomycin and PAS, the incidence of Addison's disease did not. Nor did most cases of the disease respond to antituberculous therapy. No exact statistics are available. By the late 1940s adrenocortical deficiency of whatever origin could be controlled though not cured with cortisone (much as diabetes could be controlled with insulin), and deaths from the disease became rare.[12] Textbooks also slowly and quietly began to attribute Addison's disease (or at least most cases of Addison's disease) not to tuberculosis but to autoimmunity (whatever that meant).

More common than Addison's disease was intestinal tuberculosis, including an unverifiable number of patients who must have suffered not from tuberculosis but from regional ileitis of unknown aetiology. This condition too, like autoimmune adrenocortical deficiency, was recognised as a distinct entity only in the late 1940s. It is commonly referred to nowadays as Crohn's

---

March 1849 to the South London Medical Society. This was the first indication that the adrenals were essential to life and according to many the beginning of modern endocrinology. He later expanded these observations into a book.

The adrenal glands are irregularly shaped structures, about three centimetres in diameter, perched on top of the kidneys, each consisting of two anatomically close but functionally entirely distinct parts, the medulla and the cortex. Oddly perhaps but not uniquely the atrophy in Addison's disease, whether of tuberculous or autoimmune origin, never extends to the medullae of the glands. In the same way tuberculous epidydimitis, once common, always spared the adjacent testis.

[10] As seen in the mouths of Dalmatian hounds, as Addison himself observed.

[11] It was unusual for tuberculosis to destroy paired organs symmetrically and destruction of a single adrenal cortex does not cause adrenocortical deficiency.

[12] One recent sufferer was President John F. Kennedy.

disease after the observant New York gastroenterologist who first recognised it;[13] and Crohn himself described its mode of emergence. It would never have been discovered but for the fact that, while most of the severe cases of intestinal tuberculosis got better on the newly available antituberculous treatment, some of the less severe ones did not.[14] The reason was simple: the non-responders had never had tuberculosis in the first place. How common was Crohn's disease before specific antituberculous therapy? Nobody knows. It is true that, by definition, tissue samples from Crohn's disease could never have yielded tubercle bacilli;[15] and some other features of tuberculosis, most notably caseation, are usually absent from non-specific ileitis. But even in its heyday tuberculosis was never expected to display *all* its characteristics in any one patient; and in everyday practice the demonstration of the organism was never a sine qua non of a positive diagnosis. Clinically and on examination of the lesions (both by the naked eye and microscopically) the two conditions were virtually indistinguishable. Both usually began in early adult life and tended to progress episodically. In both, recurrences after remissions were often precipitated by physical or mental stress. Both often required emergency surgery to relieve acute intestinal obstruction. In both the operations often left a legacy of more intraperitoneal adhesions, abscesses, poorly healing wounds and discharging fistulae.[16] But Crohn's disease had a greater tendency to burn itself out; and patients with intestinal tuberculosis who eventually recovered may have suffered from this slightly less crippling illness.

Closest to tuberculosis was a disease long known to dermatologist as sarcoidosis, a chronic and usually self-limiting inflammatory condition of the skin, similar to early lupus vulgaris but carrying a far better prognosis. By the late 1940s it was recognised as the localised manifestation of a general illness,[17] much as lupus vulgaris was a localised form of tuberculosis. Like tuberculosis, sarcoidosis could affect almost any organ or system, most notably the lungs, the lymph nodes, the eyes, the bones (particularly of the fingers and toes) and the kidneys. Like tuberculosis, it was often associated

[13] Crohn, B. B., *Regional Ileitis* (London, 1949); Crohn, B. B., Janowitz, H. D., *Journal of the American Medical Association*, 156 (1954), 1221.

[14] Once the entity had been established and its non-tuberculous origin accepted the hunt was on to find a plausible alternative aetiology. (The same has been true of the other successor diseases.) Suggestions have ranged from various bacteriological infections to the excessive use of toothpaste containing silica or talcum powder.

[15] Which, by definition, would have made them tuberculosis.

[16] See Chapter 29.

[17] Ricker, W., Clark, M., *American Journal of Pathology*, 19 (1949), 725; Robb-Smith, A. H. T., *Recent Advances in Clinical Pathology* (London, 1947), chapter 34.

with fever, loss of weight, tiredness and anaemia. On chest X-ray it could shiveringly reproduce the snow-storm effect of usually fatal miliary tuberculosis. On microscopic examination the lesions consisted of tubercles, complete with epitheloid cells, giant cells, small round-cell infiltration and fibrosis. What ultimately distinguished the two conditions was not the negative tuberculin test or the absence of tubercle bacilli in sarcoidosis – neither feature was essential for the diagnosis of tuberculosis – but the lack of response of sarcoidosis to antituberculous chemotherapy.[18] The last characteristic (shared with several other less well-defined chronic inflammatory conditions) created a bizarre change in perception.

Before streptomycin and PAS non-specific or autoimmune chronic inflammatory pathologies probably accounted for many of those cases of tuberculosis which, contrary to expectation and after a more or less stormy start, either recovered or settled into a slow smouldering course. They justified the description of tuberculosis as an unpredictable disease and probably explained some responses to weird and wonderful remedies. After streptomycin and PAS these same diseases became a troublesome minority, sometimes self-limiting and generally less destructive than tuberculosis used to be, but difficult since, once again contrary to expectation, they did not respond to antituberculous treatment. Only then was their non-tuberculous nature recognised.[19] Since it is impossible to believe that half a dozen comparatively common tuberculosis-like but non-tuberculous conditions suddenly emerged to coincide with the discovery of a particular group of drugs, their recognition might also have injected a note of caution, even humility, into the interpretation of early tuberculosis statistics and the pontifical diagnosis of historical cases. This has not always been a conspicuous sequel.[20]

---

[18] Today a number of laboratory tests, as well as a skin sensitivity test, are available which make a positive diagnosis (rather than a diagnosis by exclusion) possible; but these were not available in the 1940s. Clinically sarcoidosis and tuberculosis are still often indistinguishable.

[19] Today it is tuberculosis which is more likely to be missed in the Developed World.

[20] The accuracy of historical diagnoses are difficult enough to establish: the accuracy of historical misdiagnoses even more so. Nevertheless, two examples illustrate mistakes due to one off the successor diseases (probably sarcoidosis) being misdiagnosed for tuberculosis.

In May 1939 Major-General Bernard L. Montgomery was hoisted on a stretcher aboard a troopship in Haifa harbour with the firm diagnosis of pulmonary tuberculosis. There was no need to wait for the sputum cultures, as the clinical symptoms and signs and the chest X-ray were unequivocal. Escorted home by two nursing sisters and two nursing orderlies he was, by the time the ship docked in Tilbury, well enough to walk off her and was passed fit at Millbank Military Hospital. He was soon importuning the War Office to be allowed to take over his new command of 3rd Infantry Division.

In the same year Admiral (later Sir James) Somerville was bemoaning his fate of being

Turning back to the fight against real tuberculosis, the mid 1970s were the high noon of international confidence: in the Churchillian phrase, it was the beginning of the end. In 1962 the Medical Research Council had cautiously settled on an optimal course of chemotherapy – streptomycin, PAS and isoniazid lasting two years – as their considered recommendation. It was soon apparent that treatment could be given as effectively on an outpatient basis as in a hospital and that bed rest was unnecessary.[21] After a short preliminary intensive course the frequency of taking the tablets could also be reduced to three times or even twice weekly, a small but significant advance in poor countries.[22] The introduction of rifampicin opened the way to shorter treatment regimes.[23] In combination with isoniazid a nine-months course was soon shown to be as effective as the older two-year triple therapy. Another drug, pyrazinamide, had been tried a few years earlier but had been abandoned because of its toxic side-effects. Now Wallace Fox and his team at the Medical Research Council showed that in lower doses and over shorter periods than had been originally recommended it was acceptably safe.[24] Its addition to the repertory allowed a further shortening of the treatment course; and already new and even better drugs were in the offing. It was an embarrassment of riches.

Other developments added to the prevailing mood of optimism. BCG vaccination continued to be maddeningly unpredictable in different parts of the world – its protective efficacy seemed to range from 0 to 80 per cent – but even where it did not protect against the infection, it significantly reduced much-feared extrapulmonary complications.[25] It remained part of the World Health Organisation's anti-tuberculosis campaign. It was rumoured that

retired on the eve of a war with the diagnosis of active pulmonary tuberculosis. He had had a troublesome cough and loss of weight for some months; his chest X-ray showed advanced tuberculous infiltration with early miliary spread; and his sputum was query positive. On the voyage back from Aden to Portsmouth he too staged a spectacular recovery, but the Admiralty could not waive the unalterable Service rule of automatic discharge once tuberculosis had been diagnosed. Fortunately for Somerville, the unalterable rules of peacetime were soon altered by war: edging his way from an interdepartmental committee on radio-interception through various other administrative jobs, he found an excuse to visit the beleaguered garrison of Calais in May 1940 and was back in command of H Force in time for the melancholy task of blowing the French fleet out of the water at Oran in July 1940. Nothing more was heard of his tuberculosis for the rest of his distinguished wartime career.

[21] Snider, D. E., "Tuberculosis: The World Situation", in *Tuberculosis: Back to the Future*, ed. J. D. H. Porter, K. P. W. J. McAdam (Chichester, 1994).

[22] D'Esopo, N. D., *American Review of Respiratory Disease*, 125 (1982), 85.

[23] Sbarbaro, J. A., Johnson, S., *American Review of Respiratory Disease*, 97 (1968), 85.

[24] Fox, W., Mitchison, D. A. *American Review of Respiratory Disease*, 111 (1975), 325.

[25] Fox, W., *British Journal of Diseases of the Chest*, 75 (1981), 331.

other vaccines might follow. The concept of preventative chemotherapy also held out promise. In 1960 it was estimated that worldwide 10 per cent of children infected with the organism progressed to the clinical illness. New trials suggested that prophylactic isoniazid might significantly reduce that percentage.[26] It might also be useful given to close adult contacts in heavily infected households. The scent of victory generated goodwill. Even in the poorest countries co-operation between local antituberculosis agencies and international bodies was warm and the tone of papers read at international gatherings tended to be a little smug. But few begrudged the field workers their moment of glory.

Then, over a period of only two or three years, the statistics became confused. Confusion soon became certainty. By 1980, for the first time in at least a century, both the incidence of tuberculosis and mortality from it were again on the increase. This was not a blip caused by a world war or the side-effect of economic recession. In the Developed World standards of living (as measured by conventional markers and averages) had been rising without a break since the late 1940s. They were still rising. At a much lower level, almost out of sight, there had been a rise even in some developing countries. Though the upturn of the morbidity and mortality curves – "the beginning of the terrible U-shape" – was worldwide, its steepness varied. In western Europe and North America the annual increase during most of the 1980s was less than 1 per cent (starting from a very low level) , barely perceptible to ordinary people. But in several eastern European and South American countries it was nearer 5 per cent, in parts of Asia at a rough but conservative estimate 2–300 per cent, and in much of sub-Saharan Africa a frightening 500 per cent. By 1990 the number of cases diagnosed over the previous five years in the Developing World was estimated to be around seven million.[27] The comparable figure in industrialised countries was 400,000. The World Health Organisation reported that 1.3 million children under fifteen were being infected annually and that half a million died from the disease; but the greatest concentration of deaths (70–80 per cent) was in the economically most productive fifteen-to-fifty age bracket.[28] Globally tuberculosis was once again by far the biggest killer among infections, accounting for 7 per cent of all deaths and 26 per cent of all avoidable deaths.[29] The reason was at first far from clear.

It is still often said in First World countries (at least at cocktail-party level)

[26] Ferebee, S. H., *Advances in Tuberculosis Research*, 17 (1970), 28.

[27] Murray, C. J. L., Styblo, K., Rouillon, A., *Bulletin of the International Union Against Tuberculosis and Lung Diseases*, 65 (1990), 2.

[28] World Health Organisation, *Childhood Tuberculosis and BCG Vaccine* (Geneva, 1989).

[29] Kochi, A., *Tubercle*, 72 (1991), 1.

that the tuberculosis which is re-emerging is not the same disease as has been described in old medical text-books and is familiar from literature, folklore and opera. It is a reassuring notion but there is not much truth in it. Tuberculosis has always been an opportunistic infection. It increased explosively during the Industrial Revolution. It rose to sharp peaks during world wars. It has long been recognised as a sequel to many common debilitating illnesses. What has changed over the past twenty years is not the disease but its opportunities. In particular, there have been two dramatic developments. The first has been the outbreak of the human immunovirus (HIV) pandemic; the second, still only a handkerchief-size cloud on the horizon, is the emergence of multidrug resistance (MDR).

Since the natural history of the acquired immune deficiency syndrome (AIDS) is a progressive loss of of immune function and the eventual appearance of one or more opportunistic diseases, its effect on tuberculosis, critically dependent on the body's immune defences, might have been predicted. Few people did. Indeed, even after the association was recognised, the horror and novelty of AIDS distracted attention from the older infection. Tuberculosis was barely mentioned in the first clinical reports of the new disease, almost all in white homosexual males. But by the end of the 1980s post-mortem studies in Abidjan, Côte d'Ivoire, showed that tuberculosis was the commonest single cause of death in HIV positive individuals (35 per cent).[30] Other work suggested that HIV positive individuals were at least forty times more likely to contract tuberculosis than normal individuals and at least twenty times more likely to die from it.

Increased susceptibility to tuberculosis was compounded by other AIDS-related complications. Worldwide the microscopic examination of sputum is still the most generally applicable diagnostic test, even though the accuracy of a single examination is rarely higher than 75 per cent. In AIDS patients even this modest figure was significantly reduced. Clinical signs too, especially those depending on cavitation, were often atypical; and X-ray appearances could be deceptive. Extrapulmonary complications were more common. Even before the emergence of MDR, treatment with many of the generally safest drugs produced violent, sometimes fatal reactions.[31] In the Developed World the death rate from tuberculosis was three or four times higher in HIV positive than in HIV negative patients.

Just as the downward trends in the disease in the 1970s generated a feeling of confidence and co-operation, so the change in direction affected morale

---

[30] Lucas, S. B., *Lancet*, 337 (1991), 428.
[31] Small, P. M., Schecter, G. F., Goodman, P. C., Sande, M. A., Chaisson, R. E., Hopewell, P. C., *New England Journal of Medicine*, 324 (1991), 289.

in the opposite sense. All the experience gained over the previous twenty-five years began to be questioned. Should all HIV positive infants be given priority chemoprophylaxis? Or were they beyond hope? Could BCG actually *disseminate* tuberculosis in HIV positive children? What were to be the new diagnostic criteria? What treatment could be safely applied? Who should be treated? Most pressingly: where was the money to come from to cope with the new epidemic? In the campaign against AIDS tuberculosis was and would clearly remain a somewhat peripheral issue. The development of anti-HIV vaccines and drugs and, above all, sex education and prophylaxis were given priority and first call on resources. As rival claims clashed, relations between antituberculous and anti-AIDS agencies deteriorated. Almost everywhere the former were losing out. At a morbid level there are fashions in diseases as there are in swimwear, pop groups and religious cults; and by the mid 1980s in popular appeal (and royal patronage) AIDS easily outshone tuberculosis. In the long term this was probably an unrealistic bias.

AIDS-related tuberculosis did not mean that the upsurge in tuberculosis was confined to HIV positive individuals: AIDS was merely the trigger for the new dissemination. By 1990 the number of clinically tuberculous patients had probably trebled worldwide since 1980; but nowhere did the HIV positive tuberculous account for more than 20 per cent of the total. The spread of AIDS, moreover, was theoretically at least more preventable than the spread of tuberculosis: unprotected sex could be avoided, breathing could not. Against this it could be argued that AIDS was still incurable, tuberculosis was not. Unfortunately, by the mid 1990s, the bedrock of that last belief was beginning to crack.

Just as the AIDS-related upsurge of tuberculosis had its roots in the Third World, multi-drug resistance – or MDR to use its newly-minted acronym – surfaced in the Fourth. This was the world of urban squalor in the midst of unprecedented plenty, a new land in the same way as Bohemia was a new land in the Paris of the 1830s. Of course isolated cases of tuberculosis which did not respond to standard chemotherapy had been reported before; and some observers predicted that in time this would become more common and more intractable. But as a real-life – or real-death – public-health problem it did not exist until 30 August 1991, when the Morbidity and Mortality Weekly Report of the United States Centres for Disease Control and Prevention described four small outbreaks, three of them in the heart of the Fourth World, New York City.[32] All the patients were down-and-outs, many but not all were HIV positive and some were drug addicts, alcoholics

[32] Centers for Disease Control, *Mortality and Morbidity Weekly Reports*, 40 (1991), 585; Morse, D. L., in *Tuberculosis: Back to the Future*, p. 225.

or both. The mortality in the group was between 70 and 90 per cent and the period between diagnosis and death was four to sixteen weeks. In one outbreak the organism was thoroughly investigated and shown to be insensitive in culture to seven of the most commonly used chemotherapeutic agents.[33] In historic terms the disease caused by such a bacillus was as untreatable as it had been when Keats had his first haemorrhage.

Despite the alarming implications, the official response was muted. If there was one region of the globe from which the First World felt remote, it was the Fourth World. It existed – the evidence was unpleasantly obtrusive – but it was best ignored. Nor was it clear why its citizens should develop drug-resistance. The episodes were probably freakish instances: or somebody was courting publicity. But only a month after the first outbreaks the New York State Department of Health reported a cluster of cases of skin-test conversions among the *staff* of an Upstate New York Hospital. Epidemiological follow-up revealed that forty-six health-care workers had been in contact with a prison inmate who had been admitted for treatment of tuberculosis resistant to the same seven drugs as had been tested in the earlier cases. Four of the hospital staff and one of the guards who had accompanied the prisoner became clinically ill and three died within a month. This was the first hint of the unthinkable, MDR tuberculosis crossing the social barrier from derelicts to gainfully employed public servants, and it set the telephone wires humming. The Prison Officers' Association and hospital staff and other health-care unions threatened industrial action unless prompt preventative measures were taken. An emergency investigation of the prison whose inmate had started the outbreak showed a skin-test conversion rate of over 30 per cent among those who had started their term of incarceration within the previous two years. Subsequent screening of the entire 69,000 strong population of the New York State Correctional System demonstrated that the MDR strain had been introduced into at least twenty-three prisons and that at least twenty-six prisoners who may have been infected had been treated at one time or another in New York City hospitals.

Official response was swift. In Washington the Federal Tuberculosis Programme, which had been quietly mothballed a few years earlier, was recommissioned with an increase in funding from an annual $8 to $100 million. Both the New York State and New York City Health Departments inaugurated an epidemiological and clinical programme designed to detect, survey, control and if possible eradicate the new disease. There was a prompt

---

[33] Pablos-Mendez, A., Raviglione, M. C., Battan, R., Ramos-Zuniga, R., *New York State Journal of Medicine*, 90 (1990), 351; Frieden, T. R., Sterling, T. et al., *New England Journal of Medicine*, 328 (1993), 521.

though slightly less urgent response from other cities in the United States. Official interest was expressed even in Britain and continental Europe. Things American had a fearful tendency to cross the Atlantic.

Interest did not necessarily signify understanding. A number of instant and glib explanations were advanced, none entirely convincing. The basis of MDR either at the molecular or at the clinical level is still far from clear. The vast majority of tubercle bacilli either in an affected individual or in any population are still sensitive to several antituberculous drugs. These organisms are potentially lethal; but one of their subsidiary actions is to keep less vigorous strains of their own species at bay. Such strains may emerge all the time, just as genetic mutants and chromosomal abnormalities emerge in human populations; but, unable to compete with the dominant type, they tend to perish. Once, however, the dominant type has been eliminated by a particular drug, drug-resistant freaks may seize their chance. This at least in rough outline (and more or less in the classical Darwinian mould) is the currently accepted sequence of events. It does not explain many observed facts, just as many widely accepted aetiologies 200 years ago did not explain the vagaries of clinical tuberculosis. Nevertheless, it quickly led to the promulgation of two ground rules. The first was that the treatment of clinically affected individuals must continue until there was clear laboratory evidence that all organisms had been destroyed. This often did not happen for weeks or months after symptoms and signs had subsided. The second was that no drug, let alone a succession of drugs, should ever be used singly. The experimental evidence in support of the second rule was strong; but it was hard on Third World countries where international bodies had for many years vigorously promoted single-drug strategies.

The practical measure designed to apply these rules was another acronym – DOT for Direct Observation Therapy. It was later supplemented with DOTS for Direct Observation Therapy Shortened Course. Both were meant to eliminate the improper use of drugs. This could take many forms. In the Developed World Crofton singled out the addition syndrome as a particular menace, a new drug being added to the therapeutic regime whenever a patient seemed to deteriorate and, conversely, a drug being discontinued as soon as he or she showed signs of improvement.[34] In the Developing World it was easy to find other culprits – the ignorance of doctors, unscrupulous sales talk, the adulteration of drugs, endemic corruption, inadequate laboratory facilities and everywhere and most commonly sheer poverty.

Even to those not entirely clear about their meaning, DOT and DOTS had

[34] Crofton, J., *Bulletin of the International Union Against Tuberculosis and Lung Diseases*, 62 (1987), 6.

a reassuringly peremptory ring: surely no organism would dare to resist their whiplash. On paper, moreover, they were simple to implement. All that was necessary was to ensure that patients took their prescribed combination of drugs for the necessary length of time by actually observing them perform the act of putting the tablets into their mouths. In practice, the concept had several limitations.

Most obviously it was no cure for established cases. Fortunately, they were (or seemed to be for some years) almost entirely confined to the Fourth World. There an average life expectancy had to be regretfully accepted as being less than a year. (At least this would limit the spread of the MDR strain.) Secondly, experts were divided about which drug combinations to recommend and where: as with BCG, there were wide regional variations in efficacy, reflecting perhaps past local drug usage and abuse. Thirdly, as had happened with Bohemia 150 years earlier, despite the depredations of disease, outposts of the Fourth World were becoming entrenched in every major city of the First and Second World and all were potential reservoirs of MDR. A 1997 survey of those sleeping rough in the streets of London – a social phenomenon not seen between the First World War and the 1960s – showed that 5 per cent had active tuberculosis; and an estimated 10 per cent of these were probably MDR.[35] The figures most widely quoted were not significantly different in Paris, Rome or Zurich. Few meaningful statistics were available about the growing army of vagrants and beggars which was becoming part of the new cityscape in many former Communist countries. As the Fourth World expanded it also became more inaccessible. Prisons and hospitals could at least be monitored. But health workers could not be expected to carry DOT or DOTS to patients whose abode changed nightly. It was also hard to convince those sheltering in subways and entrances to department stores that they owed it to society as well as to themselves to adhere, comply or co-operate with their treatment. (Much argument centred – as it still does – on the best term to use, always an ominous sign.) The prettily coloured tablets often tasted like sweets but they relieved neither hunger nor thirst, let alone a craving for oblivion.

In what was becoming a slow but accelerating progress to the past there was another element of déjà-vu. Some of the advocacy for the rigorous application of DOT or DOTS began to resemble the tone adopted by doctors, politicians and philanthropists in touting sanatoria as the ultimate panacea a hundred years ago, a disconcerting mixture of self-delusion and high-minded bullying. Only the plethora of computer-generated graphs and statistics was new.

---

[35] Citron, K. M., *Out of the Shadow* (London, 1997).

Apart from giving birth to DOT (and DOTS), MDR tuberculosis high-lighted the need for new drugs. The prospects for this were – and are – not good. Since the intense and extraordinarily fruitful research period of the 1950s and 1960s, capital investment into the search for fresh antituberculous compounds has been declining. The suggestion that it is unlikely to start rising again until MDR crosses the social barrier and begins to strike at those who can pay for their survival tends to provoke indignant protests. Spokes-men for the pharmaceutical industry point out – correctly – that vast sums of money are still being spent on pure (or purish) research. Yet drug com-panies, however noble, are not a public service; and they must take note of the fact that in some of the world's poorest countries, where tuberculosis is both most prevalent and most menacing, 80 per cent of antituberculous medication is taken up by the private medical sector. (It looks after less than 1 per cent of the population.) Nor has the free market always dealt kindly with the pharmaceutical industries of former Communist countries which, at the cost of inefficiency, appalling pollution and not always perfect quality control, did at least provide for local needs.

The outlook seems a little brighter in the more esoteric area of basic research. The next decade will almost certainly see advances in the under-standing of the genetic material and molecular structure of the different kinds and strains of *Mycobacteria*, a potential window into the mechanism of drug resistance and perhaps a pointer to its rapid detection and even prevention.[36] (The genome of the *Mycobacterium leprae* is already complete and large chunks of it can be used to establish that of the *Mycobacterium tuberculosis*.)[37] New drugs, different in kind from existing chemotherapeutic agents, might also in the fullness of time be based on a firmer grasp on the biochemistry of the bacillus.[38] On the medical conference circuit "designer drug" is becoming a buzz word.

What then, shorn of sensationalism on the one hand and complacency on the other, are the chances – or portents – of a return to what the disease was before the antibiotic revolution? The main ground for optimism is that fundamentally the tubercle bacillus is, as it has always been, an inefficient killer. It invades easily and may be difficult to dislodge; but its further advance is precarious. For it actually to destroy the host conditions have to be almost absurdly weighted in its favour. In a perfect civilisation – or even in a

[36] Grosset, J., *Lancet*, 346 (1995), 814.

[37] This proved to be an overcautious forecast when, on 11 June 1998, the whole genome of the Mycobacterium tuberculosis was laid bare by a team of thirty-seven authors in *Nature*, 393 (1998), 537.

[38] Hershfield, E. S., *Lancet*, 346 (1995), 814; Cole, S. T., Smith, D. R. in *Tuberculosis: Pathogen-esis, Protection and Control*, edited by B. Bloom (Washington, DC, 1994).

modestly prosperous, caring and rational one – it would continue to decline without necessarily completely disappearing. That this is actually happening is, despite occasional alarming reports in the media, still the general perception in the First World. The diagnosis of tuberculosis in a schoolchild from a respectable middle-class home in a London suburb still makes television news. Doctors are exhorted in official circulars to bear the possibility of tuberculosis in mind when investigating obscure or atypical illnesses. Drug resistance remains a threat hanging over "Them" – the derelicts, the uncared-for old, the lost mentally ill, the drug underworld, the recent and illegal immigrants. To "Us", even when the disease occasionally strikes, treatment is not a problem (except for victims of AIDS). The arsenal of antituberculous weaponry remains reasonably well-stocked and the cost is not prohibitive. It is certainly cheaper than a sanatorium regime was a hundred years ago.

Outside the First World – just below the horizon – the outlook is different. A report published in 1998 of a survey carried out jointly by the United States Centers for Control and Prevention of Disease, the World Health Organisation and the International Union against Tuberculosis and Lung Diseases must be hailed as a remarkable feat of international co-operation and organisational skill. That is the only cheering feature about it. 50,000 cases of tuberculosis in thirty-five countries have been investigated both clinically and in the laboratory. "Hot spots" of the MDR situated in larger areas of "warm zones" were identified in regions as far apart as Russia, India, the Dominican Republic, Argentina, Estonia, Latvia and Côte d'Ivoire. By any single criterion the distribution makes little sense; but this should not come as a surprise. However inefficient as a killer, tuberculosis has always had an unlimited capacity to confound; and, whatever accounts for the scatter, the hot spots are strategically placed to threaten a global wave of virtually incurable tuberculosis.[39]

In the light of these findings what is needed to forestall disaster, according to the director of the Tuberculosis Elimination Division of the United States Centers for Disease Control and Prevention, is "a comprehensive programme of Directly Observed Treatment Short Course (DOTS) ... a multifaceted approach consisting of government commitment to control tuberculosis, bacterial confirmation of all diagnoses, the assurance of an adequate drug supply everywhere, the systematic review of patients' progress and a standardised treatment plan for all cases".[40] It is impossible to quarrel with the prescription but in an imperfect civilisation the chances of its implementation are remote and probably receding. The question then is if and when the new

[39] Macready, N., *Lancet*, 350 (1997), 1302.
[40] Castro, K. quoted by Macready, ibid.

epidemic can be expected to burst through social, geographic and political barriers. That it will remain locked away forever in a few conveniently remote hot spots seems as fatuous as was the hope that nuclear devices can be confined to a select club of "mature" states. To put a timetable on the event would be unwise; but with natural immunity in many technologically advanced countries as low today as it was among the Indians of the North American prairies a hundred and fifty years ago, the prospect is not a pleasant one. And yet ...

A hundred and twenty years ago, at the dawn of the bacteriological era, Pasteur declared: "It is within the power of man to eradicate all parasitic [meaning infectious] diseases from the earth". He was expressing not only his own faith but also the faith of his generation. Despite uncertainties and admitted imperfections, it was an age which firmly believed in progress. After two world wars, in the face of AIDS, genocide, man-induced famine and a new atomic arms race, it is difficult to recapture that spirit of confidence. Even narrowing the field to a small corner marked by spectacular successes over the past fifty years, not many would bet today on *Homo sapiens* outliving *Mycobacterium tuberculosis* rather than the other way round. Yet, more perhaps than many other more obvious dangers and afflictions which cast a shadow over the modern world, tuberculosis remains to many a matter of passionate concern and a spur to extraordinary individual effort.

In this respect, too, it continues to run true to form. A thin but seemingly unbreakable thread is woven into the history of the White Death. It has been alluded to several times before. The *spes phthisica*, the hope of the tuberculous has been described by Osler as the Great Delusion. Trudeau dismissed it as a folly. The Hungarian poet Csokonay apostrophised it as a most cruel and deceiving goddess. Many others have pointed out that hope is not the hallmark of any particular illness or indeed of any human predicament. This may be true. Yet such figments rarely survive for centuries without reason. Illnesses have their personalities in much the same way as nationalities and historic periods, impossible to define but, once experienced, instantly recognisable. Nor do they affect only their victims. They imprint themselves on all those with whom they come into contact – families, friends, lovers, doctors, researchers, reformers, administrators, even politicans. The hope of the tuberculous has always been of a particular kind. Without conflicting with a more transcendental faith, it has always inspired a will to live in this world, a will to fight in this world and a will to create in this world. To the eyes of one astonished observer it still does.

Bibliography

This bibliography is inevitably a personal selection. Some of the famous victims of tuberculosis referred to in the text – the Brontës, Chopin, Modigliani, Schiller – have had hundreds of books, articles and theses written about them. With the medical and scientific figures linked to tuberculosis the difficulty has been the opposite, an embarrassment of poverty rather than of riches. Even the most outstanding among them have rarely had more than one full-scale biography (none in the cases of Auenbrugger, Villemin, Bodington or Brehmer) and the ones available tend to be devotional rather than informative. (Doctors have often been deplorably indiscreet about their patients but rarely about each other.)

Works of literature touching on tuberculosis are too numerous to list. A little reluctantly short stories and plays have been excluded – even masterly ones by Tolstoy, Chekhov, Maupassant, Somerset Maugham and Kosztolányi – in favour of full-scale books, mostly autobiographies and many not widely read today. All shed light on some aspect of the illness, – often more revealing than many a learned tome.

The scientific and medical literature used to fill libraries. Around 1910 at least twenty learned journals in at least twelve languages were dedicated exclusively to the disease, discounting published proceedings of learned or charitable societies, official memoranda and collections of papers read at congresses; and there is hardly an issue of the *Lancet*, the *British Medical Journal*, the *Journal of the American Medical Association* or their German, French or Italian counterparts which does not contain at least one relevant article or news item. Even the number of new books published in English in any one year with tuberculosis in its title between 1910 and 1930 was never less than twenty. From this mountain of print most of the works chosen are the widely quoted authoritative texts of their day and ones which were recognised then or later as important; a few popular works written for the lay public and for patients and their families, as well as widely used student crammers and instruction books for nurses and social workers are also included. Only a few single items, mostly landmarks and comprehensive reviews, are on the general history of medicine, epidemiology, palaeopathology, medical sociology, immunology, geographical pathology and other topics which have helped the present writer to see – or at least to look at – tuberculosis in a wider context. Of the historical landmarks which include themselves, English translations of foreign or Latin works have been preferred where available to the original texts. (Some of the original titles are given in the text or the notes.) The list is mainly of books but a few historic and important review articles are included.

Abreu, M. de, "Collective Fluorography", *Radiology*, 33 (1939), 363. The historic beginning of screening by mass miniature chest radiography.

Ackerknecht, E. H., *Rudolf Virchow: Doctor, Statesman, Archeologist* (Madison, Wisconsin, 1953)

Agate, J., *Rachel* (London, 1928)

Aitken, K. M., *Hugh Owen Thomas: His Principles and Practice* (Oxford, 1968)

Alexander, J., *The Collapse Therapy of Pulmonary Tuberculosis* (Springfield, Illinois, 1937). The standard and most popular textbook on tuberculosis surgery for nearly two decades.

Almeida, H. de, *Romantic Medicine and John Keats* (Oxford, 1991)

Ashburn, P. M., *The Ranks of Death* (New York, 1947)

Auenbrugger, L., *A New Invention for Percussing the Human Chest to Detect Hidden Signs of Disease*, translated by J. Forbes (London, 1824). A classic.

Baillie, M., *The Morbid Anatomy of Some of the Most Important Parts of the Human Body* (London, 1793). The first description of caseation.

Bailyn, B., *Voyages to the West: A Passage in the Peopling of America* (New York, 1984)

Baldwin, E. R., Petroff, S. A., Gardner, L. U., *Tuberculosis: Bacteriology, Pathology and Laboratory Diagnosis* (London, 1947)

Bankoff, G., *The Conquest of Tuberculosis* (London, 1946)

Barker, Juliet, *The Brontës: A Life in Letters* (London, 1997)

Bardswell, N. D., *Advice to Consumptives* (London, 1910)

Barry, V. C., *Chemotherapy of Tuberculosis* (London, 1964)

Barnes, D. S., *The Making of a Social Disease: Tuberculosis in Nineteenth-Century France* (Berkeley, California, 1995)

Barnes, P., Steele, M. A., "Tuberculosis in Patients with HIV Infection", *Chest*, 102 (1992), 428

Bashkirtseva, M. K., *The Journal of a Young Artist*, translated by Mary J. Serrano (New York, 1926)

Bateman, T., *Report on the Diseases of London* (London, 1919). The beginning of modern public-health statistics.

Bayle, G. L., *Researches on Pulmonary Phthisis*, translated by W. Barrow (Liverpool, 1810)

Beddoes, T., *Essay on the Causes, Early Signs and Prevention of Pulmonary Consumption* (London, 1799). The bible of inhalation therapy.

Bennett, J. B., *The Pathology and Treatment of Pulmonary Tuberculosis* (Edinburgh, 1853)

Behring, E. von, *The Suppression of Tuberculosis* (New York, 1904)

Bickerton, T. H., A *Medical History of Liverpool* (Liverpool, 1936). What was true of Liverpool was true of many other English cities.

Bloom, B. R., *Tuberculosis* (New York, 1994)

Bloom, B. R., Murray, C. J. L., "Tuberculosis: Commentary on a Re-Emergent Killer", *Science,* 257 (1992), 1055

Bodington, G., *An Essay on the Treatment and Cure of Pulmonary Tuberculosis* (London, 1804; reprinted, London, 1906)

Bonnefoix-Demalet, P., *Traité sur la nature et la traitment de la phthisie pulmonaire* (Paris, 1904)

Boyer, G. R., *An Economic History of the English Poor Law, 1750–1850* (Cambridge, 1990)

Brieger, E. M., *The Papworth Families* (London, 1944)

Brown, L., *The Story of Clinical Pulmonary Tuberculosis* (Baltimore, Maryland, 1941)

Brothwell, D., Sandison, A. T. (eds), *Diseases in Antiquity* (Springfield, Illinois, 1967)

Bryder, L., *Below the Magic Mountain: A Social History of Tuberculosis in Twelfth-Century Britain* (Oxford, 1988). A well-researched scholarly work, especially good on the village settlements.

Bulman, B., *The House of Quiet People* (London, 1939). A savagely realistic sanatorium novel.

Bulstrode, H. T., *Report on Sanatorium for Consumption* (London, 1908). A mine of factual information and surprisingly sane comments (for its date).

Burke, R. M. N., *A Historical Chronology of Tuberculosis* (Springfield, Illinois, 1955)

Burnet, M., White D. O., *The Natural History of Infectious Diseases* (4th edn, Cambridge, 1972). A classic of modern immunology.

Burrell, L. S. T., *The Artificial Pneumothorax* (3rd edn, London, 1937)

Cabanes, A., *Poitrinaires et grandes amoreuses* (Paris, 1912). The intertwining story of tuberculosis and the demi-monde.

Cahuet, A., *Moussai: ou la vie et mort de Marie Bashkirtsheff* (Paris, 1926)

Calmette, A., *The Tubercle Bacillus: Infection and Tuberculosis in Man and Animals,* translated by W. B. Soper and H. H. Smith (Baltimore, Maryland, 1925)

Camby, H. S., *Thoreau* (Boston, 1939)

Cameron, V., Long, E. R., *Tuberculosis Research, 1904–1955* (New York, 1955)

Canetti, G., *The Tubercle Bacillus* (New York, 1955)

Carswell, R., *Pathological Anatomy: Illustrations of the Elementary Forms of Disease* (London, 1838)

Cartwright, F. F., *A Social History of Medicine* (London, 1977)

Castiglione, A., *A History of Tuberculosis* (New York, 1933)

Chadwick, H. D., Pope, A. S., *The Modern Attack on Tuberculosis* (New York, 1942)

Citron, K. M., *Coming Out of the Shadow* (London 1997). A publication by "Crisis" about tuberculosis among the homeless in English cities in the 1990s.

Clark, Sir J., *A Treatise of Pulmonary Tuberculosis* (London, 1835). A much-quoted standard textbook by Keats's tender-hearted killer.

Cobbett, L., *The Causes of Tuberculosis* (Cambridge, 1917)

Cohen, N. M., *Health and the Rise of Civilisation* (New Haven, Connecticut, 1989)

Cole, L. G., "On the Technique of the Application of the Röntgen Rays in the Diagnosis of Pulmonary Tuberculosis", *American Journal of Medical Science*, 140 (1910), 29. The foundation paper of the radiology of tuberculosis.

Coote, S., *John Keats: A Life* (London, 1895)

Courcy, C., *Grandeur et déclin d'une maladie: la tuberculose au cours des âges* (Paris, 1972)

Craig, J., *Consumption in Ireland* (Dublin, 1900)

Creighton, C., *Bovine Tuberculosis in Man: An Account of the Pathology of Suspected Cases* (London, 1881). A prophetic book.

Crick, B., *George Orwell: A Life* (London, 1988)

Crofton, J., "Chemotherapy of Pulmonary Tuberculosis", *British Medical Journal* (1959), no. 1, 1910. A ringing declaration of faith of the triumphalist decade but also a wise and prescient warning.

Crofton, J., *Science and Society* (London, 1995)

Crofton, J., Horne, N., Miller, F., *Clinical Tuberculosis* (London, 1992). A non-technical, easily readable guide designed to be available in the Developing World to village health workers as well as to doctors. It has been translated into many languages.

Crowther, M. A., *The Workhouse System, 1839–1926: The History of an English Institution* (London, 1981)

Cummins, S. Lyle, *The Fight Against Tuberculosis* (London, 1939)

Cummins, S. Lyle, *Tuberculosis in History* (London 1949). The title is somewhat misleading. The book is a collection of readable thumb-nail sketches of some of the leading figures in the history of tuberculosis.

Davies, P. D. O. (ed.), *Clinical Tuberculosis* (3rd edn, London, 1998). The currently standard and authoritative British multi-author textbook.

Dessault, P., *A Treatise on the Venereal Distemper with a Dissertation upon Consumption*, translated by J. André (London, 1738)

Dewhurst, K., *John Locke, Physician and Philosopher: A Medical Biography* (London, 1963)

Dobell, C., *Antony van Leeuwenhoek and his Little Animalcules* (London, 1932)

Dowling, H. F., *Fighting Infection* (Cambridge, Massachusetts, 1977)

Douglas, A., *Artists' Quarters: Reminiscences of Montmartre and Montparnasse* (London, 1941). Evocative background to tuberculosis in Bohemia.

Drage, M. D., *The State and the Poor* (London, 1914).

Drolet, G. J., "The Epidemiology of Tuberculosis", *Clinical Tuberculosis*, edited by B. Goldberg (Davis, California, 1946)

Dubos, R., *Man Adapting* (New Haven, Connecticut, 1965). The evolving relationship between man and microbes.

Dubos, R. and J., *The White Plague: Tuberculosis, Man and Society* (London, 1953). Written on the threshold of the antibiotic era, the first author of this book, René Dubos, French-born but a naturalised American, was a distinguished participant in the search for specific antituberculous treatment which preceded the discovery of streptomycin and PAS. He gave up active research after the death from tuberculosis of his first wife, Marie-Louise. His second wife, Jean, also developed the disease but was one of the first to recover on specific chemotherapy. Their work is inevitably out of date; but it remains a landmark in the historiography of tuberculosis. It is rich in social and philosophical insights and remains a prime source of factual information.

Duffy, J., *The Sanitarians: A History of American Public Health* (Ithaca, New York, 1953)

Ehrlich, P., *Das Sauerstoff-Bedürfnis des Organismus: eine farbenanalitische Studie* (Berlin, 1885). A classic of histopathology including the first description of the workable staining of the tubercle bacillus.

Fearis, W. H., *The Treatment of Tuberculosis by Means of the Immune Substances (IK) Therapy* (London, 1912). A sample of the vast quack literature of tuberculosis.

Ferebee, S. H., "Controlled Chemoprophylaxis Trials in Tuberculosis", *Advances in Tuberculosis Research*, 17 (1970), 28

Fine, P. E. M., "The BCG Story: Lessons from the Past and Implications for the Future", *Reviews of Infectious Diseases*, 11 (1989), supplement, 353

Flick, L. F., *Development of our Knowledge of Tuberculosis* (Paris, 1931)

Forlanini, C., "Zur Behandlung der Lungenschwindsucht durch künstlich erzeugten Pneumothorax", *Deutsche medizinische Wochenschrift*, 32 (1906), 1401

Foster, W. D., *A History of Medical Bacteriology and Immunology* (Edinburgh, 1970)

Foster, W. D., *A Short History of Clinical Pathology* (Edinburgh, 1961)

Fournet, J. *Researches on Auscultation of the Respiratory Organs and on the First Stage of Phthisis*, translated by T. Brady (London, 1841)

Fowler, J. Kingson, *Problems in Tuberculosis* (London, 1923). Ruminations by one of the hierarchs of British tuberculosis medicine.

Francis, J., *Bovine Tuberculosis: Including a Contrast with Human Tuberculosis* (London, 1947). A classic on bovine tuberculosis and other veterinary aspects of the disease. The comprehensive treatise on the subject.

Frazer, W. M., *A History of English Public Health, 1834–1939* (London, 1950)

Furesz, S., Timball, M. T., "Antibacterial Activity of Rifamycins", *Chemotherapia*, 7 (1963), 200. The beginning of rifampicin.

Fywel, T. R., *George Orwell: A Personal Memoir* (London, 1982)

Gauvain, H., *Tuberculous Cripples* (London, 1918)

Ghon, A., *The Primary Lung Focus of Tuberculosis in Children* (Prague, 1912)

Gibson, J. A., *The Nordrach Treatment* (London, 1901)

Gilman, S., *Franz Kafka: The Jewish Patient* (London, 1995)

Glasser, E., *W. C. Röntgen* (Springfield, Illinois, 1945)

Gloyne, S. R. E., *Social Aspects of Tuberculosis* (London, 1944)

Gordon, D., *Health, Sickness and Society* (San Lucia, Queensland, 1976)

Goring, C., *On the Inheritance of the Diathesis of Phthisis and Insanity: A Statistical Study based on 1500 Criminals* (London, 1909). A widely quoted compendium of almost total nonsense based on "incontrovertible" statistical evidence.

Granchet, J., *Diagnostic précoce de la tuberculose pulmonaire* (Copenhagen, 1886). The blueprint for l'Oeuvre Grancher.

Greenwood, M., *Epidemics and Crowd Diseases* (London, 1933) A canonical text of the 1930s by Calmette's self-appointed scourge.

Grellet, Isabella, Ruse, C., *Les fièvres de l'âme: histoire de la tuberculose, 1800–1940* (Paris, 1983)

Grmek, M., *A History of AIDS: The Emergence and Origin of a Modern Pandemic* (Princeton, New Jersey, 1990). So far the best monograph on the emergence of AIDS, highly relevant to tuberculosis.

Grmek, M., *Diseases in the Ancient Greek World* (Baltimore, Maryland, 1989)

Grygier, P. S., *A Long Way from Home* (Montreal, 1994). Tuberculosis among the Innuits.

Guilleaume, R., *Du désespoir au salut: les tuberculeux aux 19e et 20e siècles* (Paris, 1980). A good survey of tuberculosis in France.

Guinard, L., *La pratique des sanatoriums* (Paris, 1925)

Hale-White, W., *Keats as Doctor and Patient* (Oxford, 1938)

Harraden, B., *Ships that Pass in the Night* (London, 1893). A true mountain sanatorium story beautifully told.

Hammond, J. L., Hammond, B., *The Bleak Age* (London, 1934)

Hart, P. D'Arcy, *The Value of the Tuberculin Test in Man* (London, 1932)

Hart, P. D'Arcy, Wright, G. P., *Tuberculosis and Social Conditions: A Statistical Study* (London, 1939).

Heaf, F. R. G. (ed.), *Symposium on Tuberculosis* (London, 1957)

Helman, C., *Culture, Health and Illness* (Bristol, 1984)

Hill, A. B., "The Recent Trend in England and Wales of Mortality from Phthisis in Young Adults", *Journal of the Royal Statistical Society*, 42 (1936), 1. A classic article by the future father figure of medical statistics in Britain.

Hirsch, A., *Handbook of Geographical and Historical Pathology* (London, 1885). Widely quoted in its day and replete with weird and wonderful information.

Hodin, J. P., *Munch* (London, 1977)

Holtby, W. *The Land of Green Ginger* (London, 1927). A memorable and tragic story of the tuberculous destiny in the 1920s.

Hoyle, C., "The Brompton Hospital: A Centenary Review", *Diseases of the Chest*, 14 (1948), 269

Hutas, I., *Tuberkulozis Ma (Tuberculosis Today)* (Budapest, 1993)

Interdepartmental Committee on Tuberculosis, *Report: Sanatoria for Soldiers* (London, 1919). The beginning (and very nearly the end) of a brave new world fit for heroes.

Irvine, K. N., *BCG Vaccination in Theory and Practice* (Oxford, 1949)

Jaccoud, S., *The Curability and Treatment of Pulmonary Phthisis*, translated by M. Lubbock (London, 1855). A leading French textbook popular in England.

Kayne, G. G., Pagel, W., O'Shaugnessy, L., *Pulmonary Tuberculosis* (London, 1939). The standard English text for thirty years.

Keers, R. Y., *Pulmonary Tuberculosis: A Journey down the Centuries* (London, 1978). An elegant, important and scholarly work addressed to doctors rather than to the general reader.

Kervran, R., *Laënnec: médecin Breton* (Paris, 1955). The best biography so far (against little real competition) of one of the greatest medical figures in tuberculosis.

Kelynack, T. N., ed., *Defective Children* (London, 1915)

Kiple, K., ed., *The Cambridge World History of Diseases* (Cambridge, 1993)

Kissen, D. M., *Emotional Factors in Pulmonary Tuberculosis* (London, 1958)

Knopf, S. A., "Hermann Brehmer", *New York State Medical Journal*, 1 (1904), 98

Koch, R., "Die Aetiologie der Tuberkulose", *Berliner klinische Wochenschrift*, 19 (1882), 221. A landmark.

Laënnec, R. T. H., *A Treatise on Diseases of the Chest and on Mediate Auscultation*, translated by J. Forbes (London, 1827)

"Lancet Conference Report: Assessment of a World-Wide Tuberculosis Control", *Lancet*, 350 (1997), 642

Landis, H. R. M., "The Reception of Koch's Discovery in the United States", *Annals of Medical History*, 14 (1932), 521.

Latham, A., Garland, C. H., *The Conquest of Tuberculosis* (London, 1910). A premature trumpet call, one of many; but illuminating and compassionate.

Lawson, D., "X-Rays in the Diagnosis of Lung Disease", *Practitioner*, extra number on X-rays

Lederberg, J., Schope, R., eds, *Emerging Infections: Microbial Threats to Health in the United States* (Washington, DC, 1993). Essential background to the re-emergence of tuberculosis.

Leff, S., *The Health of the People* (London, 1950)

Lehmann, J., "Para-Aminosalicylic Acid in the Treatment of Tuberculosis", *Lancet* (1946), no. 1, 15. The historic paper announcing PAS two years after the first clinical trials.

Lehmann, J., "Twenty Years Afterwards", *American Review of Respiratory Disease*, 90 (1964), 953

Lindenboom, G. A., *Hermann Boerhaave: The Man and his Work* (London, 1968)

Lister, T. D., *Medical Examination for Life Insurance* (London, 1921)

Livingstone, J. L., Holmes-Sellors, T., eds, *Modern Practice of Tuberculosis* (London, 1952). The standard multi-author textbook on tuberculosis in Britain in the 1950s.

Loewy, A., Wittkower, E., *The Pathology of High Altitude Climate* (Oxford, 1937). Widely quoted in the last phase of altitude therapy.

Logan, W. D. P., *Mortality in England and Wales from 1849 to 1947*, iv, *Population Studies* (London, 1951)

Logan, W. P. D., Benjamin, B., *Tuberculosis Statistics for England and Wales* (London 1957)

Long, E. R., *A History of Pathology* (Baltimore, Maryland, 1928)

Long, E. R., *A History of the Therapy of Tuberculosis: Chopin's Illness* (Kansas, 1956)

Louis, P. C. A., *Recherches anatomico-pathologiques sur la phthisie* (Paris, 1887)

Luelmo, F., "BCG Vaccination", *American Review of Respiratory Disease*, 125 (1982), 70

MacDonald, Betty, *The Plague and I* (London,1948). A witty and authentic first-hand account of sanatorium life just before the antibiotic revolution.

McCourt, Frank, *Angela's Ashes* (London, 1977)

McDougall, J. B., *Tuberculosis: A Global Study in Social Pathology* (Edinburgh, 1950)

McKeown, T., *The Origin of Human Diseases* (Oxford, 1988)

McKeown, T., Lowe, R., *An Introduction to Social Medicine* (London, 1974)

McKeown, T., *The Role of Medicine* (Oxford, 1979). The spontaneous versus medicine-engineered decline of tuberculosis.

McLynn, F., *Robert Louis Stevenson* (London, 1993)

McNalty, A. S., *A Report on Tuberculosis: Including an Examination of the Results of Sanatorium Treatment* (London, 1932). A masterly exercise in sitting on the fence.

McNeill, W., *Plagues and People* (Garden City, New York, 1976)

Mann, Thomas, *The Magic Mountain*, translated by H. T. Lowe-Porter (London, 1928). A huge emblematic work, the quintessential German *Bildungsroman* about tuberculosis and Davos; or rather about Thomas Mann's thoughts inspired by his brief visit to Davos in 1912. It is either one of the monuments of European literature or the most long-winded work of fiction since *War and Peace*, perhaps both.

March, J., *The Pre-Raphaelite Sisterhood* (London, 1985)

Mariott, C. I., *Heswall* (Liverpool, 1985)

Marten, B., *A New Theory of Consumption: More Specially of Phthisis or Consumption of the Lung* (London, 1720)

Masters, D., *How to Conquer Consumption* (London, 1930). A characteristic book of exhortations of the 1930s.

Mazumdar, P. M. H., *Species and Specificity: An Interpretation of the History of Immunology* (Cambridge, 1994). Some good essays on a subject of mind-boggling complexity.

Medical Research Council, "Treatment of Pulmonary Tuberculosis with Streptomycin and Para-Amino-Salicylic Acid", *British Medical Journal* (1950), no. 2, 1073

Merquiol A., *La Côte d'Azur dans la littérature française* (Paris, 1949)

Miller, D. L., Farmer, R., eds, *Epidemiology of Diseases* (Oxford, 1982)

Miller, F. J. F., *Growing Up in Newcastle upon Tyne* (Oxford, 1960)

Motion, A., *Keats* (London, 1997)

Moore , D. F., "The History and Development of BCG", *Practitioner*, 227 (1983), 317

Morton, R., *Phthisiologia* (London, 1720)

Morton, S. G., *Illustrations of Pulmonary Consumption, its Anatomical Characters, Causes, Symptoms and Treatment* (Philadelphia, 1834). The first American textbook of tuberculosis, reflecting the sane views of Laënnec, Bayle and Louis under whom Morton studied in Paris. It quickly went into several editions.

Much, H., *Tuberculosis in Children* (New York, 1921)

Murger, H., *Vie de Bohème*, translated by N. Cameron, introduced by M. Sadler (London, 1960)

Muthu, D. J. A. C., *Pulmonary Tuberculosis and Sanatorium Treatment* (London, 1910)

Myers, J. A., *Man's Greatest Victory over Tuberculosis* (Baltimore, Maryland, 1940). The triumphalist title refers to the eradication of bovine tuberculosis in the USA.

Niemeyer, F., *Clinical Lectures on Pulmonary Consumption*, translated by C. Beumler (London, 1883)

O'Shea, J., *Music and Medicine* (London, 1990). Includes useful essays on the medical histories of Chopin, Paganini and Weber.

Packard, E. N., Hayes, J. N., Blanchet, S. F., *The Artificial Pneumothorax* (London, 1940)

Packard, R. M., *White Plague, Black Labour: Tuberculosis in the Politics and Health of South Africa* (Pietermaritzburg, 1990)

Pagel, W., Simmonds, F. A. H., McDonald, N., Nassau, E., *Pulmonary Tuberculosis* (Oxford, 1964). A much-quoted standard text.

Parker, R., *On the Road: The Papworth Story* (Cambridge, 1977)

Parrot, J. M., *The Primary Lung Focus of Tuberculosis in Children*, translated by D. B. King (London, 1876)

Pasteur-Valery-Radot, R., *La vie de Pasteur* (Paris, 1924)

Pawel, E., *The Nightmare of Reason* (London, 1988). A balanced and well-researched biography of Kafka.

Pearson, S. V., *Man, Medicine and Myself* (London, 1926). A first-hand account of the Nordrach sanatorium regime.

Pearson, S. V., *The State Provision of Sanatoriums* (Cambridge, 1913)

Pierry, A. M., Rosheim, J., *Histoire de la tuberculose* (Paris, 1931)

Pirquet, C. von, "Der diagnostische Werk der kutanen Tubekulin-Reaktion bei der Tuberkulose des Kindesalters auf Grund von 100 Sektionen", *Wienerische klinische Wochenschrift*, 20 (1907), 1123. The foundation article of skin testing.

Pollock, J. E., *The Elements of Consumption* (London, 1865)

Porter, Dorothy, ed., *The History of Public Health and the Modern State* (Amsterdam, 1994)

Porter, J. D. H., Keith, P. W., McAdam, J., *Tuberculosis: Back to the Future* (Chichester, 1994). An unusually informative collection of conference papers.

Porter, R., *Health for Sale: Quackery in England, 1650–1850* (Manchester, 1989)

Porter, R., *The Greatest Benefit to Mankind* (London, 1997). Probably the best currently available general one-volume history of medicine from antiquity to the present, with a useful bibliography.

Powell, D., Hartley, P. H. S., *Diseases of the Lungs and Pleurae* (London, 1921)

Pratt, J. H., "The Development of the Rest Treatment of Pulmonary Tuberculosis",. *New England Journal of Medicine*, 206 (1932), 64. A historic refutation of Paterson's half-baked autoinoculation theory and work therapy.

Pulver, J., *Paganini: The Romantic Virtuoso* (London, 1936)

Ranke, K. E., "Primäres, Sekundäres und Tertiäres Stadium der Menschlichen Tuberkulose", *Berliner klinisch-therapeutische Wochenschrift*, 54 (1917), 397. The revered paper establishing the widely adopted "staging" of tuberculosis, almost entirely based on the misinterpretation of pathological evidence.

Ratledge, C., Stanford, J., *The Biology of the Mycobacteria* (London, 1983)

Rayfild, D., *Anton Chekhov* (London, 1996)

Reichman, L. B., "The U-Shaped Curve of Concern" (editorial), *American Review of Respiratory Diseases*, 144 (1991), 741

Reid, T., *An Essay on the Nature and Cure of Pulmonary Phthisis* (London, 1785)

Rich, A. R., *The Pathogenesis of Tuberculosis* (Springfield, Illinois, 1944)

Rivers, D. et al., "The Prevalence of Tuberculosis at Necropsy in Progressive Massive Fibrosis in Coalworkers", *British Journal of Industrial Medicine*, 9 (1957)

Roberts, Charlotte, Manchester, K., *The Archeology of Disease* (2nd edn, Ithaca, New York, 1995). An authoritative introduction to the archaeology of tuberculosis (and other diseases).

Robinson, V., *Robert Koch* (New York, 1932)

Rogers, F. B., "The Rise and Decline of Altitude Therapy in Tuberculosis", *Bulletin of the History of Medicine*, 43 (1969), 3

Rollier, A., *The Healer: How to Fight Tuberculosis*, translated by E. Glogue and M. Yearsley (London, 1925)

Rosenkrants, B. G., *From Consumption to Tuberculosis: A Documentary History* (New York, 1994)

Rosenthal, R. R., *BCG Vaccination* (Boston, 1957)

Rotberg, R., *The Founder: Cecil Rhodes and the Pursuit of Power* (Oxford,1988)

Rothman, S. M., *Living in the Shadow of Death* (Baltimore, Maryland, 1995). An evocative work about tuberculosis in the United States in the age before chemotherapy based largely on the authentic first-hand accounts of patients.

Ryan, F., *The Greatest Story Never Told: The Human Story of the Search for the Cure of Tuberculosis and the New Global Threat* (Bromsgrove, Worcestershire, 1992). A well researched and stylishly written book which lives up to its subtitle. In the Paul de Kruif tradition (looking at history through the lives of outstanding individuals), but less breathlessly adulatory and far more informative, it is *the* book for anyone interested in the personalities involved in the chemotherapy-antibiotic revolution: Domagk, Waksman, Lehmann, Dubos, Feldman and others.

Sand, George, *Un hiver en Majorque* (Paris, 1852)

Sandstone, D. A., *Saranac Diary* (New York, 1914)

Sauerbruch, F., *A Surgeon's Life*, translated by G. Renier and A. Cliff (London, 1953)

Savage, W. G., *Milk and the Public Health* (London, 1912). A pioneering work to which nobody in authority paid any attention.

Savage, W. G., *The Prevention of Human Tuberculosis of Bovine Origin* (London, 1929)

Schatz, A., Bugie, E., Waksman, S. A., "Streptomycin: A Substance Exhibiting Antibiotic Activity against Gram-Positive and Gram-Negative Bacteria", *Proceedings of the Society for Experimental Biology and Medicine*, 55 (1944), 66. The beginning of antituberculous chemotherapy.

Science, "Resistance to Tuberculosis" (a collection of eleven articles), *Science*, 359 (1994), 393

Seibert, F. B., "The History of the Development of Purified Protein Derivative", *American Review of Tuberculosis*, 44 (1941), 328

Shennan, D. H., *Tuberculosis Control in Developing Countries* (Edinburgh, 1969). The end of the Optimistic Decade.

Sigerist, H. E., *Civilisation and Disease* (Ithaca, New York, 1943)

Smith, F. B., *The People's Health, 1830–1910* (London, 1979)

Smith, F. B., *The Retreat of Tuberculosis, 1850–1950* (London, 1988). This wonderfully angry, as well as thoroughly researched, book is an essential corrective to the slightly smug medical histories written by doctors which tend to overflow with notable advances and other invaluable contributions.

Smith, T., "A Comparative Study of Bovine Tubercle Bacilli and of Tubercle Bacilli from Sputum", *Journal of Experimental Medicine*, 3 (1898), 451. A landmark paper distinguishing human from bovine tuberculosis.

Smollett, T., *Travels through France and Italy*, edited by F. Felsenstein (Oxford, 1979)

Smyth, J. C., *The Works of the Late William Stark* (London, 1788)

Snider, D. E., Roper, W. L., "The New Tuberculosis", *New England Journal of Medicine*, 326 (1992), 703

Spink, W. E., *Infectious Diseases: Prevention and Treatment in the Eighteenth and Nineteenth Centuries* (Minneapolis, Minnesota, 1978)

Squire, J. E., *The Hygienic Prevention of Consumption* (London, 1893)

Stern, B. F., *Society and Medical Progress* (Princeton, 1983)

Stanley, N. F., Joske, R. A., eds, *Changing Disease Patterns and Human Behaviour* (New York, 1947)

Styblo, K., "Overview and Epidemiological Assessment of the Current Global Tuberculosis Situation with an Emphasis on Control in Developing Countries", *Review of Infectious Diseases*, 11 (1989), supplement, 339

Sutherland, H. G., ed., *The Control and Eradication of Tuberculosis* (Edinburgh, 1911). A Festschrift compiled in honour of R. W. Philip with contributions by thirty-one workers from five continents. The volume is a useful conspectus of the dispensary-sanatorium movement approaching its peak.

Sydenham, T., *The Works of Thomas Sydenham*, translated by R. G. Latham (London, 1850)

Tauber, A. I., Chernyak, L., *Metchnikof and the Origin of Immunology* (New York, 1991)

Taylor, R., *Saranac: America's Magic Mountain* (Boston, 1985)

Thérèse, Saint, of Lisieux, *Story of Soul*, translated by John Clarke (3rd edn, Washington, DC, 1996). Tuberculosis at its most spiritual: one of the most influential religious works of the century and a masterpiece.

Thomson, H. H., *Tuberculosis and Public Health* (London, 1920)

Thomson, W., *The Germ Theory of Disease* (Melbourne, 1882)

Tomson, W. B., *Notes and Suggestions on the Finding of Employment for the Tuberculous* (London, 1926)

Tomson, W. B., *Some Methods for the Prevention of Tuberculosis* (London, 1929)

Toussaint, P., *Marie Dupléssis, la vrai Dame aux Camélias* (Paris, 1958).

Trousseau, A., Pidoux, H., *Traité du therapeutique de la tuberculose* (Paris, 1855). French academic orthodoxy for nearly half a century.

Trudeau, E. L., *Autobiography* (New York 1912)

Underwood, E. A., *A Manual of Tuberculosis, Clinical and Administrative* (Edinburgh, 1945)

Underwood, E. A., *A Manual of Tuberculosis for Nurses* (Edinburgh, 1931)

Uplekar, M. W., Rangan, S., *Tackling TB: The Search for a Solution* (Bombay, 1996)

Varrier-Jones, P. J., *Papers of a Pioneer*, edited by P. Fraser (London, 1943)

Voigt, J., *Tuberkulose: Geschichte einer Krankheit* (Köln, 1994). Good on German victims of tuberculosis.

Waksman, S. A., *My Life with Microbes* (London, 1958)

Waldenburg, I., *Die Lungenschwindsucht und Skrofulose* (Berlin, 1869). A monument of nineteenth-century continental medical scholarship.

Warner, J. H., *Therapy and Perspective: Medical Knowledge and Identity in America, 1820–1885* (Cambridge, Massachusetts, 1986)

Warrack, J., *Carl Maria von Weber* (London, 1968)

Webb, G. B., *Tuberculosis* (New York, 1946)

Weber, Sir H., *Sea Voyages in the Therapy of Tuberculosis* (London, 1899)

Webster, C., *Health: Historical Issues* (London, 1984)

Weeks, G., *California Copy* (Washington, 1928). Reprint of an historical best-seller.

Weintraub, S., *Aubrey Beardsley: Imp of the Perverse* (Philadelphia, 1977)

Weiss, R., "On the Track of Killer Tuberculosis", *Science*, 225 (1922), 148

Wherrett, G. J., *The Miracle of the Empty Bed* (Toronto, 1977)

Whorton, J. C., *Crusaders for Fitness: The History of American Health Reformers* (Princeton, 1982)

Wilkinson, L., *Animals and Disease* (Cambridge, 1992). A good introduction to comparative tuberculosis.

Wilkinson, W. C., *The Treatment of Consumption* (London, 1908). The English defence of tuberculin.

Williams, C. T., "The Contagion of Phthisis", *British Medical Journal* (1882), p. 618. An authoritative refutation of the infection hypothesis by a leading light of the Brompton Hospital.

Williams, F. H., "The Röntgen Ray in Thoracic Disease", *American Journal of Medical Science*, 114 (1897), 665. A pioneering paper on the application of X-Rays to tuberculosis.

Williams, H. I., Herbert, I., *Social Work for the Tuberculous* (London, 1945)

Willis, T., *The Practice of Physic* (London, 1684)

Wilson, G. S., *The Pasteurisation of Milk* (London, 1942)

Wilson, L. G., "The Historical Decline of Tuberculosis in Europe and America", *Journal of the History of Medicine and Allied Sciences*, 45 (1990), 366

Wimslow, C. E. A., *The Life of Hermann M. Biggs* (Philadelphia, 1929)

Wittkower, E., *A Psychiatrist Looks at Tuberculosis* (2nd edn, London, 1955)

Wohl, A., *Endangered Lives: Public Health in Victorian Britain* (London, 1983)

Wood, C., *Tissot* (London, 1984)

Wood, Corinne, *Human Sickness and Health: A Biocultural View* (Mountain View, California, 1979). An excellent introduction to medical anthropology.

Woodhead, Sir G., Varrier-Jones, P. C., *Industrial Colonies and Village Settlements* (Cambridge, 1920)

World Health Organisation, *Mass Health Examination* (Geneva, 1971)

World Health Organisation, *Report on the Tuberculosis Epidemic* (Geneva, 1996)

Zamoyski, A., *Chopin* (London, 1979)

Index

Illustrations are shown in bold